Multiple Pregnancy

Edited by

Mark Kilby, Philip Baker,
Hilary Critchley and David Field

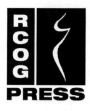

Mark D Kilby MD MRCOG
Professor of Maternal and Fetal Medicine, Department of Fetal Medicine, Floor 3, Birmingham Women's Hospital, Birmingham B15 2TG

Philip N Baker DM FRCOG
Professor of Maternal and Fetal Health, Maternal and Fetal Health Research Centre, The University of Manchester, St Mary's Hospital, Hathersage Road, Manchester M13 0JH

Hilary OD Critchley MD FRCOG FRANZCOG
Professor of Reproductive Medicine and Consultant Gynaecologist, Centre for Reproductive Biology, University of Edinburgh, The Chancellor's Building, 49 Little France Crescent, Edinburgh EH16 4SB

David J Field MBBS DCH FRCPCH FRCP(Ed) DM
Professor of Neonatal Medicine, University of Leicester, Neonatal Unit, Leicester Royal Infirmary, Infirmary Square, Leicester LE1 5WW

Published by the **RCOG Press** at the Royal College of Obstetricians and Gynaecologists, 27 Sussex Place, Regent's Park, London NW1 4RG

www.rcog.org.uk

Registered charity no. 213280

First published 2006

ISBN 1-904752-22-5

RCOG Editor: Andrew Welsh
Design/typesetting by Karl Harrington, FiSH Books, London
Index by Liza Furnival
Printed by Henry Ling Ltd, The Dorchester Press, Dorchester DT1 1HD

Contents

Participants

Philip Baker
Convenor of RCOG Study Groups and Professor of Maternal and Fetal Health,
Maternal and Fetal Health Research Centre, The University of Manchester,
St Mary's Hospital, Hathersage Road, Manchester M13 0JH, UK.

Jon FR Barrett
Associate Professor of Obstetrics and Gynaecology, Gynaecology, Women's College
Hospital, 60 Grosvenor Street, Toronto, Canada, M5S 1B6.

Phillip Bennett
Professor of Obstetrics and Gynaecology, Imperial College Parturition Research
Group, Institute of Reproductive and Developmental Biology, Hammersmith
Hospital Campus, Du Cane Road, London W12 0NN, UK.

Siladitya Bhattacharya
Reader and Honorary Consultant, Acting Head of Department of Obstetrics and
Gynaecology, University of Aberdeen, Foresterhill, Aberdeen AB25 2ZD, UK.

Isaac Blickstein
Professor of Obstetrics and Gynecology, High-risk Pregnancy Unit, Department of
Obstetrics and Gynecology, Kaplan Medical Center, Rehovot, 76100, Israel.

David Chitayat
Professor and Head, The Prenatal Diagnosis and Medical Genetics Program,
Department of Obstetrics and Gynecology, Mount Sinai Hospital, 700 University
Avenue, Ontario Power Generation Building, Room 3292, Toronto, Ontario,
Canada M5G 1Z5.

Hilary OD Critchley
Professor of Reproductive Medicine and Consultant Gynaecologist, Centre for
Reproductive Biology, University of Edinburgh, The Queen's Medical Research
Institute, 47 Little France Crescent, Edinburgh EH16 4TJ, UK.

David Field
Professor of Neonatal Medicine, University of Leicester, Neonatal Unit, Leicester Royal Infirmary, Infirmary Square, Leicester LE1 5WW, UK.

Nicholas M Fisk
Professor of Obstetrics and Fetal Medicine, Institute of Reproductive & Developmental Biology, Imperial College London, Hammersmith Campus, Du Cane Road, London W12 0NN, UK.

Khalid S Khan
Professor of Obstetrics, Gynaecology and Clinical Epidemiology, Birmingham Women's Hospital, Birmingham B15 2TG, UK.

Mark D Kilby
Professor of Maternal and Fetal Medicine, Department of Fetal Medicine, Division of Reproduction and Child Health, Floor 3, Birmingham Women's Hospital, Birmingham B15 2TG, UK.

Jennifer J Kurinczuk
Consultant Clinical Epidemiologist, National Perinatal Epidemiology Unit, University of Oxford, Old Road Campus, Headington, Oxford OX3 7LF, UK.

Neil Marlow
Professor of Neonatal Medicine, Academic Division of Child Health, University Hospital, Queen's Medical Centre, Nottingham NG7 2UH, UK.

James Neilson
Professor of Obstetrics and Gynaecology, Developmental Medicine, University of Liverpool, Liverpool Women's Hospital, Crown Street, Liverpool L8 7SS, UK.

Kypros H Nicolaides
Professor and Director, Harris Birthright Research Centre for Fetal Medicine, 9 Jubilee Wing, King's College Hospital, Denmark Hill, London SE5 9RS, UK.

Peter GJ Nikkels
Pathologist, Department of Pathology, University Medical Centre Utrecht, PO Pox 85500, Utrecht 3508 GA, The Netherlands.

Stephen Ong
Subspecialty Trainee in Fetal Medicine, Department of Fetal Medicine, Birmingham Women's Hospital, Birmingham B15 2TG, UK.

Neil J Sebire
Consultant in Paediatric Pathology, Department of Paediatric Pathology, Great Ormond Street Hospital, Great Ormond Street, London WC1N 3JH, UK.

Debbie Sen
Senior Research Nurse Manager, Clinical Research Facility, 4th Floor, Leazes Wing, Royal Victoria Infirmary, Newcastle upon Tyne, NE2 4LP, UK.

Yves Ville
Professor of Obstetrics and Gynaecology and Head of Department,
Service de Gynécologie Obstétrique, CHI Poissy Saint Germain en Laye,
Université de Paris-Ouest Versailles-St. Quentin en Yvelines,
10 Rue de Champ Gaillard, Poissy 78300, France.

Ruwan C Wimalasundera
Consultant Obstetrician and Fetal Medicine Specialist, Centre for Fetal Care,
Queen Charlotte's and Chelsea Hospital, Du Cane Road, London W12 0HS, UK.

Additional contributors

Andrew Carlin
Subspecialty Trainee in Fetal-Maternal Medicine, Liverpool Women's Hospital,
Crown Street, Liverpool L8 7SS, UK.

William JB Dennes
Senior Registrar, Centre for Fetal Care, Queen Charlotte's and Chelsea Hospital,
Du Cane Road, London W12 0HS, UK.

Caroline Fox
Senior House Officer, Birmingham Women's Hospital, Birmingham B15 2TG, UK.

Judith G Hall
Professor Emeritus of Pediatrics and Medical Genetics, British Columbia's
Children's Hospital, Department of Pediatrics, Room L408, 4480 Oak Street,
Vancouver, British Columbia, Canada V6H 3V4.

Pradeep M Jayaram
Senior House Officer, Birmingham Women's Hospital, Birmingham B15 2TG, UK.

Sheri Lim
Imperial College Parturition Research Group, Institute of Reproductive and
Developmental Biology, Hammersmith Hospital Campus, Du Cane Road,
London W12 0NN, UK.

Zabeena Pandian
Specialist Registrar, Department of Obstetrics and Gynaecology, Aberdeen
Maternity Hospital, Cornhill Road, Aberdeen AB25 2ZL, UK.

Stephen Robson
Professor of Fetal Medicine, School of Surgical and Reproductive Sciences,
3rd Floor, Leech Building, Medical School, University of Newcastle, Newcastle
NE2 4HH, UK.

Waldo Sepulveda
Professor of Fetal Medicine, Fetal Medicine Unit, University of Santiago, Chile.

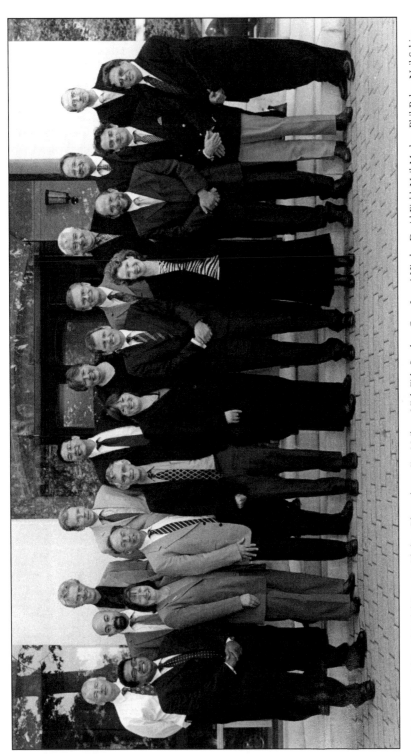

Back row (from left to right): **Phil Bennett, Siladitya Bhattacharya, Jim Neilson, Nick Fisk, Stephen Ong, Jacqui Hiesler, David Field, Neil Marlow, Phil Baker, Neil Sebire**

Front row (from left to right): **Ruwan Wimalasundera, Jenny Kurinczuk, Peter Nikkels, David Chitayat, Debbie Sen, Mark Kilby, Hilary Critchley, Jon Barrett, Yves Ville, Isaac Blickstein**

Mark FH Sullivan
Senior Lecturer in Reproductive Biochemistry, Institute of Reproductive and
Developmental Biology, Imperial College London, Hammersmith Campus,
Du Cane Road, London W12 0NN, UK.

TG Teoh
Consultant Obsterician, St Mary's Hospital, Praed Street, Paddington, London, UK.

Jeroen PHM van den Wijngaard
Research Scientist, Laser Centre, Academic Medical Centre, University of
Amsterdam, Meibergdreef 9, Amsterdam 1105 AZ, The Netherlands.

Martin JC van Gemert
Director, Laser Centre, Academic Medical Centre, University of Amsterdam,
Meibergdreef 9, Amsterdam 1105 AZ, The Netherlands.

Masami Yamamoto
Unidad de Medicina Materno Fetal, Clinica Alemana de Santiago y Hospital Padre
Hurtado, Universidad del Desarrollo, Manquehue Norte 1407, Vitacura, Santiago,
Chile.

Javier Zamora
Medical Statistician, Clinical Biostatistics Unit, Hospital Ramon y Cajal, Madrid
28034, Spain.

Discussant

Jacqui Hiesler
Lay Member, RCOG Consumer's Forum, Royal College of Obstetricians and
Gynaecologists, 27 Sussex Place, Regent's Park, London NW1 4RG, UK.

DECLARATION OF INTEREST

All contributors to the Study Group were invited to make a specific Declaration of Interest in relation
to the subject of the Study Group. This was undertaken and all contributors complied with this
request. Philip Bennett holds a patent on the inhibition of nuclear factor kappa B in the prevention
of preterm labour and acts as a consultant to pharmaceutical companies that are developing drugs for
the prevention of preterm labour. Nicholas Fisk has consultancies with Ferring International,
EUMOM Ltd, the Gerson-Lehrman Group and IC Consultants. He is a member of the Ferring UK
Obstetric Advisory Board and the Scientific Advisory Board of Omnicyte Ltd, and is an independent
member of the Data Safety and Monitoring Board of the US NICHHD Twin–Twin Transfusion
Syndrome Trial. He has a medico-legal consultancy and undertakes private practice on behalf of the
Institute of Obstetrics and Gynaecology Trust, a registered charity. He is a member of the MRC
College of Experts. He has written numerous chapters, editorials and reviews, generating modest
editorial fees. He holds one patent, and his department holds numerous patents related to obstetrics
and gynaecology. Neil Marlow is President of the British Association of Perinatal Medicine and a
working member of the Nuffield Council on Bioethics.

Preface

It has been over ten years since the Royal College of Obstetricians and Gynaecologists commissioned a study group to investigate the multidisciplinary aspects of multiple pregnancy. The book arising from that study group was edited by Mr R Humphrey-Ward and Professor Martin Whittle.

Despite the passing of over ten years, multiple pregnancy continues to be responsible for considerable perinatal morbidity and mortality compared with singleton pregnancy. Over that time the various challenges associated with the management of subfertility have, if anything, increased. Avoiding multiple pregnancy, with the potential pathologies of intrauterine growth restriction, increased risk of congenital anomalies and premature delivery, is currently a matter of considerable debate, in particular whether careful monitoring of ovulation induction and limitation in the number of embryos replaced during *in vitro* fertilisation treatment will be sufficient to reduce iatrogenic twinning.

Although all twins and multiple pregnancies have relatively increased perinatal morbidity and mortality compared with singleton pregnancies, it is twins with monochorionic placentation that have the most significant risk factors and that present challenges in obstetric management. Over the last 10–15 years, scientific understanding of the pathogenesis of twin-to-twin transfusion syndrome has increased and fetal therapy such as fetoscopic laser ablation has been proven by randomised controlled studies to be efficacious in severe disease.

All healthcare professionals involved in women's health need to have an awareness of the special antenatal and postnatal problems for the mother having twins or indeed a higher order multiple pregnancy. There are also particular challenges facing those caring for neonates born from multiple pregnancies.

Contributions to this volume come from multidisciplinary healthcare professionals who are leaders in both the scientific understanding and the clinical management of multiple pregnancy. Their chapters address not only issues related to pathophysiology and delivery in multiple pregnancy but also the various potential implications and long-term sequelae for the children. The continuing need to support mothers who give birth to multiple pregnancies is also recognised and addressed.

The editors wish to thank all those who so willingly contributed to the 50th Study Group and shared their considerable expertise. We believe that this volume will provide a useful overview of the current literature to those healthcare professionals working within obstetrics, midwifery and paediatrics.

At the end of this book are the consensus views arising from the 50th Study Group on Multiple Pregnancy. These should stimulate debate, which will lead to improvements in clinical care for both the mother and her children.

Mark Kilby • Phil Baker • Hilary Critchley • David Field

Chapter 1
Epidemiology of multiple pregnancy: changing effects of assisted conception

Jennifer J Kurinczuk

The vast majority of human pregnancies result in the birth of a single infant; as a consequence, multiple births have often been regarded as something of a curiosity. Historically, many customs and beliefs about multiples, particularly twins, emerged around the world, with twins being abhorred in some places and highly prized in others.[1] Twins have figured prominently in history, mythology and literature. For example, Shakespeare, himself the father of boy–girl twins Hamnet and Judith, developed the theme of twins in both Twelfth Night and The Comedy of Errors.[1]

The incidence of multiples, especially twins, varies both within and between populations, and over time. This variation is largely confined to dizygous twinning with monozygous twinning remaining relatively constant, although, because of variations in dizygous twinning, the balance in the proportion of each also varies between populations. This chapter describes the epidemiology of twinning, including the variations in twinning rates seen between and within populations, variations over time, and the influence of factors known to affect twinning rates. The effects of assisted reproductive technologies (ART) are specifically highlighted, particularly in relation to the UK population. Perinatal morbidity and mortality rates for twins are then described with reference to rates in singletons. The chapter concludes with consideration of these issues in relation to triplets and higher order multiples.

The rates of twins, triplets and higher order multiples are quantified using maternities as the denominator. The term 'maternities' refers to the number of women delivered of twins (or triplets and higher order multiples) and is thus analogous with the terms 'deliveries' and 'confinements' used by some authors; it does not refer to total conceptions or the total number of babies born. The denominators used are thus a count of women and not babies. The term maternities is used in keeping with the terminology employed by the majority of authors in this field and with the Office for National Statistics (ONS) in England and Wales.

Population differences in the incidence of twins

Spontaneous twinning rates vary between populations, from generally low rates in Japan, Taiwan and Hawaii (between 2 and 7 per 1000 maternities; that is, 1 in 500 to 1 in 143 maternities), with intermediate rates (9–20 per 1000; 1 in 111 to 1 in 50) in

Europe and most countries in Africa, America, Asia and Oceania, through to higher rates in some specific African populations and in parts of America into which there was forced migration from West Africa (rates in excess of 20 per 1000; 1 in 50).[2] In 1988, Little and Thompson[2] estimated that prior to the introduction of ovulation induction treatment and ART there was a fifteen-fold variation in global twinning rates.

The Yoruba population, who live predominantly in south-west Nigeria, have one of the highest documented dizygous twinning rates in the world although, interestingly, they have monozygous rates comparable with European populations. When originally described by Nylander in 1969,[3] one set of twins was delivered for every 22 maternities (45 per 1000 maternities) which effectively meant that one person in every 11 in the Yoruba population was a twin. The triplet rate was also very high. In addition to possible cultural and social reasons for the perpetuation of a high twinning rate, aspects of the diet of this isolated rural population were also postulated as a cause.[4] Subsequent migration to urban centres and changes in diet were followed by a decline in twinning rates in the migrating Yoruba, although presumably a change in diet associated with urbanisation may also have been accompanied by a change in social and cultural practices that may have affected marriage arrangements and disrupted the genetic isolation of the Yoruba.

In contrast to the Yoruba, the Japanese and other South-East Asian populations have relatively low rates of spontaneous dizygous twinning. For example, from the mid-1950s to the mid-1960s, prior to the introduction of ovulation induction therapies for the treatment of infertility, the twinning rate in Japan was about 6.4 per 1000 births.[5] Within Japan, geographical variations in dizygous twinning are evident. For example, in 1974 there was a higher dizygous twinning rate in the north-east

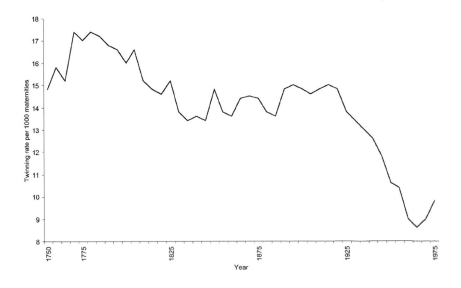

Figure 1.1.   Twinning rates per 1000 maternities in five year averages, Sweden, 1756–1976; data adapted from Eriksson *et al.*[7]

compared with the south-west, whereas monozygous twinning rates remained essentially constant. One consequence of the relatively low spontaneous dizygous twinning rate in Japan, which contrasts with twinning seen in Western populations, is that monozygous twins constitute a much higher proportion of twins overall, with monozygous twinning occurring at twice the rate of dizygous twinning.[5] The latter low rate is thought to be due to lower gonadotrophin levels in Japanese women compared with European, American and African women.[6]

European populations have intermediate and fairly similar spontaneous twinning rates, although there is some between-country variation that, as in Japan, appears to be related to latitude, with a south-west/north-east gradient from low to high.[2] In their 1988 review, Little and Thompson concluded that, in the period prior to the introduction of ovulation induction treatment, twinning rates across Europe varied from 9 to 20 per 1000 maternities with a general variation of between 1.5-fold and two-fold.[2]

Secular trends in twinning rates

Remarkable though it might seem given current concerns about twinning rates, the available evidence suggests that the rate of spontaneous twinning actually declined in many Western populations over most of the 20th century. For example, Swedish records that go back to 1750 describe twinning rates of about 17 per 1000 (1 in 59) maternities in the second half of the 18th century (Figure 1.1) with a decline to around 9 per 1000 (1 in 110) by the mid-1970s.[7] The reasons for the originally high Swedish rates and subsequent decline, which was particularly marked from 1920 onwards, remain unclear but are postulated to be due to the effects of endogamy

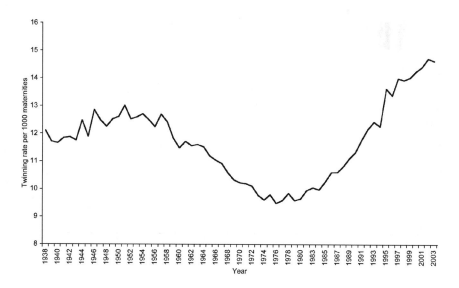

Figure 1.2.   Twinning rate per 1000 maternities by year, England and Wales, 1938–2003; data from the Office for National Statistics (ONS) (1981 data not available)

(intermarriage within small, isolated communities) and its subsequent disappearance with industrialisation and urbanisation.[8]

This general decline in the twinning rate was replicated in other European countries. Following a further rapid decline during the 1960s, the nadir was reached in the mid-1970s,[9] as illustrated for England and Wales between 1938 and 2003 in Figure 1.2 and described by Wood in 1997.[10] The twinning rate in England and Wales from 1938 to 1956 was between 11.7 (1 in 85) and 13.0 (1 in 77) per 1000 maternities. The rate then declined steeply from 12.7 twin pregnancies per 1000 maternities (1 in 79) in 1957 to 9.5 per 1000 (1 in 105) in 1976. This was followed by a marked upturn and steady increase to 14.6 per 1000 maternities (1 in 68) by 2003. This U-shaped relationship has been replicated in many European countries over the same period. In 1995 Derom *et al.*[9] described a similar U-shaped change over the same period in Denmark, the Netherlands, West Germany, England and Wales, Luxembourg and Belgium. The reasons for such a widespread and remarkably consistent pattern are complex and not yet fully understood. However, the relationship between twinning rates, maternal age and fertility treatment undoubtedly plays a large part. Furthermore, while the relative contribution of the two effects of the increase in births to older mothers and of fertility treatment varies between countries, the effects of both are evident in most Western populations.

The association between increasing maternal age (up to about the age of 40 years) and an increase in the probability of spontaneous dizygous twinning is well established. Derom *et al.*[9] used data from the Netherlands to plot the twinning rate and overlaid the proportion of births to mothers aged 29 years and over. The results of a similar analysis using data from England and Wales from 1938 to 2003 are illustrated in Figure 1.3.

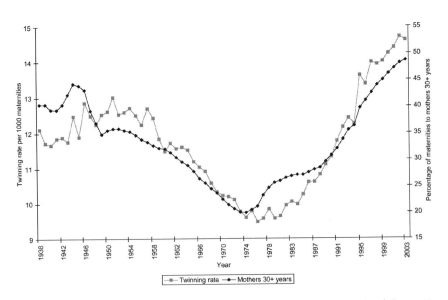

Figure 1.3.   Relationship between the twinning rate per 1000 maternities and the proportion of all maternities to mothers age 30 years and over by year, England and Wales, 1938–2003; data from the ONS (1981 data not available)

Factors influencing the twinning rate

Maternal age

As long ago as 1865, the Scottish obstetrician Matthews Duncan recognised the relationship between increasing maternal age and the increased risk of twinning.[11] He also noted that from the age of 40 years fertility diminishes and with it there is a decline in the twinning rate. Figure 1.4 illustrates the relationship between maternal age and the probability of delivering twins in England and Wales in more recent times and extends the analysis carried out by Wood in 1997.[10]

Figure 1.4 clearly delineates the separate rates of twinning experienced by mothers of different ages, with the lowest twinning rate (5.1–6.9 per 1000 maternities; 1 in 196 to 1 in 145) experienced by women aged less than 20 years and the highest rate experienced by women aged 35–39 years at delivery (13.1–21.5 per 1000; 1 in 76 to 1 in 47), with a relative decline in twinning in women aged 40 years and over, except in the most recent years (9.4–21.4 per 1000; 1 in 106 to 1 in 47). Figure 1.4 also shows the increase in age-specific twinning rates observed over time, with an increase from the early 1980s onwards in women aged 25 years and over but particularly in those women aged 30 years and over.

The consequences of the difference in the probability of twinning by maternal age and the change in the age-specific twinning rate over time have combined to profoundly affect the relative proportion of twins born to women of different ages (Figure 1.5). In 1974 only 29% of twin maternities were to women aged 30 years and older and only 9% were to women aged 35 years and older. By 2003 the former proportion had more than doubled to 63% and the latter had increased three-fold to 27%. There was also a three-fold increase in the proportion of twin maternities to women aged 40 years and over, from 1.5% in 1974 to 4.5% in 2003.

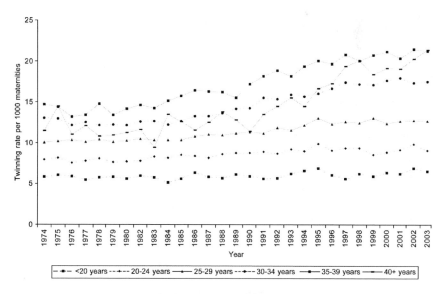

Figure 1.4. Maternal age group specific twinning rate per 1000 maternities by year, England and Wales, 1974–2003; data from the ONS (1981 data not available)

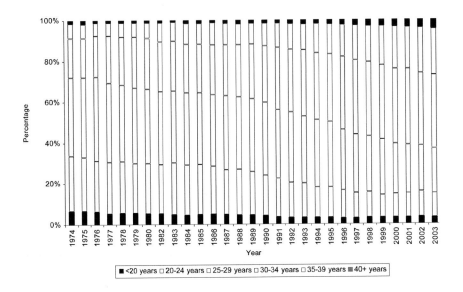

Figure 1.5.   Maternal age group specific proportion of twins by year, England and Wales, 1974–2003; data from the ONS (1981 data not available)

Parity

Matthews Duncan was also probably the first person to recognise that the probability of twinning is associated with parity as well as maternal age.[11] Figure 1.6 shows the relationship between the increased risk of twinning and increasing parity in Aberdeen in the pre-ART treatment era; an effect almost certainly confined to dizygous twinning.[11]

The reasons for the relationship between parity and risk of twinning are unclear. In 1970 Allen and Schachter[12] proposed the theory that women who conceive twins are more 'fertile' and conceive more easily than other women. If this were the case then in the period before the widespread availability of effective contraception the higher rates of twinning associated with higher parity could simply have been an effect of these more 'fertile' women having more pregnancies than other women and thus forming a high proportion of older high-parity mothers. Allen investigated this theory indirectly using US data and demonstrated that such a parity effect could indeed account for most of the observed variation in parity-specific twinning.[13]

An alternative theory relating to the confounded relationship between parity, maternal age and risk of twinning was investigated by MacGillivray et al.[11] They used data from Aberdeen City District from 1951 to 1983 that enabled them to investigate the parity–maternal age relationship in the era when large families and thus higher levels of parity were still relatively common and before the widespread introduction of ART. Using a logistic regression model to simultaneously adjust for the effects of parity, maternal age, maternal height, time period and occupation on the risk of twinning, they were able to examine the interaction between maternal age and parity.

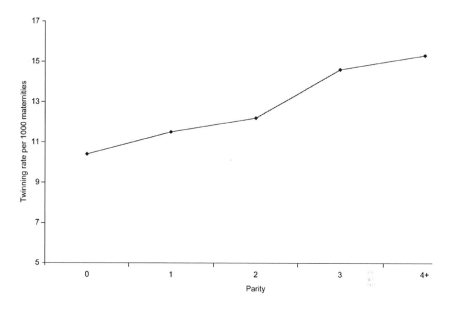

Figure 1.6.   Twinning rate per 1000 maternities by parity, Aberdeen City District, 1951–83; data adapted from MacGillivray *et al.*[11]

The relationship between increasing parity and increasing risk of twinning disappeared once maternal age was included in the model and they concluded that the apparent association between twinning and parity is largely a maternal age effect.[11]

Even if parity were a substantial contributor to modern twinning rates, the effects of parity are unlikely to have made a substantial contribution to the recent changes in twinning rates which are discussed in the next section. This is because, in contrast to the increase in average maternal age, since the mid-1970s average parity has declined. For example, in Scotland in 1995 compared with 1976, there was a 26% reduction in the rate of women having a fourth child and over a 40% reduction in the rate of women having a fifth or subsequent child.[14]

Fertility treatment

The lowest level of twinning in England and Wales since 1938 (when documentation allowed the calculation of twinning rates) was in 1976 (Figure 1.2).[10] This low level was almost certainly related to the relatively high proportion of births to younger women who are, as demonstrated in Figure 1.4, at lowest risk of conceiving twins. Figure 1.7 illustrates the change in the age-specific distribution of all maternities since 1938 in England and Wales.

With 80% of all maternities being in women under 30 years of age, 1974–76 had the highest proportion of all maternities to women of this age group for the whole 65 year period from 1938 to 2003. The mid-1970s represented the peak in a trend, which, apart from in the immediate post World War II years, had shown a consistent increase in the percentage of maternities to women under 30 from 1938 onwards (the

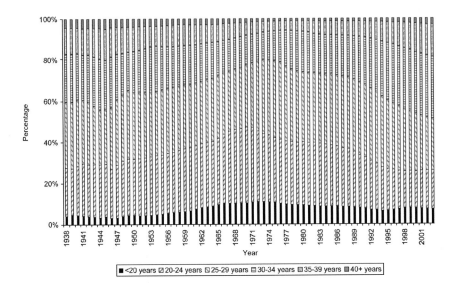

Figure 1.7.   Maternal age group specific proportion of all maternities by year, England and Wales, 1938–2003; data from the ONS

proportion was 60% in 1938). The peak in the mid-1970s was the consequence of several demographic and social phenomena, the most important of which was probably the effects of the post-war 'baby boomer' generation embarking upon parenthood. Other factors likely to have influenced the relative proportions of births by maternal age were the availability of the oral contraceptive pill primarily to older married women rather then younger women when first introduced and, while termination of pregnancy was legalised in 1968, accessibility for many sections of the pregnant population remained very limited in the early 1970s.

Since the mid-1970s there has been a steady and marked decline in the proportion of births to women under the age of 30 years. In contrast to the mid-1970 when 80% of maternities were to women younger than 30 years, by 2003 only 51% of all maternities were to women in this age group. Because the risk of twinning varies with maternal age, had all other things remained unchanged, an increase in the overall twinning rate through the 1980s, 1990s and into the 21st century, compared with the mid-1970s, would have been expected simply because of the change in maternal age distribution during this period.

Figure 1.8 illustrates an analysis, which includes the most recent UK-based data, of what would have happened to the twinning rate through the late 1970s to 2003 if the maternal age distribution had remained as in 1974, compared with the actual rate of twinning. This extends the analysis carried out by Wood in 1997.[10] The former rate was estimated using indirect standardisation to the 1974 maternal age specific rate of twinning. During this period there was actually a 1.5-fold increase in the twinning rate from 9.8 per 1000 maternities (1 in 102) in 1974 to 14.6 per 1000 maternities (1 in 68) in 2003. Had the maternal age distribution of births of 1974 prevailed, there

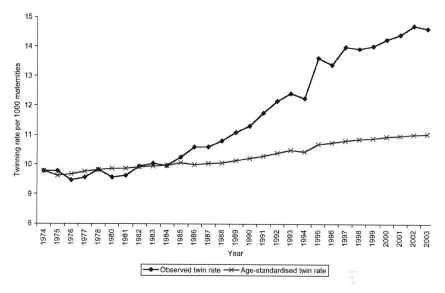

Figure 1.8.   Twinning rate age-standardised to the maternal age distribution of the 1974 maternity population by year, England and Wales, 1974–2003; data from the ONS (1981 data not available)

would have been a much smaller change from 9.8 to only 11.0 per 1000 maternities (1 in 91), a 1.12-fold increase.

Using the data derived to produce Figure 1.8, the proportion of twin maternities delivered in the period 1974–2003 that can be attributed to the change in maternal age distribution of all births was estimated. By subtraction from the proportion of twins equivalent to the 1974 twinning rate, the proportion due to 'other' influences was also estimated. These estimates are illustrated in Figure 1.9.

While the 1974 equivalent twinning rate preceded the introduction of ART such as *in vitro* fertilisation (IVF), it cannot be completely regarded as the 'natural' twinning rate as fertility treatments such as ovulation induction agents, including clomifene citrate, were available and being prescribed in the UK from the mid-1960s onwards. As can be seen from Figure 1.9, as the change in maternal age distribution and 'other' influences started to have an effect, the proportion of twins attributable to the 1974 equivalent twinning rate declined from 100% in 1974 to 67% by 2003. The change in the age distribution was responsible for 1% of twins in 1981 compared with 1974 and the proportion increased steadily from 1981 onwards to just less than 10% in 2003, with only recent evidence of a slowing in the rate of increase (Figure 1.10). By 2003 the 1974 equivalent twinning rate and the change in maternal age distribution combined accounted for an estimated 75% of all twin maternities. In 1997 Wood[10] described a similar analysis and calculated that '37% of the overall rise in the twinning rate … since 1975 could be accounted for by the rise in age of mothers'. This is equivalent to the change in maternal age accounting for 9.9% of all twins maternities.

Current projections from the ONS indicate that the mean age at the completion of childbearing for women born in the UK, which has risen in all cohorts of women

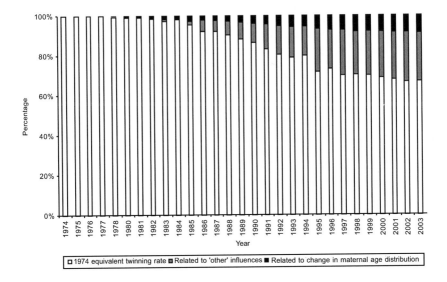

Figure 1.9. Estimated proportion of twins equivalent to the 1974 twinning rate, the change in maternal age distribution and the effect of 'other' influences on the twinning rate by year, England and Wales, 1974–2003; data from the ONS (1981 data not available)

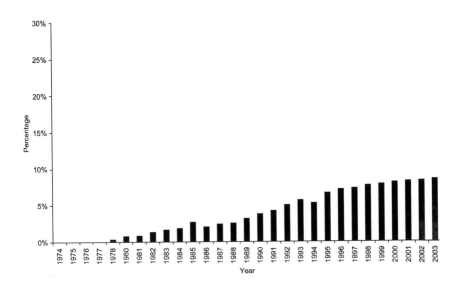

Figure 1.10. Estimated proportion of twins attributable to the change in maternal age distribution compared with the maternal age distribution in 1974 by year, England and Wales, 1974–2003; data from the ONS (1981 data not available)

born since the mid–1940s, is likely to continue to increase in all groups of women up to those born in 1990; figures for birth cohorts after 1990 were not projected.[15] This suggests that the maternal age contribution to the twinning rate is likely to continue to rise into the foreseeable future, although the rate of increase may slow down.

If the reasonable assumption is made that the largest contributor to the proportion of twins due to 'other' influences is the treatment of infertility additional to that being carried out in 1974, it can be seen from Figure 1.11 that this proportion is estimated to have increased from about 1% of all twin maternities in 1983 to about 25% by 2003; there is some evidence of a slowing in the rate of increase since about the year 2000.

Given the reasonable assumption that the largest contributor to the proportion of twins due to 'other' influences is the treatment of infertility, the questions that arise are what are the relative contributions of the different types of treatment and to what extent will moving from three to two embryo transfer IVF influence the overall twinning rate. There are, however, few data available in the UK to answer the former question and thus predict the latter.

The Millennium Cohort Study involved a survey of 18 553 UK families conducted over a 16 month period from 2000 to 2002. Just over a quarter of the twins (26%) in the study were conceived following fertility treatment,[16] a finding that concurs with the proportion estimated for the same period (23% to 25%) using the indirect standardisation method and illustrated in Figures 1.9 and 1.11. About three-quarters of the 26% of the Millennium Cohort Study twin pairs born following fertility treatment were conceived by IVF or a related procedure; just less than a quarter were conceived following ovulation induction alone; and fewer than 1% followed non-ART-related surgery.[16] This suggests that in the UK at the beginning of the 21st century about 20%

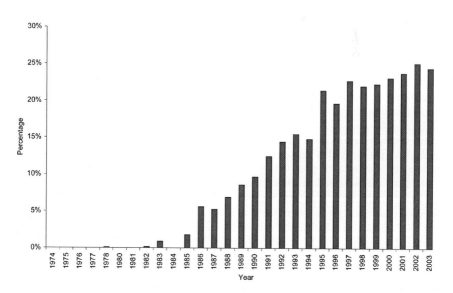

Figure 1.11.   Estimated proportion of twins attributable to 'other' influences by year, England and Wales, 1974–2003; data from the ONS (1981 data not available)

of all twin maternities were conceived following ART and about 6% were conceived following ovulation induction alone. Bergh *et al.*[17] estimated that in Sweden in 1994–95 IVF was responsible for 17% of twin deliveries and Derom *et al.*[18] estimated that in 1992 30% of all twins in the East Flanders Prospective Twin Survey were iatrogenic. The variations between countries will be in part due to the differences in rates of IVF usage and number of embryos transferred per cycle, and how both of these factors have changed over time.

Thus, all other things being equal, a halving in the rate of IVF-related twins would result in a return to a twinning rate equivalent to that seen in 1956 and last seen in 1995. The introduction of a single-embryo transfer policy as in Sweden and all other things being equal would result in a return to about the twinning rate last seen in 1991. However, 'all other things' are unlikely to be equal since, as noted above, the proportion of twins due to the increase in average maternal age is likely to continue to increase, as the average maternal age is projected to continue to rise.[15] Thus, any effect of changes in ART treatment on the twinning rate is likely to be masked, at least in part, by the continuing trend related to the maternal age effects.

Perinatal mortality and morbidity of twins

Twin pregnancies in general have a higher rate of most complications and adverse outcomes than singleton pregnancies. Much of this additional pathology arises because of the increased risk of preterm delivery and low birthweight associated with twins, both of which are important determinants of perinatal mortality and morbidity. Furthermore, morbidity in the perinatal period can have serious and severe long-term health consequences for the affected children.

Overall perinatal morbidity and mortality

The perinatal mortality rate is defined in the UK as the total number of stillbirths at 24 weeks of gestation or greater plus live births who die in the first week (seven days) after birth divided by the total number of live births and stillbirths. This represents a change in definition as prior to 1993 stillbirths were only included if they occurred at 28 weeks of gestation or greater. As can be seen from Figure 1.12, the perinatal mortality rate for both singleton and twin births has decreased since 1993. In this period the highest perinatal mortality rate for singletons was 8.1 per 1000 total births in 1993, following which the rate declined to its lowest rate ever of 7.2 per 1000 in 2001, with the rate in 2002 being 7.6 per 1000. During the same period the perinatal mortality rate for twins decreased from 40.4 per 1000 total births in 1994 to the lowest rate ever of 29.6 per 1000 in 2002.

In 1993 the perinatal mortality rate for twin births was over five times (rate ratio 5.1) higher than the rate for singletons (Figure 1.13). As the overall decrease in mortality has been greater in twins than singletons, the difference in the rate between the two has decreased over the ten year period to 2002. Nevertheless, by 2002 the perinatal mortality rate for twins was still nearly four times (rate ratio 3.9) that of singletons. The risk of perinatal death is strongly influenced by a history of pregnancy complications, preterm delivery and low birthweight. It is therefore not surprising that twin pregnancies, which tend to experience higher rates of all these factors, have a higher rate of perinatal mortality.

Because twins are at higher risk of preterm delivery and low birthweight they make a disproportionate contribution to the rates of both perinatal morbidity and

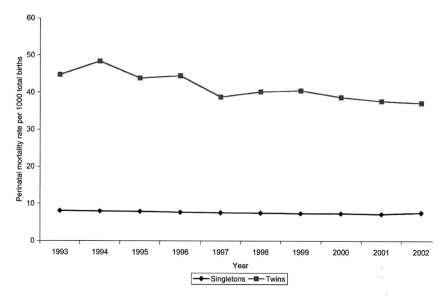

Figure 1.12. Perinatal mortality rate per 1000 total births for singleton and twin births by year, England and Wales, 1993–2002 (perinatal mortality is defined in the UK as all stillbirths born at 24 weeks of gestation or greater plus all live births who die in the first week after birth); data from the ONS

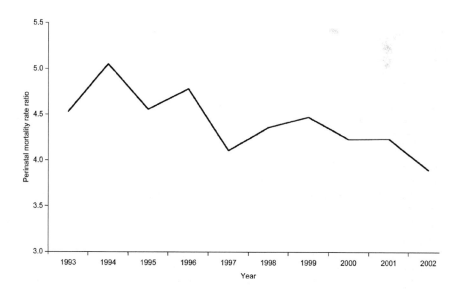

Figure 1.13. Rate ratio of the perinatal mortality rate per 1000 total births for twin births compared with singleton births by year, England and Wales, 1993–2002 (perinatal mortality is defined in the UK as all stillbirths born at 24 weeks of gestation or greater plus all live births who die in the first week after birth); data from the ONS

mortality. Blondel *et al.*[19] quantified this contribution in the mid-1990s as 10–19% of the preterm delivery rate, 17–21% of the low birthweight rate and about 20% of the very preterm delivery and very low birthweight rates. This is against the background rate of twins at about 3% of all births.

The other complications experienced at a higher rate in twins include antepartum haemorrhage, polyhydramnios and pre-eclampsia.[20] Specific twin-related complications also account for some deaths and this is particularly so for monozygous twins who have a higher mortality rate than dizygous twins.[21] For example, twin-to-twin transfusion and cord accidents occur in monozygous twins and can lead to the *in utero* demise of one or both babies. Monozygous twins also have a higher rate of non-deformational congenital anomalies than dizygous twins and a higher overall rate of congenital anomalies compared with singletons.[22]

Interestingly, however, mortality rates for twins are not uniformly greater than those of singletons across the entire gestational age and birthweight range. In 1995 Powers *et al.*[23] analysed gestational age specific neonatal mortality rates for singletons and twins in the USA from 1983 to 1985. The data relating to the white US population are illustrated in Figure 1.14.

While neonatal mortality is higher overall for twins than singletons, as can be seen from Figure 1.14, the rates are lower for twins than singletons who were born between 31 and 36 weeks of gestation. Powers *et al.*[23] postulated two explanations for this apparently counterintuitive finding. The first explanation is that potentially higher levels of stress are experienced by twins *in utero* leading to increased endogenous steroid production resulting in accelerated pulmonary maturation and thus lower rates of respiratory distress syndrome at birth. The second explanation relates to the probability that singletons born preterm are more likely to have a pathological reason for their

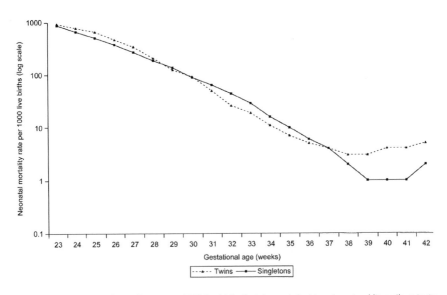

Figure 1.14.   Neonatal mortality rate per 1000 live births for twins and singletons born to white mothers in the USA, 1983–85 (neonatal mortality is defined here as all live births who die in the first month (28 days) after birth); data adapted from Powers *et al.*[23]

early delivery whereas twins are more likely to deliver at these earlier gestations simply because the uterus can no longer physically contain two fetuses and labour is precipitated without any specific underlying pathological cause.

As well as higher rates of perinatal complications, twins also experience higher rates of long-term health problems, such as cerebral palsy. Using Western Australian perinatal and infant mortality data linked to the Western Australian Cerebral Palsy Register, Petterson et al.[24] were able to combine population-based data about deaths and cerebral palsy. They demonstrated that in the 1980s overall one in ten Western Australian women who delivered a twin pregnancy experienced one of the following outcomes which affected at least one of her babies: a stillbirth, an infant death or a child who was subsequently diagnosed with cerebral palsy.

Perinatal morbidity and mortality of twins born following ART

Given that a relatively high proportion of ART conceptions (currently about 1 in 4) result in twin deliveries, quantification of the risk of perinatal mortality and morbidity for this specific group is needed to enable couples to embark upon treatment with realistic expectations of the outcome.

Perinatal mortality rates for twins born following IVF treatment in the UK in 1994–99 have been published by the Human Fertilisation and Embryology Authority (HFEA).[25–30] These rates are compared with the overall England and Wales perinatal mortality rates in Figure 1.15. In 1994 the perinatal mortality rate for IVF twins was 58.3 per 1000 total births and by 1998 the rate had decreased to 43.8 per 1 000. This is in comparison with the overall England and Wales rates for twins which were 40.4 and 32.7 per 1000 live births, respectively. These results suggest that the risk of perinatal death in this period was between 1.2-fold and 1.4-fold higher for twins born following IVF than for twins overall.

A recent meta-analysis carried out by Helmerhorst et al.[31] showed that, having matched for a range of potential confounding factors, for example maternal age and parity, the risk of perinatal mortality for ART twins was in fact significantly less than that of spontaneously conceived twins (rate ratio 0.58; 95% CI 0.44–0.77). They concluded that these findings suggest that the excess mortality experienced by ART twins is due to the characteristics associated with receipt of ART treatment, including older maternal age. They also postulated that the reduction in twin mortality associated with ART may also relate to the relatively low proportion of monozygotic twins (estimated 3–5%) conceived following ART compared with spontaneous twins where monozygosity, with its attendant higher rates of morbidity and mortality, accounts for about 30% of twins in European populations.

Population differences in the rate of triplets and higher order multiples

Prior to the introduction of fertility treatment the occurrence of triplet pregnancies, and indeed higher order multiples, was very uncommon indeed. For example, from 1938 to 1995 there were between 50 and 100 sets of triplets born each year in England and Wales. This relative rarity is reflected in the general lack of information about triplets in the medical literature. As an illustration of this, a simple Medline search was conducted in August 2005 for publications relating to human triplets in the period 1966–68. This generated only 27 references and 20 years later in 1996–98 the number had risen to only 332, which is only just over 100 papers per year.

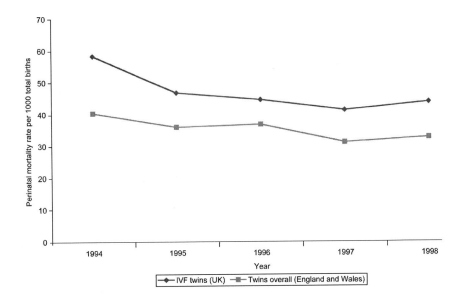

Figure 1.15. Perinatal mortality rate per 1000 total births for twins overall in England and Wales and twins born following IVF in the UK by year, 1994–98 (perinatal mortality is defined in the UK as all stillbirths born at 24 weeks of gestation or greater plus all live births who die in the first week after birth); data from the ONS (overall statistics) and the HFEA (IVF statistics)[27–30]

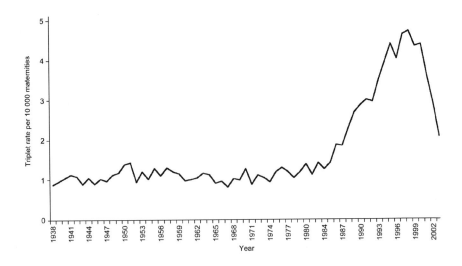

Figure 1.16. Triplet rate per 10 000 maternities by year, England and Wales, 1938–2003; data from the ONS (1981 data not available)

Because of the rarity of triplets and higher order multiples, the rates quoted in the following section for triplets are per 10 000 maternities and for higher order multiples are per million maternities. This is in contrast to twinning rates, which are quoted per 1000 maternities.

As expected from the general lack of information about triplets and higher order multiples, population estimates of the rates of triplet and higher order multiple maternities are scarce. Macfarlane *et al.*[32] summarised the few available data concerning the rate of triplet and higher order multiples across Europe in 2000 and demonstrated that in 1960 there was a four-fold difference in the rate of triplet and higher order multiple maternities across Western Europe. The figures ranged from 0.39 per 10 000 maternities (1 in 25 640) in Sweden to 1.6 per 10 000 (1 in 6250) in Portugal. Following a relatively steady rate of triplets and higher order multiples through the 1960s and early 1970s in most European countries, the rate generally increased from the mid- to late 1970s onwards. From the early 1980s onwards, however, the rates began to rise almost exponentially through to the late 1990s.[32] For example, in 1990 the triplet and higher order multiple rate in the Netherlands reached 6.1 per 10 000 maternities (1 in 1663) compared with a rate of 0.75 per 10 000 (1 in 13 300) in 1975, a nearly ten-fold increase in just 15 years.

Secular trends in the rate of triplets and higher order multiples

Figure 1.16 illustrates the triplet rate per 10 000 maternities in England and Wales from 1938 to 2003. The triplet rate remained relatively constant at around one triplet pregnancy per 10 000 maternities (1 in 10 000) from 1938 until the early 1980s; the year-on-year variation simply reflects the relative rarity of a triplet maternity and thus small-number random variation.

The triplet rate subsequently doubled such that the rate was about 2 per 10 000 (1 in 5000) in the period 1985–89; it trebled in 1990–94 to over 3 per 10 000 (1 in 3000); and quadrupled in the following period, reaching a peak rate of 4.7 per 10 000 or one triplet pregnancy in every 2130 maternities in 1998. A rapid decline followed the 1998 peak such that by 2003 the triplet rate had fallen to 2.1 per 10 000 (1 in 4760) and was roughly equivalent to the rate in the late 1980s.[33]

The rate of higher order multiple maternities in England and Wales from 1938 onwards is shown in Figure 1.17. Apart from the expected wide year-on-year variation due to small numbers, the overall rate was relatively stable, with between zero and five higher order multiple sets born each year, from 1938 until the early 1970s, following which there was a general increase in the rate. The rate of increase became more marked in the early 1980s, with a peak in the rate of higher order multiple maternities in 1993 at 19.4 per million (1 in 51 500). The rate subsequently declined during the 1990s. With the delivery of only three sets of quadruplets in England and Wales in 2003, the rate in this year was just less than five per million, which is equivalent to the rate last seen in the 1970s. Figure 1.18 illustrates the number of higher order multiple maternities delivered since 1938 in England and Wales; the vast majority were quadruplets, with quintuplets, sextuplets and septuplets accounting for only 12%. It is notable that of all maternities resulting in quintuplets and greater in the last 65 years, about 60% of them were born in the last 25 years.

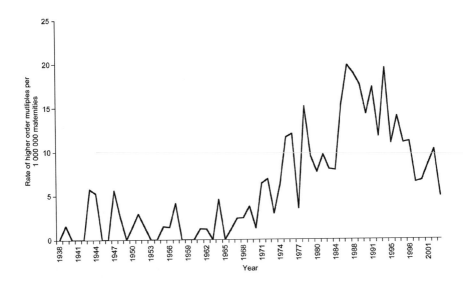

Figure 1.17. Higher order multiple (quadruplet, quintuplet, sextuplet and septuplet) rate per 1 000 000 maternities by year, England and Wales, 1938–2003; data from the ONS (1981, 1987 and 1994 data not available)

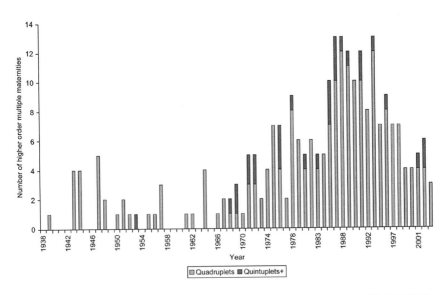

Figure 1.18. Number of higher order multiple (quadruplet, quintuplet, sextuplet and septuplet) maternities by type of plural pregnancy by year, England and Wales, 1938–2003; data from the ONS (1981, 1987 and 1994 data not available)

Factors influencing the rate of triplets and higher order multiples

Maternal age

Although the effect is not as marked as with twinning, the probability of delivering a triplet pregnancy varies with maternal age. As can be seen in Figure 1.19, in England and Wales in the era prior to the introduction of ART women aged 25 years and over experienced triplet maternities at a rate that was about three times higher than their younger counterparts. For example, the triplet rate for women aged 20–24 years was 0.59 per 10 000 maternities (1 in 16 950) compared with a rate of 1.45 per 10 000 (1 in 6900) for women aged 35–39 years. As with twinning, the probability of delivering a triplet pregnancy after the age of 39 years, while still high relative to younger women, is lower than the probability for women aged 25–39 years.

Again, in a pattern similar to that seen for twinning, the age-specific triplet rate in England and Wales has changed profoundly over the last 30 years (Figure 1.20). The triplet maternity rate for women aged 24 years and under remained essentially unchanged between 1974 and 2003. In contrast, from about 1985 onwards, the rates for women aged 25 years and older all increased markedly, and particularly so for women aged 30 years and over. The rate peaked for women aged 25–29 years at 3.6 per 10 000 maternities (1 in 2 780) in 1995, it peaked for women aged 30–34 years at 7.3 per 10 000 (1 in 1370) in 1998, and the rate peaked in 1998 at 12.1 per 10 000 maternities (1 in 826) for women aged 40 years and over.

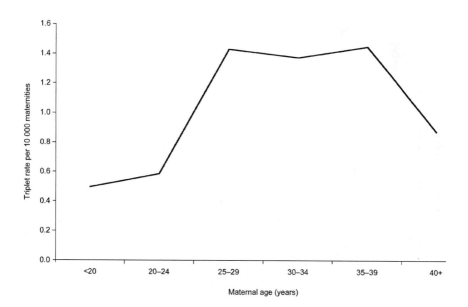

Figure 1.19. Triplet rate per 10 000 maternities by maternal age group, England and Wales, 1974–78; data from the ONS

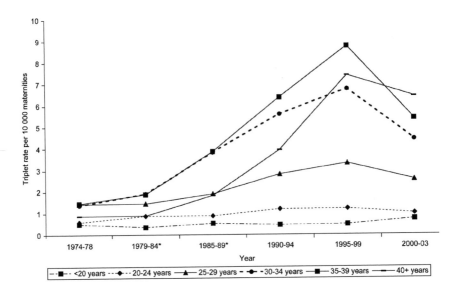

Figure 1.20. Maternal age group specific triplet rate per 10 000 maternities by grouped years, England and Wales, 1974–2003; data from the ONS (1981 and 1988 data not available)

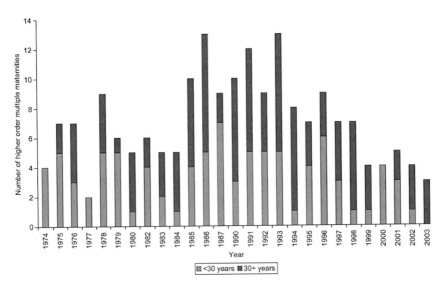

Figure 1.21. Number of higher order multiple (quadruplet, quintuplet, sextuplet and septuplet) maternities by maternal age group and year, England and Wales, 1974–2003; data from the ONS (1981, 1988 and 1989 data not available)

From the early 1980s to the end of the 1990s, women aged 30–34 years experienced nearly a four-fold (relative risk 3.8) increase in the probability of a triplet maternity, for women aged 35–39 years the risk increased 4.7-fold, and for women aged 40 years and over the increased risk was over eight-fold (RR 8.3). The triplet rate for all groups of women subsequently declined, although it is interesting that the decline has been at a slower rate for women aged 40 years and over who now have the highest age-specific triplet rate, having exceeded the rate of their younger counterparts aged 35–39 years. The respective rates in the 2000–03 period were 6.4 and 5.4 per 10 000.

With only a total of 190 higher order multiple maternities delivered in England and Wales since 1974, it is not possible to estimate the maternal age specific higher order multiple maternity rate reliably. However, it is of note that in the period 1974–2003 53% of all higher order maternities were to women aged 30 years and over (Figure 1.21) whereas only 32% of maternities during this whole period were to women in this age group.

Fertility treatment

There is little doubt that the 'epidemic' of triplet and higher order multiple pregnancies seen between the mid-1980s and the turn of the century is largely a direct result of the effects of fertility treatment.[10,19,33] The rapid and almost exponential rise in the triplet rate was mostly confined to women aged 30 years and over and coincided with the widespread and expanding use of ART. The subsequent decline in the rate coincided with a reduction in the proportion of ART treatment cycles that involved the transfer of three embryos. Of all IVF treatment cycles started in 1993,

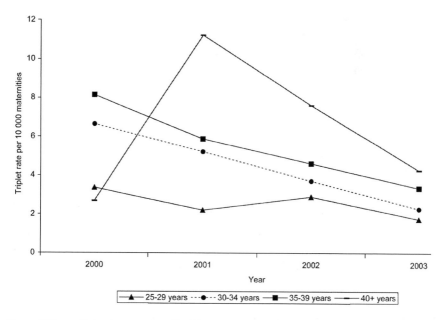

Figure 1.22. Maternal age group specific triplet rate per 10 000 maternities for women aged 25 years and older by year, England and Wales, 2000–2003; data from the ONS

57% involved the transfer of three embryos and 31% involved the transfer of two.[26] By 1997–98 these figures had changed to 48% and 40%, respectively.[30]

Figure 1.22 illustrates in more detail what has happened to the triplet rate in the last four years for which data are currently available in England and Wales. It will be interesting to monitor the effect of the recent Human Fertilisation and Embryology Authority (HFEA) policy change, launched in January 2004, that no more than two embryos should be transferred in women under the age of 40 years.[34] An acceleration in the rate of decline in the triplet and higher order multiples rate for women under the age of 40 can be expected, although the same may not be true for women aged 40 years and over.

Because the risk of triplets varies by maternal age (although the variation is not as marked as for twinning), had all other things remained unchanged, as with twinning some increase in the triplet rate from the mid-1970s onwards would have been expected simply because of the change in the age distribution of women having babies over this period. Figure 1.23 shows an estimate of what would have happened to the rate of triplets from the late 1970s onwards had the same maternal age distribution as in 1974 continued, compared with the actual rate of triplets delivered. Again, as for twinning (Figure 1.8), and extending the analysis carried out by Wood in 1997,[10] the triplet rate was estimated using the method of indirect standardisation. During this period there has actually been a four-fold increase in the triplet rate overall from 1.1 per 10 000 maternities (1 in 9090) in 1974–78 to an overall rate of 4.4 per 10 000 (1 in 2270) in 1995–99. Had the maternal age distribution of births in 1974 prevailed, only a 1.1-fold increase would have been expected, from 1.1 per 10 000 (1 in 9090) in 1974–78 to 1.2 per 10 000 (1 in 8300) in 2000–2003.

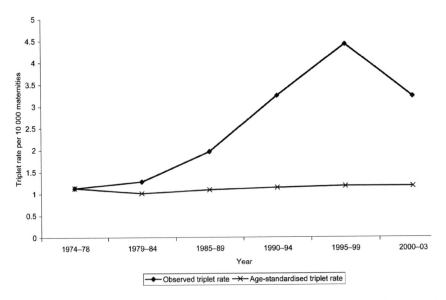

Figure 1.23.   Triplet rate age-standardised to the maternal age distribution of the 1974 maternity population by year, England and Wales, 1974–2003; data from the ONS (1981 and 1988 data not available)

Using the data derived to produce Figure 1.23, the proportion of triplet maternities delivered in the period 1974–2003 that can be attributed to the change in maternal age distribution of all births was estimated. By subtraction from the proportion of triplets equivalent to the 1974 triplet rate, the proportion due to 'other' influences was also estimated. These estimates are illustrated in Figure 1.24. The effects of the change in maternal age distribution from 1974 has, in contrast to the situation for twins, only had a very small effect on the change in the triplet maternity rate. The largest impact was the 'other effects' category, which it seems reasonable to assume largely represents the effects of fertility treatment. Again, in contrast to the situation for twins (Figure 1.9), there is evidence of a decline in the proportion of triplet maternities related to the contribution of these 'other' (likely fertility treatment) effects.

Perinatal mortality and morbidity of triplets and higher order multiples

The pregnancy complications experienced by women pregnant with twins are also experienced by women pregnant with triplets and higher order multiples. Again, as with twins, much of the additional burden of pathology arises because of the increased risk of preterm delivery and low birthweight associated with triplet and higher order pregnancies, both of which are important determinants of perinatal morbidity and mortality and longer term problems. Blondel et al.[19] quantified the contribution of triplets to the preterm delivery rate in the mid-1990s as about 1.2%, as 3% of the very preterm delivery rate, 2% of the low birthweight rate and 4% of the

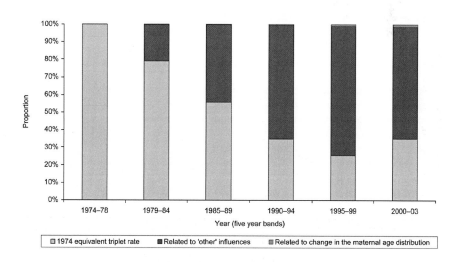

Figure 1.24. Estimated proportion of triplets equivalent to the 1974 triplet rate, the change in maternal age distribution and the effect of 'other' influences on the triplet rate by grouped years, England and Wales, 1974–2003; data from the ONS (1981 and 1988 data not available)

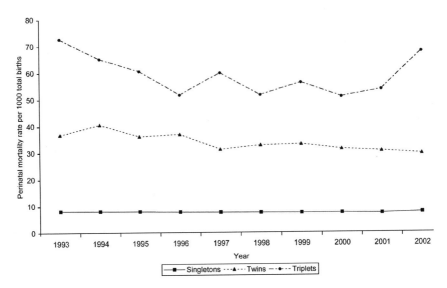

Figure 1.25. Perinatal mortality rate per 1000 total births for singleton, twin and triplet births by year, England and Wales, 1993–2002 (perinatal mortality is defined in the UK as all stillbirths born at 24 weeks of gestation or greater plus all live births who die in the first week after birth); data from the ONS

very low birthweight rate. This was in the context of triplets contributing only 0.13% of all births.[19] The data of Petterson *et al.*[24] are useful to illustrate one aspect of the increased risks of adverse longer term outcomes experienced by triplets. They found that in the 1980s overall one in five Western Australian women who delivered a triplet pregnancy experienced one of the following outcomes that affected at least one of her babies: a stillbirth, an infant death or a child who was subsequently diagnosed with cerebral palsy.[24]

Overall perinatal morbidity and mortality

As noted previously, the perinatal mortality rate is defined in the UK as the total number of stillbirths at 24 weeks of gestation or greater plus live births who die in the first week after birth, divided by the total number of live births and stillbirths. This represents a change in definition, as prior to 1993 stillbirths were only included if they occurred at 28 weeks of gestation or greater.

As can be seen from Figure 1.25, the England and Wales perinatal mortality rate for triplets in the 10-year period 1993–2002 declined initially to the lowest rate in 2000 at 51 per 1000 total births. This was followed by an increase to a rate of 68 per 1000 total births in 2002. This increase was due to an increase in the stillbirth rate (Figure 1.26) rather than deaths in the first week. Over this period the perinatal mortality rate of triplets was between 1.5 and 2.3 times that of twins and between 6.5 and 9.0 times that of singletons.

The perinatal mortality rate of higher order multiples has also declined over the last 10 years with a pattern similar to that of triplets of a decrease followed by a more recent increase, although, with the extremely small numbers involved, the overall change is not statistically significant.

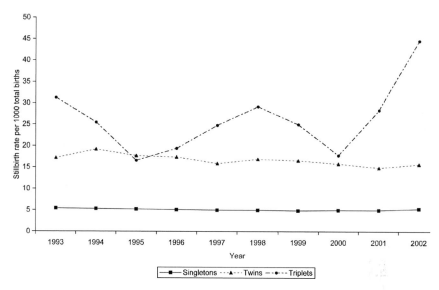

Figure 1.26.   Stillbirth rate per 1000 total births for singleton, twin and triplet births by year, England and Wales, 1993–2002 (the stillbirth rate is defined in the UK as all stillbirths born at 24 weeks of gestation or greater divided by the total number of stillbirths and live births); data from the ONS

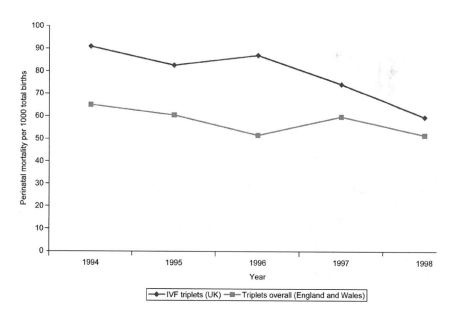

Figure 1.27.   Perinatal mortality rate per 1000 total births for triplets overall in England and Wales and for triplets born following IVF in the UK by year, 1994–1998 (perinatal mortality is defined in the UK as all stillbirths born at 24 weeks of gestation or greater plus all live births who die in the week after birth); data from the ONS (overall statistics) and the HFEA (IVF statistics)[25–30]

Perinatal morbidity and mortality of triplets born following ART

UK-based perinatal mortality rates for triplets born following IVF in 1994–99 have been published by the HFEA.[27–30] These rates are compared with the overall England and Wales perinatal mortality rates in Figure 1.27. In 1994 the perinatal mortality rate for IVF triplets was 90.9 per 1000 total births and by 1998 the rate had decreased to 59.6 per 1000. This is in comparison with the overall England and Wales rates which were 65.1 and 51.6 per 1000 total births, respectively. The risk of perinatal death in this period was thus between 1.2-fold and 1.7-fold higher for triplets born following IVF than for triplets overall.

Conclusions and recommendations

Recent variations in the rate of twins, triplets and higher order multiples, both between and within populations, are strongly influenced by age at motherhood and the effects of treatment for infertility. It is estimated that, compared with the situation in 1974, by 2003 the change in maternal age distribution accounted for 10% of all twin maternities. The effects of fertility treatment over and above the effects experienced in the mid-1970s are estimated to account for about 25% of all twin maternities. There is some evidence of a slowing in the rate of change of the influences of these two factors and the recent change in policy from three to two embryo transfer for most women undergoing IVF is likely to assist in reducing the proportion of twins attributable to this source of conception. However, current projections by the ONS suggest that the mean maternal age at completion of childbearing, which has risen in all cohorts of women born since the mid-1940s in the UK, is likely to continue to increase in all groups of women up to those born in 1990. This suggests that the maternal age contribution to the twinning rate is likely to continue to rise into the foreseeable future, although the rate of increase may slow down. Thus, any effect of changes in ART treatment on the overall twinning rate is likely to be masked by the continuing trend related to maternal age effects. It is therefore recommended that the effects of both maternal age and fertility treatment on the rate of twins, triplets and higher order multiples continue to be closely monitored to enable the influence of these two factors to be disentangled.

While the proportion of iatrogenic multiples attributable to fertility treatments other than IVF is relatively small, the data to enable this estimate to be made in the UK are extremely limited. It is therefore recommended that a mechanism be set up which would allow the monitoring of the impact of non-IVF-related fertility treatment on the multiple maternity rate alongside the monitoring of the effects of IVF treatment.

The differences in mortality rate between multiples and singletons have narrowed in recent years but twins, triplets and higher order multiples continue to experience considerably higher mortality and morbidity than singletons. While there is some evidence that, having adjusted for factors such as maternal age and parity, iatrogenic twins have lower mortality rates than spontaneous twins, they nevertheless experience mortality rates that are well in excess of the rates seen in singletons. For this reason it is recommended that, where possible, iatrogenic multiple conceptions should be avoided and the HFEA should strongly consider moving to a policy of single-embryo transfer for those women at highest risk of conceiving a multiple pregnancy following IVF treatment.

Acknowledgements

Jennifer Kurinczuk is partially funded by a National Public Health Career Scientist award from the Department of Health and NHS R&D (PHCS 022) and partially funded by the grant from the Department of Health to the National Perinatal Epidemiology Unit.

References

1. MacGillivray I. Introduction. In: MacGillivray I, Campbell DM, Thompson B, editors. *Twinning and Twins*. Chichester: John Wiley & Sons; 1988. p. 1–5.

2. Little J, Thompson B. Descriptive epidemiology. In: MacGillivray I, Campbell DM, Thompson B, editors. *Twinning and Twins*. Chichester: John Wiley & Sons; 1988. p. 37–66.

3. Nylander PPS. The frequency of twinning in a rural community in western Nigeria. *Ann Hum Genet* 1969;33:41–4.

4. Hardman R. Pharmaceutical products from plant steroids. *Trop Sci* 1969;11:196.

5. Imaizumi Y. Twinning rates in Japan, 1951–1990. *Acta Genet Med Gemellol (Roma)* 1992;41:165–75.

6. Yoshida K. Soma H. A study of twin placentation in Tokyo. *Acta Genet Med Gemellol (Roma)* 1984;33:115–20.

7. Eriksson AW, Eskola MR, Fellman JO. Retrospective studies on the twinning rate in Scandinavia. *Acta Genet Med Gemellol (Roma)* 1976;25:29–35.

8. Eriksson AW, Fellman JO. Differences in the twinning trends between Finns and Swedes. *Am J Hum Genet* 1973;25:141–51.

9. Derom R, Orlebeke J, Eriksson A, Thiery M. The epidemiology of multiple births in Europe. In: Keith LG, Papiernick E, Keith DM, Luke B, editors. *Multiple Pregnancy, Epidemiology, Gestation and Perinatal Outcome*. New York: The Parthenon Publishing Group; 1995. p. 145–62.

10. Wood R. Trends in multiple births; 1938–1995 *Popul Trends* 1997;87:29–35.

11. MacGillivray I, Samphier M, Little J. Factors affecting twinning. In: MacGillivray I, Campbell DM, Thompson B, editors. *Twinning and Twins*. Chichester: John Wiley & Sons; 1988. p. 67–92.

12. Allen G, Schachter J. Do conception delays explain some changes in twinning rates? *Acta Genet Med Gemellol (Roma)* 1970;19:30–4.

13. Allen G. The parity effect and fertility in mothers of twins. In: Nance WE, Allen G, Parisi P, editors. *Twin Research 3, Biology and Epidemiology*. New York: Alan R Liss; 1978. p. 89–97.

14. Information and Statistics Division, Scottish Health Services. *Births in Scotland*. Edinburgh: ISD Publications; 1997. p. 10.

15. *Fertility: women are having children later*. Office for National Statistics; 2005 [www.statistics.gov.uk/cci/nugget_print.asp?ID=762].

16. Kurinczuk JJ, Quigley MA, Hockley C, Henderson J, McVeigh E, Barlow DH, *et al*. The contribution of infertility treatment to births in the UK at the turn of the millennium. Unpublished data.

17. Bergh T, Ericson A, Hillensjö T, Nygren K-G, Wennerholm UB. Deliveries and children born after in-vitro fertilisation in Sweden; 1982–95: a retrospective cohort study. *Lancet* 1999;354:1579–85.

18. Derom C, Derom R, Vlientinck R, Maes H, Van den Berghe H. Iatrogenic multiple pregnancies in East Flanders, Belgium. *Fertil Steril* 1993;60:493–6.

19. Blondel B, Kogan MD, Alexander GR, Dattani N, Kramer MS, Macfarlane AJ, *et al*. The impact of the increasing number of multiple births on rates of preterm birth and low birthweight: an international study. *Am J Public Health* 2002;92:1323–30.

20. MacGillivray I, Campbell DM. Management of twin pregnancies. In: MacGillivray I, Campbell DM, Thompson B, editors. *Twinning and Twins*. Chichester: John Wiley & Sons; 1988. p. 111–41.

21. Lopez-Zeno JA, Navarro-Pando J. The intrauterine demise of one fetus. In: Keith LG, Papiernick E, Keith DM, Luke B, editors. *Multiple Pregnancy: Epidemiology, Gestation and Perinatal Outcome*. New York: The Parthenon Publishing Group; 1995. p. 407–10.

22. Allan MC. Factors affecting developmental outcomes. In: Keith LG, Papiernick E, Keith DM, Luke B, editors. *Multiple Pregnancy: Epidemiology, Gestation and Perinatal Outcome*. New York: The Parthenon Publishing Group; 1995. p. 599–612.

23. Powers WF, Kiely JL, Fowler MG. The role of birth weight, gestational age, race and other infant characteristics in twin intrauterine growth and infant mortality. In: Keith LG, Papiernick E, Keith

DM, Luke B, editors. *Multiple Pregnancy: Epidemiology, Gestation and Perinatal Outcome*. New York: The Parthenon Publishing Group; 1995. p. 163–74.

24. Petterson B, Nelson KB, Watson L, Stanley FJ. Twins, triplets and cerebral palsy in births in Western Australia in the 1980s. *BMJ* 1993;307:1239–43.

25. Human Fertilisation and Embryology Authority. *Human Fertilisation and Embryology Authority Third Annual Report 1994*. London: HFEA; 1994. p. 41.

26. Human Fertilisation and Embryology Authority. *Human Fertilisation and Embryology Authority Fourth Annual Report 1995*. London: HFEA; 1995. p. 31.

27. Human Fertilisation and Embryology Authority. *Human Fertilisation and Embryology Authority Fifth Annual Report 1996*. London: HFEA; 1996. p. 32.

28. Human Fertilisation and Embryology Authority. *Human Fertilisation and Embryology Authority Sixth Annual Report 1997*. London: HFEA; 1997. p. 26.

29. Human Fertilisation and Embryology Authority. *Human Fertilisation and Embryology Authority Seventh Annual Report and Accounts 1998*. London: HFEA; 1998. p. 12.

30. Human Fertilisation and Embryology Authority. *Human Fertilisation and Embryology Authority Eighth Annual Report and Accounts 1999*. London: HFEA; 1999. p. 16.

31. Helmerhorst FM, Perquin AM, Donker D, Keirse MJNC. Perinatal outcomes of singletons and twins after assisted conception: a systematic review of controlled studies. *BMJ* 2004;328:261.

32. Macfarlane AJ, Mugford M, Henderson J, Furtado A, Stevens J, Dunn A. *Birth Counts: Statistics of Pregnancy and Childbirth. Volume 2: Tables*, 2nd ed. London: The Stationery Office; 2000.

33. Simmons R, Doyle P, Maconochie N. Dramatic reduction in triplet and higher order births in England and Wales. *BJOG* 2004;111:856.

34. Human Fertilisation and Embryology Authority. *Facing up to the Challenge. Human Fertilisation and Embryology Authority Annual Report; 2003/2004*. London: HFEA; 2004. p. 19–20.

Chapter 2

Assisted conception and multiple pregnancies: methods of reducing multiples from assisted reproduction

Siladitya Bhattacharya and Zabeena Pandian

Introduction

Between 1996 and 2002, the number of assisted reproductive technology (ART) cycles performed in the USA increased by 78% from 64 681 to 115 392 (Figure 2.1). The number of live birth events over the same period increased by 128% from 14 507 to 33 141. The increase in the use of ART over the past two decades has led to a significant increase in the incidence of multiple pregnancy and higher order births.[1] Following *in vitro* fertilisation (IVF), the chance of conceiving twins is 20 times higher and that of higher order multiples is 400 times higher than in the general population.[2] Thus, in many cases a live birth delivery yields more than one infant. There was an absolute increase of 120% in the number of ART infants delivered in the USA between 1996 and 2002, from 20 840 to 45 751.[3] Worldwide, about 50 000 children are born annually as a result of IVF treatment. In Sweden they account for 2% of all infants born,[4] while in Denmark the figure is even higher at 5%.[5] This number is set to rise further in the next few years. As more than half of all babies born following ART are twins or higher order multiples, there are serious concerns about the impact of the global growth in assisted reproduction techniques on future healthcare needs.

This chapter describes the risks of iatrogenic multiple pregnancy (including higher order multiples) in assisted conception, examines the factors that encourage multiples and reviews the literature on the effect of embryo number on IVF outcome. Finally, it explores suggested ways of reducing unwanted multiple pregnancies, including regulation of assisted reproduction.

Risk of multiple pregnancies in ART

Figures from the Society for Assisted Reproductive Technology Registry for the year 2002[3] indicate that out of a total of 29 423 non-donor ART pregnancies in the USA, 58% were singletons, 29% were twins and 7% were triplets or higher order multiples (Figure 2.2). Comparable figures from Europe in 2001 based on 289 690 cycles show that 75% of babies conceived through ART births were singletons, 24% were twins and 1.5% were triplets. Quadruplets occurred in seven cases (Figure 2.3).

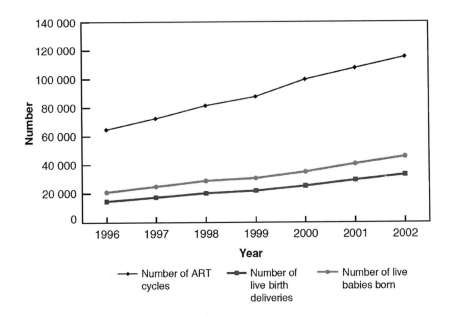

Figure 2.1. Trends in ART in the USA; adapted with permission from the Centers for Disease Control and Prevention[3]

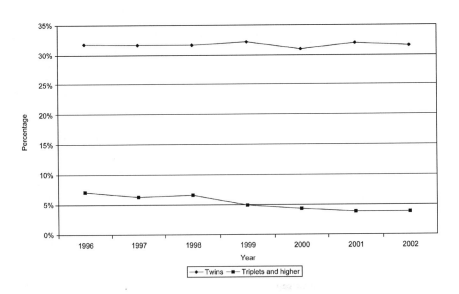

Figure 2.2. Trends in multiple births in the USA; data from the Centers for Disease Control and Prevention[3,51] and the American Society for Reproductive Medicine/Society for Assisted Reproductive Technology Registry[52-56]

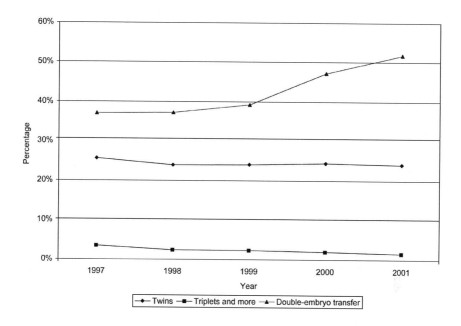

Figure 2.3.   Trends in multiple births in Europe; data from the European IVF-Monitoring Programme (EIM)[23,57-60]

Data from IVF cycles in the UK published by the Human Fertilisation and Embryology Authority (HFEA)[6] for the year 2000–01 show a twin birth rate of 25% and a triplet birth rate of 1.7%. Historical data from this national database during the periods 1994–95, 1995–96, 1996–97 and 1997–98 demonstrate a fairly stable trend (25%, 27%, 25% and 25% for twins and 4%, 3%, 3% and 3% for triplets, respectively).[2]

In comparison with singletons, twins have a six-fold and triplets a 10-fold to 20-fold increased risk of mortality.[2] In 1995 the overall perinatal mortality rate in England and Wales was 8.7 per 1000 live births. The corresponding figure was 46.8 per 1000 for IVF twins, and 82.6 per 1000 for IVF triplets. There are also concerns about increased maternal risks in multiple pregnancies.[7] There has traditionally been a tacit acceptance that iatrogenic multiple pregnancy is a necessary price that couples and clinicians must pay in order to ensure the success of invasive, expensive and emotionally demanding fertility treatment. Twins, in some cases, are even perceived to be desirable end products of ART by couples as well as by healthcare providers.[8] It has only been in recent years that there has been a growing awareness that the aim of fertility treatment is not merely to achieve conception but to ensure the birth of a healthy infant.

Risk of multiple pregnancies with specific ART techniques

While IVF remains the most common cause, other assisted conception techniques such as superovulation and intrauterine insemination (IUI) are also responsible for iatrogenic multiple pregnancies. In fact, gonadotrophin stimulation of the ovaries in non-IVF treatment cycles is a major cause of higher order multiples.[9] Among quadruplets or higher order multiples in the USA, 50–72% are caused by ovarian stimulation, 42% are due to IVF, while 6–7% occur spontaneously.[10] IUI with or without ovarian stimulation is commonly used in couples with either unexplained infertility or male factor problems. Both IUI and ovarian stimulation independently increase the probability of conception.[11] When used in combination, the chance of pregnancy increases further – as does the risk of multiples. A large randomised controlled trial (RCT) in the USA[12] has shown that in couples undergoing IUI, gonadotrophin stimulation increases pregnancy rates (OR 1.7, 95% CI 1.2–2.6), but at a significant cost. Among the 77 women in the trial who conceived following IUI with gonadotrophin stimulation, the twin rate was 22%, the triplet rate was 4% and the quadruplet rate was 3%. In contrast, there were no multiple pregnancies among the 42 pregnancies in the unstimulated IUI group. The risk of multiple pregnancies associated with stimulated IUI depends on the aggressiveness of the stimulation regimen. An unpublished multicentre observational study[13] conducted in the UK reported the outcome of 1580 stimulated IUI cycles. Among the 126 pregnancies reported, there were 11 twins (9%), two triplets (1.6%) and one higher order (quadruplet) pregnancy (0.8%). A randomised trial conducted in the Netherlands on 120 couples found that 36% of the couples who had stimulated IUI achieved a live birth compared with 24% of couples who received unstimulated IUI (RR 1.52, 95% CI 0.86–2.68). In the stimulated IUI group, 17 out of 59 pregnancies were multiples (OR 0.63, 95% CI 0.27–1.47).

Unlike IVF, there are few effective practical measures for the prevention of multiple pregnancies in association with stimulated IUI. Peak serum oestradiol and number and size of ovarian follicles have been suggested as predictors of higher order multiple pregnancy. Cancellation of treatment cycles where the peak serum oestradiol concentration is high or where there is sonographic evidence of multiple large follicles has been suggested. In a large retrospective cohort study of 3137 gonadotrophin-stimulated ovarian cycles, Gleicher et al.[14] confirmed that the peak serum oestradiol concentration and the total number of follicles were independent predictors of higher order multiple pregnancy. As the total number of follicles is often difficult to determine by ultrasonography, and the predictive value of the number of large follicles (those > 16 mm in diameter) was low, the authors concluded that sonographic assessment of ovarian stimulation was of limited value in reducing the risk of multiple pregnancies. Their analysis revealed that stimulation up to a maximal serum oestradiol concentration of 1385 pg/mL could reduce the incidence of higher order multiple pregnancy. A lesser degree of stimulation, with lower peak serum oestradiol levels, could potentially reduce the incidence of higher order multiple pregnancy but could also compromise pregnancy rates by increasing the number of cycles cancelled. It is evident from these findings that the correlation between ultrasonographic and hormonal parameters of ovarian stimulation and clinical outcome is not sufficiently clear to guide clinical practice. The authors concluded that the options to minimise the risk of multiple pregnancy were either to choose a regimen with milder ovarian stimulation or to consider IVF as a substitute.

A systematic review[15] of five RCTs ($n = 231$) compared oral (anti-oestrogens) and injectable (gonadotrophin) drugs for stimulated IUI in couples with unexplained infertility. In some of the RCTs, the oral anti-oestrogen treatment group received human chorionic gonadotrophin (hCG) as an ovulation trigger. This review found no significant difference in multiple birth rates per couple (OR 1.08, 95% CI 0.16–7.03) between the two groups. However, the pregnancy rate per couple was significantly lower with oral anti-oestrogen-stimulated IUI than with gonadotrophin-stimulated IUI

(OR 0.41, 95% CI 0.17–0.80). An RCT[16] ($n = 97$) compared various gonadotrophin regimens with IUI and found no difference with conventional follicle-stimulating hormone (FSH) and IUI when compared with low-dose and step-up FSH and IUI on the multiple pregnancy rate (28.6% versus 14.3%, RR 2.0, 95% CI 0.23–17.34).

Pre-ovulatory vaginal ultrasound-guided aspiration of supernumerary follicles has been advocated as an effective strategy to control the multiple pregnancy rate in superovulation and IUI cycles.[2] However, it is argued that conversion of the treatment to IVF/embryo transfer would provide a higher level of clinical control over the prevailing risks of multiple pregnancy. Avoiding ovarian stimulation and providing unstimulated IUI alone where indicated appears to be the safer option at present.

Based on the results of the above studies, the National Institute for Health and Clinical Excellence (NICE) guidelines published in the UK in 2004[17] recommended that routine use of ovarian stimulation in IUI should be avoided (even though it may be associated with higher pregnancy rates) because of the substantial risk of multiple pregnancies.

IVF and multiple pregnancies: how many embryos should be transferred?

Triplets and higher order multiples

The number of embryos transferred in IVF/intracytoplasmic sperm injection (ICSI) treatment is crucial in determining the risk of multiple births (Table 2.1). By the end of the 1990s, it became clear that a policy of replacing three or more embryos needed to be modified if the rate of triplets and higher order multiples was to be checked. Determining the optimum number of embryos for transfer in IVF requires identifying the point at which transfer of an extra embryo will increase the risk of multiple pregnancy without a corresponding benefit in terms of live birth rates.[18] Analysis of the HFEA National Database in the United Kingdom has revealed that in women under 40 years who have four or more embryos available, transferring two rather than three embryos reduces the risk of triplets without affecting the live birth rate.[19] Tables 2.2 and 2.3 show the relationship between the number of fertilised eggs, the actual number of embryos transferred and the IVF outcome (live births as well as multiples). Although data on embryo quality were not available in this study, the assumption was that availability of a number of embryos for transfer was a surrogate marker of embryo quality. A second study[20] based on a large national dataset from the USA confirmed that the risk of multiple pregnancy was related to maternal age and the number of embryos replaced. In younger women (under 35 years), high live birth rates were achieved by transferring two embryos. In older women, increasing the number of embryos resulted in an increase in live birth rates (not statistically significant) which was accompanied by a highly significant rise in multiple birth rates from 12% to 29%. Younger women thus have an increased chance of live births as well as of multiple births. Table 2.4 shows the relationship between the number of embryos transferred, live births and multiple births in women younger than 35 years of age who chose to set aside some embryos for future use rather than transfer all available embryos at one time. In this group, the chance for a live birth was about 50% when only two embryos were transferred and there was no additional advantage in transferring three embryos. The risk of multiple-infant births was nil with transfer of one embryo, but very high at 40% with two embryos and 47% with three embryos. Transferring three or more embryos also created an additional risk for higher order multiple births.

Table 2.1. Live births and multiple pregnancies for ART cycles using fresh non-donor eggs or embryos, by number of embryos transferred; data from the Centers for Disease Control and Prevention[3]

Embryos transferred	Rate (%)			
	Live birth rate per transfer	Singletons	Twins	Triplets or more
1	12.8	98.0	2.0	–
2	39.5	66.7	32.6	0.7
3	37.7	61.7	32.6	5.7
4	32.8	62.3	32.1	5.6
≥5	28.9	63.2	31.3	5.6

Apart from the quality of the embryo/s transferred,[2] other factors that influence the success of IVF treatment, such as duration of infertility and number of previous IVF attempts, also appear to affect the risk of multiple pregnancy.[19] These factors should thus be taken into account when planning an individualised treatment strategy. For example, in women with prolonged infertility and multiple previous IVF failures, it may be reasonable to allow a three-embryo transfer.

Despite the absence of randomised trials comparing a three versus two embryo policy, the available evidence, based on analyses of large national datasets, is compelling. The British Fertility Society, the Royal College of Obstetricians and Gynaecologists and the HFEA have recommended a double-embryo transfer policy in the UK except in exceptional cases.[2] A number of other observational studies have confirmed the fact that an elective double-embryo transfer policy substantially reduces the risk of triplets without affecting overall live birth rates.[21,22] Confirmation of the effectiveness of a double-embryo transfer policy comes from a comparison of European and American data. In 2001 64% of all transfers in Europe involved one or two embryos.[23] In the USA, the corresponding figure was 37%.[3] The proportion of IVF-related triplet deliveries in Europe during this period was 1.5% compared with 3.8% in the USA.[3,23]

Table 2.2. Effect of number of embryos transferred on live births and multiple births; data from Templeton and Morris[19]

Eggs fertilised	Embryos transferred	Odds of live birth (95% CI)	Odds of multiple birth (95% CI)
2	2	0.5 (0.4–0.5)	0.5 (0.4–0.7)
3–4	2	0.6 (0.5–0.7)	0.7 (0.6–0.9)
3–4	3	0.7 (0.7–0.8)	1.3 (1.1–1.4)
>4	2	1.0 (0.9–1.1)	1.0 (0.9–1.1)
>4	3	1.0 (0.9–1.1)	1.6 (1.5–1.8)

Table 2.3. Number of singleton, twin and triplet births according to number of eggs fertilised and embryos transferred; data from Templeton and Morris (1998)[19]

Number of eggs fertilised and embryos transferred	Number of live births (% of total live births in brackets)			
	0	1	2	3 or more
2 eggs fertilised, 2 embryos transferred	3918	434 (84%)	82 (16%)	2 (0.4%)
> 2 eggs fertilised, > 2 embryos transferred	8297	1647 (73%)	586 (26%)	8 (0.4%)
> 2 eggs fertilised, > 3 embryos transferred	23171	3980 (65%)	1755 (29%)	356 (6%)

Strategies for prevention of twins

European data from 2001[23] show that 52% of women undergoing IVF received a double-embryo transfer, resulting in a twin delivery rate of 24%. Thus, while the problem of triplets and higher order multiples has been largely addressed, almost half of all IVF babies continue to be twins. While the actual risks are lower in comparison with higher order multiples, the sheer number of twin pregnancies raises substantial concerns about maternal and fetal wellbeing. Suggested options for reducing the risk of twins include:

- selective fetal reduction
- single blastocyst transfer
- elective single-embryo transfer.

Selective fetal reduction in twins carries a risk of miscarriage and poses serious ethical and legal questions.[24] Blastocyst transfer (i.e. replacing embryos on day 5 rather than day 2–3 post oocyte retrieval), involves transferring fewer but higher quality embryos that have survived in culture up to the blastocyst stage. This technique needs special expertise and cannot be routinely offered by all laboratories. Failure to grow to blastocyst stage limits the number of embryos available for transfer and can compromise the live birth rate per cycle started. In addition, universally agreed criteria for the selection of blastocysts for transfer have yet to be clarified.[25] A Cochrane review[26]

Table 2.4. Live births and multiple pregnancies for ART cycles in women younger than 35 years; data from the Centers for Disease Control and Prevention[3]

Embryos transferred	Rate (%)			
	Live birth rate per transfer	Singletons	Twins	Triplets or more
1	47.4	100.0	–	–
2	51.8	60.4	38.8	0.9
3	49.6	52.8	39.1	8.1
4	45.5	49.7	40.3	10.0
≥5	45.7	51.1	40.2	8.8

has failed to demonstrate any advantage of blastocyst transfer over conventional (day 2–3) transfer in terms of pregnancy rate per woman. The combined odds ratio in favour of day 2–3 transfer was 0.80 (95% CI 0.57–1.29).

Elective single-embryo transfer

Initial anxieties about the effectiveness of single-embryo transfer were not dispelled by early reports showing poor pregnancy rates when only one embryo was available (i.e. non-elective single-embryo transfer).[2] Data from observational studies on selected subgroups of women at increased risk of twins suggested that elective single-embryo transfer could virtually eliminate the risk of twins without sacrificing pregnancy and live birth rates.[27]

A systematic review of RCTs comparing elective double-embryo transfer with elective single-embryo transfer using the search strategy developed for the Cochrane Menstrual Disorders and Subfertility Group (MDSG) has been undertaken recently.[28]

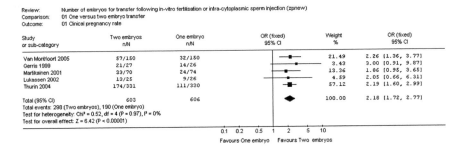

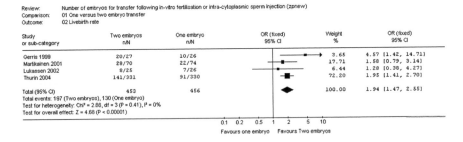

Figure 2.4. Outcome following elective single-embryo transfer versus double-embryo transfer: (a) pregnancy rate per woman per treatment; (b) live birth rate per woman per treatment

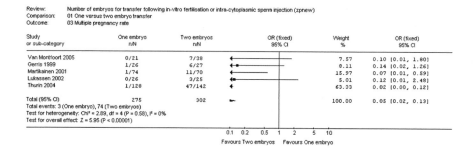

Figure 2.5. Multiple pregnancy rate associated with elective single- and double-embryo transfer

Since then, results of a further trial, which presents pregnancy rates, but not live birth rates, have become available in abstract form.[29] The literature currently includes five trials where single-embryo transfer was compared with double-embryo transfer.[29–33] In all except one, the women included were of good prognosis, i.e. younger women without a history of multiple failed IVF cycles, and with a number of embryos available for transfer. Only one trial reported live birth rates and cumulative live birth rates after a fresh elective single-embryo transfer followed by single frozen embryo transfer.[33]

In comparison with single-embryo transfer, double-embryo transfer in a fresh IVF/ICSI treatment cycle led to a significantly higher pregnancy rate (OR 2.18, 95% CI 1.72–2.77, test for overall effect $P < 0.00001$) and live birth rate (OR 1.94, 95% CI 1.47–2.55, test for overall effect $P < 0.00001$) per woman after a fresh IVF treatment cycle (Figure 2.4). The multiple pregnancy rate was significantly lower in women who had elective single-embryo transfer (OR 0.05, 95% CI 0.02–0.13, $P = 0.00001$) (Figure 2.5). The largest and most recent trial[33] compared two policies: transferring two fresh embryos versus transferring a single fresh embryo followed by a single frozen thawed embryo. There were no significant differences in the cumulative live birth rates (OR 1.19, 95% CI 0.87–1.62, $P = 0.3$) between the two groups (Figure 2.6). Multiple pregnancy rates were significantly higher in women who had elective double-embryo transfer (OR 62.83, 95% CI 8.52–463.57, $P = 0.00005$).

Review:	Number of embryos for transfer following in-vitro fertilisation or intra-cytoplasmic sperm injection (zpnew)					
Comparison:	03 One+Cryo versus Two embryo transfer					
Outcome:	03 Livebirth rate					
Study or sub-category	DET n/N	SET+1FZET n/N	OR (fixed) 95% CI	Weight %	OR (fixed) 95% CI	
Thurin 2004	142/331	128/330		100.00	1.19 [0.87, 1.62]	
Total (95% CI)	331	330		100.00	1.19 [0.87, 1.62]	
Total events: 142 (DET), 128 (SET+1FZET)						
Test for heterogeneity: not applicable						
Test for overall effect: Z = 1.08 (P = 0.28)						

0.1 0.2 0.5 1 2 5 10
Favours SET + 1FZET   Favours DET

Figure 2.6. Cumulative live birth rate per woman following fresh and frozen elective single-embryo transfer versus fresh double-embryo transfer

These results indicate that following fresh IVF treatment, the risk of multiple pregnancy, including twins, is lower following elective single-embryo transfer than after elective double-embryo transfer, as are the live birth and pregnancy rates. However, a single-embryo transfer policy involving a fresh IVF cycle followed by a frozen embryo replacement cycle reduces the risk of multiples while achieving a live birth rate comparable to that achieved by transferring two fresh embryos. There are, however, no data on cumulative live birth rates associated with fresh followed by subsequent frozen single-embryo transfer versus fresh and subsequent frozen double-embryo transfer.

How many embryos should be transferred in IVF?

Reduction in the number of embryos transferred in the course of IVF treatment is a certain way of limiting multiple pregnancies. Current evidence suggests that this can be achieved without compromising live birth rates per woman. In women under 40 years (who constitute the majority of patients receiving IVF), there is little justification for transferring more than two embryos at a time.[19] In women under 38 years with a good prognosis (first or second IVF cycle, a number of good-quality embryos available for transfer) elective single-embryo transfer should be considered as a way of avoiding twins without compromising treatment success.[27] In Europe, double-embryo transfers accounted for 51.7% of all transfers in 2001 (Figure 2.3). Three embryos were transferred in 31% of cases while four-embryo transfers accounted for 5.5%. In the USA, 2002 figures indicate that 33.6% of transfers involved three embryos and 28.3% involved four or more embryos.[3] The consequences of the different policies are reflected in the different rates of multiple pregnancies on either side of the Atlantic (Figures 2.2 and 2.3).

Double-embryo transfer is the default in many clinics in Europe and a significant minority of centres in the USA. Uptake of an elective single-embryo transfer policy has been much slower. In 2001, single-embryo transfers accounted for only 12% of IVF cycles in Europe (6.2% in the USA).

Regulation of IVF: limiting the number of embryos transferred

Any change in health strategy can be either voluntary or enforced by legislation. Voluntary change is possible only if service providers and consumers are convinced that the new policy offers advantages that outweigh any potential disadvantages. In the context of reducing the number of embryos transferred in IVF, a number of barriers need to be overcome before this can happen.

Convincing proof of effectiveness and acceptability in all settings

Evidence from randomised trials conducted in Northern Europe supports the hypothesis that replacing embryos singly, in a combination of fresh and frozen cycles, will virtually eliminate the risk of twins and yet offer live birth rates comparable to a single fresh double-embryo transfer. Although prevention of twin pregnancies is a certainty, there are not sufficient trial data on cumulative live birth rates per woman following either policy. There are also few data from prospective trials on the cumulative cost per live birth, including costs of cryopreservation and patient costs. Most importantly, there are no data on couples' views on the acceptability of the alternative strategies or their perceptions of whether single-embryo transfer offers 'value for money'. This is a crucial issue, as the majority of IVF treatments worldwide are self-funded.

Selectivity of an embryo replacement policy

Current evidence does not support a universal policy of single-embryo replacement in all women undergoing IVF. Elective single-embryo transfer should be reserved for women who are at significant risk of multiple gestation.[27] This includes those who are relatively young, are in their first or second IVF cycle and who possess a number of good-quality embryos.[34] Other women should receive two embryos, and many would argue for a three-embryo transfer policy in women over 40 years. Accurate determination of embryo quality is also a crucial component of a selective single-embryo transfer policy. A constant source of frustration is failure of implantation despite the replacement of 'good-quality' embryos. Suggested methods of improving the quality of transferred embryos include culturing embryos to the blastocyst stage[35] and pre-implantation genetic screening.[36,37] Currently, there is little convincing evidence from randomised trials to support routine use of either technique.

Cryopreservation

The outcome of a single-embryo transfer policy can be substantially improved when used in conjunction with an efficient and reliable embryo cryopreservation programme.[38,39] While human IVF embryos can be frozen successfully, the rates of survival after thawing vary substantially from clinic to clinic and live birth rates are reduced in frozen cycles. There are few controlled data to show that the protocol favoured by most clinics is optimal. Most clinics freeze pronucleate and early cleavage stage embryos and report that 30–80% survive thawing. Such damage is not inconsistent with development to term but intact embryos have a greater potential for implantation and development.[40] There is a need to develop alternative cryopreservation protocols that will lead to improved outcome in frozen cycles.

Perception of success in IVF

The decision to opt for single-embryo transfer must be influenced by the perception of success associated with treatment. It is the definition of 'success' in this context that has generated a degree of controversy. Outcomes in IVF are conventionally expressed in terms of a *live birth per fresh cycle*. Outcomes of subsequent frozen cycles are reported separately. It comes as no surprise that expressing outcomes per fresh cycle can underestimate the success of single-embryo transfer by half. It has been suggested that expressing outcomes as *live birth per woman*, makes better practical, and statistical, sense.[41] Proponents of single-embryo transfer have argued that the best outcome should be either *singleton live birth* or *term singleton live birth*.[42] While both underline the importance of a healthy singleton birth as the desired outcome of fertility treatment, they still focus on cycle (treatment) rather than the woman as the denominator.

Consumer choice

Clinicians may feel that a high twin rate in IVF is unacceptable,[43] but many couples have different views. Some women, especially mothers of IVF twins, may actually see twins as a desirable outcome.[44,45] Others who are paying for their treatment, may feel that having twins represents a cost-effective way of completing their family. Improved methods of communicating risks to couples does not always change couples' opinions.[46] Fewer than one-third of UK women in their early thirties embarking on their first IVF cycle felt that a hypothetical policy of elective single-embryo transfer was acceptable if it meant slightly reduced pregnancy rates.[46] Just over half would consider elective single-embryo transfer, provided they were not charged for cryopreservation and subsequent replacement of spare embryos.

Financial arrangements

Couples who are charged either for multiple fresh IVF cycles (resulting in a transfer of the single best embryo) or for freezing and thawing embryos are understandably reluctant to consider single-embryo transfer. In contrast, this policy has worked well in European settings where IVF is subsidised. On 1 July 2003, the Belgian government agreed to reimburse IVF/ICSI costs for all women under 43 years for a maximum of six cycles provided all women at risk of twins were given single-embryo transfers.[47] Assuming 1750 pregnancies from 7000 cycles in Belgium, the additional costs of treatment would be €8.4 million. These costs would be offset completely by €9.1 million saved by eliminating the risk of triplets and minimising twins. Early results suggest that this policy has been successful without compromising pregnancy and live birth rates.[27,47] Belgian figures show a steady decline in the number of embryos transferred and in the proportion of IVF-related multiple deliveries (from 34% in 1996 to 24% in 2001). In other countries, especially where IVF is self-funded, couples might prefer multiple-embryo transfer in order to maximise the chance of a live birth at their first attempt. The financial argument is stronger in healthcare systems where the source of funding for IVF is the same as that for obstetric and neonatal costs. The existing system in the UK, whereby many couples pay for IVF, while the cost of neonatal care is borne by the National Health Service, is apt to discourage some couples from accepting elective single-embryo transfer.

Legislation

It is clear from the European experience that legislation is a potent factor in changing practice in IVF.[48] This is backed up by the results of a qualitative study[49] which suggest that, while many couples undergoing IVF do not have a preference for elective single-embryo transfer, they would comply with any law enforcing it. From a practical perspective, it is clear that any such legislation will need to be backed up with adequate funding for multiple treatments.[45] Since 2002, new legislation in Sweden has led to a single-embryo transfer policy in couples treated within the public sector. From 2003, the law applied to all women in the country. Saldeen and Sondstrom[50] have presented data comparing the effect of this on IVF success rates during three periods – pre-legislation, a transitional period and post-legislation (Table 2.5). The results suggest that moving from a 25% to a 72% single-embryo transfer rate within a single clinic in Sweden dramatically reduced twin rates but without detriment to pregnancy rates.

Conclusion

There is a need to improve the safety of ART by reducing the rate of iatrogenic multiple pregnancies. Where IUI is indicated, withholding concurrent gonadotrophin use should be considered. In IVF, limiting the number of embryos transferred appears

Table 2.5. Effect of moving to a policy of mandatory single-embryo transfer in Sweden; data from Saldeen and Sondstrom (2005)[50]

	2001–02 (pre-legislation) n = 609	2002 (transitional) n = 320	2003 (post-legislation) n = 433	P value
Single-embryo transfer rate	25%	56%	72%	< 0.01
Clinical pregnancy per embryo transfer	33%	33%	37%	0.4
Viable pregnancy per embryo transfer	30%	30%	31%	0.4
Twin rate	23%	16%	6%	< 0.01

to be the most effective way of avoiding unwanted multiples. In the majority of women, the default position should be a double-embryo transfer policy. In women at high risk of twins, elective single-embryo transfer can lead to high cumulative live birth rates. The current body of evidence, based on the limited number of randomised trials, is unlikely to change existing clinical practice. There is a need for more multicentre RCTs evaluating single-embryo transfer as well as unstimulated IUI. Regulation of assisted reproduction is more likely to be successful in the presence of adequate funding arrangements.

Recommendations

- The risk of multiple pregnancies in IUI should be reduced by means of conservative use of gonadotrophin ovarian stimulation.
- No more than two embryos should be transferred in women undergoing IVF except in exceptional circumstances.
- Single-embryo transfer should be considered in women at high risk of twins.
- There is a need for more multicentre RCTs evaluating effectiveness and cost-effectiveness of a single-embryo transfer policy.

References

1. Luke B. The changing pattern of multiple births in the United States: maternal and infant characteristics, 1973 and 1990. *Obstet Gynecol* 1994;84:101–6.
2. Ozturk O, Templeton A. Multiple pregnancy in assisted reproduction techniques. In: Vayena E, Rowe PJ, Griffin PD, editors. *Current Practices and Controversies in Assisted Reproduction.* Geneva: World Health Organization; 2002. p. 220–34.
3. U.S. Department of Health and Human Services, Centers for Disease Control and Prevention. *2002 Assisted Reproductive Technology Success Rates. National Summary and Fertility Clinic Reports.* Atlanta: CDC; 2004 [www.cdc.gov/ART/ART02/PDF/ART2002.pdf].
4. Anonymous. Assisted reproduction: results of treatment; 1994–1997. In: *Statistics: Health and Diseases – the National Board of Health and Welfare Centre for Epidemiology.* Stockholm: Nordstedts; 2000.
5. Pinborg A, Loft A, Schmidt L, Greisen G, Rasmussen S, Andersen AN. Neurological sequelae in twins born after assisted conception: controlled national cohort study. *BMJ* 2004;329:311.
6. Human Fertilisation and Embryology Authority. *The Patient's Guide to IVF Clinics. IVF National Data Statistics.* London: HFEA; 2001.

7. Campbell D, Templeton A. Maternal complications of twin pregnancy. *Int J Gynaecol Obstet* 2004;81:71–3.

8. Buckett W, Tan SL. What is the most relevant standard of success in assisted reproduction? The importance of informed choice. *Hum Reprod* 2004;19:1043–5.

9. Evans MI, Littmann L, St. Louis L, Leblanc L, Addis J, Johnson MP, *et al*. Evolving patterns of iatrogenic multifetal pregnancy generation: implications for aggressiveness of infertility treatment. *Am J Obstet Gynecol* 1995;172:1750–3.

10. Norwitz ER. Multiple pregnancy: trends past, present, and future. *Infert Reprod Med Clin North Am* 1998;9:351–69.

11. Hughes EG. The effectiveness of ovulation induction and intrauterine insemination in the treatment of persistent infertility: a meta-analysis. *Hum Reprod* 1997;12:1865–72.

12. Guzick DS, Carson SA, Coutifaris C, Overstreet JW, Factor-Litvak P, Steinkampf MP, *et al*. Efficacy of superovulation and intrauterine insemination in the treatment of infertility. National Cooperative Reproductive Medicine Network. *N Engl J Med* 1999;340:177–83.

13. Subspeciality Trainees in Reproductive Medicine and Surgery. A multicentre analysis of 1580 cycles of superovulation with intra-uterine insemination: what is the impact on multiple pregnancy rates? [Unpublished data].

14. Gleicher N, Oleske DM, Tur-Kaspa I, Vidali A, Karande V. Reducing the risk of high-order multiple pregnancy after ovarian stimulation with gonadotrophins. *N Engl J Med* 2000;343:2–7.

15. Athaullah N, Proctor M, Johnson NP. Oral versus injectable ovulation induction agents for unexplained subfertility. *Cochrane Database Syst Rev* 2002;(3):C003062.

16. Sengoku K. The clinical efficacy of low dose step up follicle stimulating hormone administration for treatment of unexplained infertility. *Hum Reprod* 1999;14:349–53.

17. National Collaborating Centre for Women's and Children's Health (NICE). *Fertility: Assessment and Treatment for People with Fertility Problems. Clinical Guideline*. London: RCOG Press; 2004.

18. Martin PM, Welch HG. Probabilities for singleton and multiple pregnancies after *in vitro* fertilisation. *Fertil Steril* 1998;70:478–81.

19. Templeton A, Morris JK. Reducing the risk of multiple births by transfer of two embryos after *in vitro* fertilization. *N Engl J Med* 1998;339:573–7.

20. Schieve LA, Peterson HB, Meikle SF, Jeng G, Danel I, Burnett NM, *et al*. Live birth rates and multiple birth risk using in-vitro fertilisation. *JAMA* 1999;282:1832–8.

21. Staessen C, Janssenswillen C, Van den Abbeel E, Devroey P, Van Steirteghem AC. Avoidance of triplet pregnancies by elective transfer of two good quality embryos. *Hum Reprod* 1993;8:1650–3.

22. Licciardi F, Berkeley S, Krey L, Grifo J, Noyes N. A two- versus three-embryo transfer: the oocyte donation model. *Fertil Steril* 2001;75:510–13.

23. Andersen AN, Gianaroli L, Felberbaum R, de Mouzon J, Nygren G. Assisted reproductive technology in Europe; 2001. Results generated from European registers by ESHRE. *Hum Reprod* 2005;20:1158–76.

24. Berkowitz RL, Lynch L, Stone J, Alvarez M. The current status of multifetal pregnancy reduction. *Am J Obstet Gynecol* 1996;174:1265–72.

25. Bavister BD, Boatman DE. The neglected human blastocyst revisited. *Hum Reprod* 1997;12:1606–18.

26. Blake D, Proctor M, Johnson N, Olive D. Cleavage stage versus blastocyst stage embryo transfer in assisted conception. *Cochrane Database Syst Rev* 2005;(4):CD002118.

27. Gerris JMR. Single embryo transfer and IVF/ICSI outcome: a balanced appraisal. *Hum Reprod Update* 2005;11:105–21.

28. Pandian Z, Templeton A, Serour G, Bhattacharya S. Number of embryos for transfer after IVF and ICSI: a Cochrane review. *Hum Reprod* 2005;20:2681–7.

29. Van Montfoort P, Fiddelers AA, Janssen JM, Derhaag G, Dirksen CD, Dunselman GAJ, *et al*. Single embryo transfer (SET) in unselected patients: a randomized controlled trial (RCT). *Hum Reprod* 2005;20:O-150,i55.

30. Gerris J, De Neubourg D, Mangelschots K, Van Royen E, Van de Meerssche M, Valkenburg M. Prevention of twin pregnancy after in-vitro fertilisation or intracytoplasmic sperm injection based on strict embryo criteria: a prospective randomized clinical trial. *Hum Reprod* 1999;14:2581–7.

31. Martikainen H, Tiitinen A, Candido T, Tapanainen J, Orava M, Tuomivaara L, *et al*. One versus two embryo transfer after IVF and ICSI: a randomised study. *Hum Reprod* 2001;16:1900–3.

32. Lukassen HGM, Braat DDM, Zeilhuis GA, Adang EM, Kremer JAM. 2X1 versus 1X2, a randomized study. *Hum Reprod* 2002;17. Abstract book 1;1.

33. Thurin A, Hausken J, Hillensjo T, Jablonowska B, Pinborg A, Strandell A, *et al*. Elective single embryo transfer in IVF, a randomized study. *N Engl J Med*. 2004;351:2392–402.

34. Hunault CC, Eijkemans MJC, Pieters MHEC, te Velde ER, Habbema JDF, Fauser BCJM, *et al*. A

prediction model for selecting patients undergoing *in vitro* fertilisation for elective single embryo transfer. *Fertil Steril* 2002;77:725–32.

35. Gardner MK, Lane M. Culture and selection of viable human blastocysts: a feasible proposition for human IVF? *Hum Reprod Update* 1997;3:367–82.

36. Gianaroli L, Magli MC, Munné S, Fiorentino A, Montanaro N, Ferraretti AP. Will pre-implantation genetic diagnosis assist patients with a poor prognosis to achieve pregnancy? *Hum Reprod* 1997;12:1762–7.

37. Gianaroli L, Magli MC, Ferraretti AP, Munne S. Pre-implantation diagnosis for aneuploidies in patients undergoing *in vitro* fertilisation with a poor prognosis: identification of the categories for which it should be proposed. *Fertil Steril* 1999;72:837–44.

38. Tiitinen A, Halttunen M, Harkki P. Elective single embryo transfer: the value of cryopreservation *Hum Reprod*;2001;16:1140–4.

39. Tiitinen A, Hyden-Granskog C, Gissler M. What is the most relevant standard of success in assisted reproduction? The value of cryopreservation on cumulative pregnancy rates per single oocyte retrieval should not be forgotten. *Hum Reprod* 2004;19:1–3.

40. Van den Abbeel E, Camus M, Van Waesberghe L, Devroey P, Van Steirteghem AC. Viability of partially damaged human embryos after cryopreservation. *Hum Reprod* 1997;12:2006–10.

41. Vail A, Gardener E. Common statistical errors in the design and analysis of subfertility trials. *Hum Reprod* 2003;18:1000–4.

42. Min JK, Breheny SA, MacLachlan V, Healy DL. What is the most relevant standard of success in assisted reproduction? The singleton, term gestation, live birth rate per cycle initiated: the BESST endpoint for assisted reproduction. *Hum Reprod* 2003;19:3–7.

43. Hazekamp J, Bergh C, Wennerholm UB, Hovatta O, Karlstrom PO, Selbing A. Avoiding multiple pregnancies in ART: consideration of new strategies. *Hum Reprod* 2000;15:1217–19.

44. Gleicher N, Campbell DP, Chan CL, Karande V, Rae R, Balin M, Pratt D. The desire for multiple births in couples with infertility problems contradicts present practice patterns. *Hum Reprod* 1995;10:1079–84.

45. Pinborg Loft A, Schmidt L, Andersen AN. Attitudes of IVF/ICSI-twin mothers towards twins and single embryo transfer. *Hum Reprod* 2003;18:621–7.

46. Murray S, Shetty A, Rattray A, Taylor V, Bhattacharya S. A randomized comparison of alternative methods of information provision on the acceptability of elective single embryo transfer. *Hum Reprod* 2004;19:911–16.

47. Ombelet W, De Sutter P, Van der Elst J, Martens G. Multiple gestation and infertility treatment: registration, reflection and reaction – the Belgian project. *Hum Reprod Update* 2005;11:3–14.

48. Olofsson JI, Borg K, Hardarson T, Hillensjo T, Reismer U, Selleskog U, et al. Effects of novel legislation on embryo transfer policy, results and pregnancy outcome in a Swedish IVF unit. *Abstracts of the 20th Annual Meeting of the ESHRE, Berlin, Germany, 2004.* O-169,i59.

49. Porter M, Bhattacharya S. Investigation of staff and patients' opinions of a proposed trial of elective single embryo transfer. *Hum Reprod* 2005;20:2523–30.

50. Saldeen P, Sondstrom P. Would legislation imposing single embryo transfer be a feasible way to reduce the rate of multiple pregnancies after IVF treatment? *Hum Reprod* 2005;20:4–8.

51. U.S. Department of Health and Human Services, Centers for Disease Control and Prevention. *2002 Assisted Reproductive Technology Success Rates. National Summary and Fertility Clinic Reports.* Atlanta: CDC; 2004 [www.cdc.gov/ART/ART01/PDF/ART2001.pdf].

52. Anonymous. Assisted reproductive technology in the United States: 1996 results generated from the American Society for Reproductive Medicine/Society for Assisted Reproductive Technology Registry. *Fertil Steril* 1999;71:798–807.

53. Anonymous. Assisted reproductive technology in the United States: 1997 results generated from the American Society for Reproductive Medicine/Society for Assisted Reproductive Technology Registry. *Fertil Steril* 2000;74:641–53.

54. Anonymous. Assisted reproductive technology in the United States: 1998 results generated from the American Society for Reproductive Medicine/Society for Assisted Reproductive Technology Registry. *Fertil Steril* 2002;77:18–31.

55. Anonymous. Assisted reproductive technology in the United States: 1999 results generated from the American Society for Reproductive Medicine/Society for Assisted Reproductive Technology Registry. *Fertil Steril* 2002;78:918–31.

56. Anonymous. Assisted reproductive technology in the United States: 2000 results generated from the American Society for Reproductive Medicine/Society for Assisted Reproductive Technology Registry. *Fertil Steril* 2004;81:1207–20.

57. Nygren KG, Andersen AN. Assisted reproductive technology in Europe, 1997. Results generated from European registers by ESHRE. European IVF-Monitoring Programme (EIM), for the

European Society of Human Reproduction and Embryology (ESHRE). *Hum Reprod* 2001;16:384–91.

58. Nygren KG, Andersen AN; European IVF-monitoring programme (EIM). Assisted reproductive technology in Europe, 1998. Results generated from European registers by ESHRE. European Society of Human Reproduction and Embryology. *Hum Reprod* 2001;16:2459–71. Erratum in: *Hum Reprod* 2002;17:2781.

59. Nygren KG, Andersen AN. Assisted reproductive technology in Europe, 1999. Results generated from European registers by ESHRE. *Hum Reprod* 2002;17:3260–74.

60. Nyboe Andersen A, Gianaroli L, Nygren KG; European IVF-monitoring programme; European Society of Human Reproduction and Embryology. Assisted reproductive technology in Europe, 2000. Results generated from European registers by ESHRE. *Hum Reprod* 2004;19:490–503.

Chapter 3

Monochorionic twin placentas: clinical outcome and computer modelling of a high-risk pregnancy

Peter GJ Nikkels, Jeroen PHM van den Wijngaard and Martin JC van Gemert

Introduction

Twins can be dizygotic or monozygotic. Dizygotic twins always have a dichorionic placenta and are diamniotic, whereas monozygotic twins can have a dichorionic or a monochorionic placenta. Twins with a monochorionic placenta can be diamniotic or monoamniotic. Seventy percent of all twins are dizygotic and 30% are monozygotic. Three-quarters of these monozygotic placentas are monochorionic and 1% of all monochorionic twin placentas are monoamniotic.[1] A monochorionic twin placenta is a single placenta and is not fused.

Monochorionic twin pregnancies are high-risk pregnancies that carry a relatively high mortality of 10–25%.[1] Vascular anastomoses between the fetal circulations can be found in almost all monochorionic twin placentas.[2] These can be superficial (i.e. arterio-arterial (AA) or veno-venous (VV)) with a low resistance or deep (i.e. arterio-venous (AV) or opposite (AV)) with a high resistance. An unbalanced unidirectional feto-fetal transfusion can develop through these anastomoses from one twin (the donor) to the other (the recipient). This may cause an imbalance between their fetoplacental circulations of varying severity, affecting each twin in different ways and at different times. Twin-to-twin transfusion syndrome (TTTS) comprises the most severe phenotype of circulatory imbalance,[3] with a wide variation in complications in both twins.[4] Because these complications differ from those in dichorionic twins in both severity and type, the placental vascular connections are considered to be responsible for this morbidity. Unfortunately, these complications are complex in their clinical presentation. The underlying causes, i.e. the net feto-fetal transfusion, the abnormal blood pressures and the intercompartmental fluid flows (e.g. from blood to interstitium), are largely inaccessible for assessment by ultrasonography and there are no animal models. Therefore, mathematical models of the pathophysiology of monochorionic twin pregnancies and TTTS have been developed.[5–8]

The purpose of this chapter is to review various aspects and consequences of the pathology of monochorionic twin placentas and to correlate these with the consequential pathophysiological development of the twin fetuses using our mathematical computer model.[8]

Anastomoses

An AV anastomosis connects branches from the umbilical artery of the donor with the umbilical vein of the recipient. The AV connections may occur at the capillary level within a cotyledon that receives its blood from a donor chorionic artery and drains it by a recipient chorionic vein. On the chorionic plate surface, an AV anastomosis presents as a donor chorionic artery that meets 'nose-to-nose' with a recipient chorionic vein. These two vessels penetrate into the placental parenchyma through the same foramen to perfuse the cotyledon. An oppositely directed AV anastomosis (recipient to donor) often exists next to a primary AV anastomosis. Opposite AV anastomoses, denoted by VA, are defined as having the smaller diameter (higher resistance) compared with the primary AV anastomosis. AA or VV anastomoses directly connect the two umbilical arterial or venous circulations by chorionic arteries or veins of the two twins.

Recently, our group, as well as those of others such as Rubén Quintero,[9] has reported the existence of anastomoses where one or more vessels lack a direct connection with the umbilical circulation of each twin.[10] These so-called 'bridge vessels' are connected by a cotyledon to the feeding vessel and by another cotyledon to the draining vessel. Because a cotyledon is estimated to have a 20 times higher resistance than the feeding plus draining vessels together,[11] these anatomical structures connecting the umbilical circulations have an estimated 40 times higher resistance than normal, i.e. a 40 times lower feto-fetal transfusion at equal pressure gradient. Their haemodynamic capacity to mitigate the effects of the primary AV anastomosis is thus virtually zero. We have so far described three of these cases, and others have previously noted two others.[10] The third case included a pseudo-AA anastomosis that failed to compensate for the deleterious effects of the AV anastomosis in a monoamniotic placenta, resulting in severe monoamniotic TTTS.[12]

Another vascular anastomosis that occurs naturally in placentas is Hyrtl's anasto-mosis,[13–15] named after the famous Austrian anatomist Joseph Hyrtl (1810–1894). This anastomosis connects the two umbilical arteries of the fetus close to the placental surface. Hyrtl's anastomosis is sometimes absent, such as in four of 65 singleton placentas (two more had one umbilical artery) in the series reported by Ullberg et al.[14] In the series reported by Raio et al.[15] no absent Hyrtl's anastomosis was found in 41 placentas. In our series of 350 monochorionic placentas we demonstrated three cases of an absent Hyrtl's anastomosis in one of the twins.

Another group of anastomoses has recently gained considerable attention and is referred to here as 'hidden' anastomoses, i.e. anastomoses not visible on the chorionic plate but present below the surface of the plate. Identification requires the technique of vascular casting. This technique was originally used for studying placental vascular morphology in singleton placentas,[16] and subsequently in monochorionic-diamniotic twin placentas.[17] When investigating whether visual inspection of monochorionic twin placentas can quantify all vascular anastomoses between the two fetal circulations, Wee et al.[18] used a modern resin monomer as a way to obtain solid vascular casts after tissue corrosion. In eight of 15 monochorionic placentas they reported communications between cotyledons that were unnoticed before tissue digestion. A different technique whereby cord vessels were injected with barium dye before digital X-ray imaging revealed only two deep anastomoses in 16 placentas.[19]

Assuming that selective fetoscopic laser treatment of TTTS ablates only those anastomoses that are visible on the chorionic plate surface, the existence of deep anastomoses may affect the efficacy of laser therapy if the remaining flow through the deep anastomoses is uncompensated and surpasses the fetal compensatory mechanisms. The effect of deep anastomoses on treatment of TTTS remains elusive and deserves further investigation (see Chapters 11 and 12).

The result of an anastomosis is a feto–fetal transfusion of blood (and its constituents) between the twins, where the amount of transfusion is dependent on the driving pressure gradient divided by the resistance to blood flow (Ohm's law). Obviously, AV feto–fetal transfusion is the principal flow here and the combined VA, AA and VV transfusions return part of the AV flow back to the donor, owing to gradients between recipient and donor vascular pressures. The net volume of feto–fetal transfusion is thus defined as

$$\text{Net feto–fetal transfusion} = \text{AV flow} - (\text{VA flow} + \text{AA flow} + \text{VV flow}) \quad (1)$$

The direction is from donor to recipient. We emphasise that the assumed normal direction of VA, AA and VV flows is from recipient to donor – these flows will be negative in the equation if their direction is from donor to recipient (impossible for the VA flow, but possible for the AA and VV flows). Furthermore, because the fetal arterial pressure is much higher than the venous pressure, deviations from normal are likely to produce much larger inter-twin arterial pressure gradients than venous pressure gradients. This implies that an AA anastomosis has a much greater efficacy than a VV one of identical length and diameter to compensate for the AV feto–fetal transfusion. Without a hydropic recipient twin, we estimate that a VV anastomosis of identical length requires a 1.7 times larger diameter than an AA anastomosis for equal compensation of AV transfusion.[6] However, in severe TTTS with a hydropic recipient twin, the recipient venous pressure is significantly elevated, implying a VV anastomosis has better compensating capacity than without a hydropic twin.[8]

In our models, the AV, VA, AA and VV anastomoses are represented by tubes that connect directly with the two umbilical circulations without branches to the normal placental chorionic vessels. The length of all anastomotic tubes is the distance between the two cord insertions, which is taken as 15 cm at 40 weeks of gestation.[6] The individual radii at 40 weeks are variable parameters (one of the input parameters of the models). The length and radii are assumed to be proportional to gestational age, so their values at 40 weeks determine their values at all other gestations. We use Poiseuille's law of laminar blood flow to define the vascular resistance of the anastomoses, which is a function of blood viscosity, length and radius of the tube:

$$\text{resistance} = (8/\pi) \times \text{viscosity} \times (\text{length}/\text{radius}^4) \quad (2)$$

Note that the radius is included to the fourth power, which implies that radius has an exceedingly strong influence on resistance, e.g. a radius increase by a factor of two decreases the resistance by a factor of $2^4 = 16$, at constant viscosity and length.

Although a joint cotyledon (AV or VA anastomosis) is anatomically not a tube, their resistances are nevertheless equivalent because of their identical growth behaviour during pregnancy.[6] Briefly, anastomoses increase their length and radius linearly. As Equation (2) includes the ratio of length and radius to the fourth power, the resistances decrease according to an inverse proportionality of gestational age to the third power. On the other hand, in a cotyledon, the radius of the capillaries does not vary with gestational age. Instead, the number of capillaries increases proportionally with the placental volume, which is assumed to be proportional to gestational age to the third power.[6] By approximating the vascular resistance of a cotyledon to the parallel circuit of identical capillary resistances, the overall cotyledonic resistance is inversely proportional to the number of capillaries, and is thus inversely proportional to the third power of gestation (i.e. identical to the behaviour of AV and VA resistances). In previous work,[11] we used a fractal geometry model for the vascular tree to simulate how AV and VA resistances relate to the diameter of their feeding and draining vessels. In this model, the cotyledon has a 20–24 times higher resistance than the feeding artery plus draining vein. Thus, the tube used in our models to represent AV or VA resistances also has a 20–24 times higher resistance than the feeding artery plus draining vein. The AV and VA anastomotic tube radii in the model can thus not represent the actual radii of feeding and draining AV and VA vessels.

Several unidirectional AV anastomoses are equivalent to a circuit of parallel AV tube resistances and can thus be expressed using the law of parallel resistances:

$$1/R_{AVoverall} = 1/R_{AV1} + 1/R_{AV2} + 1/R_{AV3} + \dots \quad (3)$$

This holds for VA, AA and VV resistances too and thus multiple AV, VA, AA and VV anastomoses are equivalent to a set of overall single AV, VA, AA and VV resistances. We emphasise that in real monochorionic twin placentas, the anastomotic pattern is not exactly a set of tubes between the umbilical cord insertions because the connection between the umbilical circulations is always via branches to other chorionic vessels. Nevertheless, we examined the overall resistance of a monochorionic twin placental circulation, obtained from a dye-injected placenta, and have confirmed from a circuit analysis that the concept of parallel resistances is at least approximately valid. Thus, any multiple placental anastomoses of particular types are approximately equivalent to a set of overall single anastomotic resistances of the same type.

Acardiac twinning

An acardiac twin is the most severe phenotype that develops as a consequence of anastomotic vessels in monochorionic twin placentas. Its incidence is about 1% of monochorionic twins, or about 1 in 35 000 pregnancies[20] (see Chapter 13). Acardiac twins require two preconditions to exist. First, a set of AA and VV placental anastomoses must be present so the twin with a functional heart, the pump twin, can perfuse the acardiac twin's body, allowing growth despite lack of cardiac function. Second, there must be some kind of circulatory failure in one of the twins, the future acardiac twin, because its cardiac development is severely disturbed. This twin can be either anatomically normal or abnormal. Perfusion of the acardiac twin's umbilical arteries (or artery) and aorta is by reversed flow, hence the syndrome's name of twin reversed arterial perfusion (TRAP) sequence. Most likely, the reversed arterial perfusion occurring in the acardiac twin's upper body causes the great variety of malformations and lack of organs seen in acardiac twins, usually including complete lack of cardiac remnants. Typical pump twin development is an initially normal growth, then rapid onset of complications that often include plethora, cardiac decompensation and hydrops, followed by intrauterine fetal death, usually occurring in the second trimester.

One of the authors (PGJN) and an experienced obstetrician (Philip Stoutenbeek, University Medical Centre, Utrecht) observed by serial ultrasound that both monochorionic twins were normally formed at very early gestation at 8–10 weeks. At 14 weeks of gestation, hydrops and a nuchal translucency were observed in the smaller twin and colour Doppler flow revealed a superficial AA anastomosis with reversed flow in the umbilical artery and aorta of the smaller twin. A few weeks later the normal cranial and thoracic structures were no longer visible by ultrasound and the umbilical artery of the smaller twin was clipped *in utero* to prevent damage, cardiac overload or decompensation of the normal pump twin.

Recently, the authors quantified a pump twin's excess cardiac output and reduced blood oxygenation, caused by the presence of an acardiac twin, and related these parameters to the ratio of pump twin and acardiac twin umbilical blood flows or umbilical vein diameters.[21] Five clinical cases were described, four from pathology data and one just before laser therapy. Interestingly, the four cases where the pump twin had died *in utero* or had had to be haemodynamically disconnected by laser showed a decreasing pump twin to acardiac twin umbilical vein diameter ratio as a function of gestation. The fifth case, where perfusion of the acardiac mass spontaneously ceased, clearly had a much larger diameter ratio. We have since encountered two more cases. One occurred very early (at 14 weeks of gestation), where the pump twin died *in utero*, probably not much earlier than at 14 weeks, implying that the influence of a perfused acardiac mass on pump twin adaptation may not have occurred yet because the diameter ratio was about one. The other was a late case where the pump twin survived at 37 weeks (the acardiac mass was 1315 g and the pump twin birthweight was 2315 g). Figure 3.1 shows the results with the two later cases added, suggesting that a trend line may exist that separates a region of umbilical vein diameter ratio versus gestation where pump twins are likely to die or require therapy from a region where they are likely to survive. However, many more data are needed, preferably serial measurements of umbilical vein diameter ratios to assess the validity of this hypothesis.[21]

Acardiac twin pregnancies occur about three times less frequently in monoamniotic than in diamniotic-monochorionic twin placentas, based on 30 cases reported by Benirschke and Kaufmann,[20] 22 of which involved diamniotic-monochorionic placentas and eight involved monoamniotic placentas, and 86 cases reported by Healey,[22] where 65 occurred in diamniotic-monochorionic placentas and 21 in monoamniotic placentas. Thus, of the total of 116 cases, 87 (75%) occurred in diamniotic-monochorionic and 29 (25%) in monoamniotic placentas. However, the incidence of monoamniotic to diamniotic-monochorionic twins is only about 3% to 97% whereas acardiac twin pregnancies constitute about 1% of monochorionic twin placentas. For the analysis, consider 2000 monochorionic twin placentas, which therefore include 20 (1%) acardiac twin pregnancies. Of these 20 acardiac pregnancies, 25% (5/20) are monoamniotic and 75% (15/20) are diamniotic. Of the 2000 monochorionic twin placentas, 3% (60) are monoamniotic and 97% (1940) are diamniotic. Acardiac twins thus have an 8% (5/60) predicted incidence in monoamniotic and 0.8% (15/1940) in diamniotic-monochorionic twins. Because a set of AA and VV anastomoses is a prerequisite for acardiac twins to develop, the question is whether such a set of anastomoses occurs ten times (8/0.8) more frequently in monoamniotic than in diamniotic-monochorionic twins. In 238 diamniotic-monochorionic dye-injected placentas, 48 (20.2%) included this set of AA-VV anastomoses versus 10/26 (38.5%) in 26 monoamniotic placentas (excluding the two conjoint twin placentas).[23] This difference has statistical significance ($P = 0.032$, $\chi^2 = 4.576$, χ^2 analysis with one degree of freedom). The ratio of 1.9 (38.5/20.2) is significantly smaller than the factor of 10 (8/0.8). However, the distance between cord insertions is on average three times

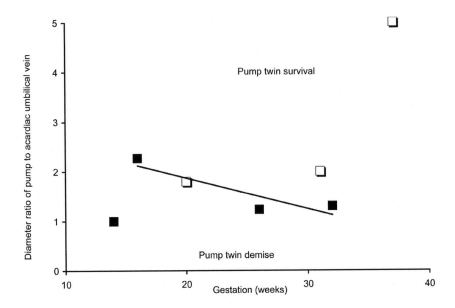

Figure 3.1. Ratio of pump twin to acardiac twin umbilical vein diameters of seven available cases (five were presented in Figure 4 of van Gemert *et al.*[21]); the open symbols represent surviving pump twins (with the one at 20 weeks of gestation being a result of successful laser therapy); the trend line through the four cases at 16, 20, 26 and 32 weeks of gestational may separate a region of umbilical vein diameter ratios versus gestation where pump twins are likely to survive from a region where they are likely to die or require therapy

smaller in monoamniotic than in diamniotic-monochorionic twins,[23] hence the AA and VV flow resistances are on average three times smaller at equal diameter in monoamniotic twin placentas. We propose that the combination of an increased incidence of a set of AA and VV anastomoses and their reduced anastomotic resistances may explain this difference in incidence of acardiac twinning between monoamniotic and diamniotic-monochorionic twins. An interesting prediction then is that one acardiac twin develops per 25 monochorionic-diamniotic placentas (20.2/0.8) that include a set of AA and VV anastomoses. In monoamniotic twin placentas this estimated ratio is as large as one per five of such placentas (38.5/8). We observed two acardiac twins in 238 diamniotic-monochorionic placentas of which 48 had an AA-VV set, confirming the predicted one per 25 such placentas, and one in the 26 monoamniotic placentas of which ten had a set of AA-VV anastomoses, not statistically different from the predicted one in five.

Monochorionic placentas: inter-twin growth discordance

In 206 monochorionic twin placentas, we investigated whether a combination of different anastomoses and placental sharing determines growth discordance between monochorionic twins. Full-blown TTTS cases that developed before 26 weeks of gestation were treated with laser therapy and were not included in this study. Vascular anastomoses in monochorionic twin placentas can be visualised by injecting the veins and arteries of the two umbilical cords with different dyes.[1,24,25] In our experience, air cannot visualise the small AV connections that can be very important, especially when there is no superficial anastomosis. A high mortality was found in the group without superficial AA anastomoses and in the group with a growth discordance of more than 25% (growth discordance was defined as the difference between largest and smallest birthweight divided by the average birthweight). VV anastomoses were rare and in this series were usually found in combination with an AA and several bidirectional AV anastomoses. In more than half of the cases in the group with superficial AA anastomoses a non-anastomosis-related death of the donor was found with subsequent exsanguination of the recipient. In most cases it was an obstetric non-twin-related problem, i.e. chorioamnionitis, placental abruption or placental infarction. In these cases the smaller donor twin died first *in utero* and the recipient exsanguinated via the superficial low-resistance AA anastomosis into the donor. When the fetuses were born, paradoxically the smaller donor twin was red and plethoric with congested internal organs and the larger recipient twin was pale. Growth discordance in this group with a superficial AA anastomosis was related to placental sharing. Larger growth discordance correlated with a smaller part of the placental parenchyma for the smaller twin based on separation of the placental parenchyma at the vascular equator (however, see also the 2nd paragraph of the model simulations section below). In the group without superficial anastomoses growth discordance and development of polyhydramnios occurred after 24 weeks of gestation.[24,25] In contrast with the group with a superficial AA anastomosis, in the group with only deep AV anastomoses in both directions (AV and VA) growth discordance was not related to placental sharing and was more severe. The mortality in this group was high and related to severe TTTS with anaemia of the donor and a plethoric status of the recipient and premature birth. In the group with a superficial VV anastomosis growth discordance was even more pronounced, as was also observed by Denbow *et al.*[2] The group with a VV anastomosis also had a remarkably high mortality of one of the two fetuses with survival of the other twin. In one case, after the death of the co-twin, the survivor perfused the entire placenta and received blood that also perfused the placental part of the dead co-twin via the AA and AV anastomoses. The blood returned to the survivor via the VV anastomosis (without perfusing the dead fetus, as is the case in the TRAP sequence). In almost all cases studied (five out of six) the death of the co-twin could not be explained by abnormalities in the fetus or in the placenta (such as chorioamnionitis, placental abruption or placental infarction). Amniotic fluid reduction was performed in one-third of the cases (with bidirectional AV anastomoses without superficial anastomoses) to treat polyhydramnios to prolong pregnancy. In this study amniotic fluid reduction was not necessary and was not performed in the group with superficial anastomoses. Late-occurring chronic TTTS was more often found in the absence of a superficial AA anastomosis.

The histology of the placental villi in the group without superficial anastomoses (even in the group without TTTS) showed larger and oedematous villi in the donor compartment and small villi in the recipient compartment. This is also indicative of a chronic process of net blood transfusion from donor to recipient. In addition, a lower haemoglobin level was found in these fetuses compared with the recipient. In the group with a superficial AA anastomosis no significant difference was found in haemoglobin levels between donor and recipient. Interestingly, in three TTTS cases caused by unidirectional or single AV anastomoses[11,24,25] the neonatal criteria of TTTS were found to be valid, i.e. at least 20% discordance in birthweight and at least 5 g/dL discordance in haemoglobin concentration. This may suggest that these neonatal criteria may still apply in TTTS caused by bidirectional AV but not by AV-AA.

The different sizes of the donor and recipient villi imply different perfusion lengths of oxygen from maternal to fetal blood. The larger (more immature) donor villi result in a lower donor blood oxygenation than the smaller size (normal to accelerated matured) recipient villi that cause a more normal blood oxygenation. Combining these different oxygenation levels in donor versus recipient blood with differences in the optical scattering of haemoglobin and oxygenated haemoglobin[26] (oxygenated blood scatters strongly at red wavelengths, causing its more reddish colour) also suggests recipient arterial blood is more reddish than donor arterial blood in severe TTTS. We have proposed that natural differences between donor and recipient blood oxygenation cause the colour differences between darker and lighter red in AA anastomoses of severe TTTS observed during fetoscopy for laser therapy.[27,28] Our suggestion was based on applying the theory of colour perception, which is standard in physics, of a volume of whole blood combined with simplified photon transport theory to calculate the back-scattered (i.e. observed) spectrum of visible light.[9] We recently confirmed our conclusion and quantified the minimum difference in arterial blood oxygenation that shows an observable colour difference by including a realistic theoretical model of the placenta, based on placental anatomy at about 23 weeks of gestation, and then calculating the back-scattering spectrum of the observed visible light from this model using advanced Monte Carlo modelling of photon transport.[29] Our predictions showed a small but clearly visible colour difference of darker red donor versus brighter red recipient arterial blood, in excellent agreement with the colour difference observed in a video of the phenomenon that was kindly provided to us by Rubén Quintero.

Thrombosis of anastomoses

Thrombosis of anastomoses that caused severe TTTS in a previously normal developing monochorionic twin pregnancy has been reported twice.[25,30] Mark Denbow[30] reported a case of thrombosis of an AA anastomosis during a meeting in London that was also attended by one of the authors (MJCvG). When, a few years later, a case with a similar clinical history occurred in the Netherlands and our group received the placenta, thrombosis was observed. However, this case[25] included further thrombosis of a chorionic vein that obliterated various oppositely directed AV anastomoses, which had previously perfectly compensated for the AV anastomoses.

Model simulations

A summary of our modelling efforts, without mathematics and presenting only the equations (in word) necessary for understanding the pathophysiology, will be published as a book chapter.[31]

One of the outcomes of our first model was the finding that a combination of deep and superficial anastomoses can produce strong but stable discordant fetal development.[6] This poses an obstetrics problem but these cases do not deteriorate into TTTS. Although the placenta is often severely unequally shared, as discussed above, unequal sharing is not required for this model. In 12 such cases, three were virtually equally shared (one 0.5:0.5 and two 0.45:0.55) with the ratio of weight difference and average weight varying between 0.21 and 0.63.[32] Our model predicts that the anastomotic pattern is the main cause of this effect, but that unequal placental sharing augments it if the donor has the smaller placenta and delays discordance if the donor has the larger placenta.[24]

For single (and unidirectional) AV anastomoses, the predicted gestational age at TTTS onset increases with increasing resistance values, i.e. at smaller diameter AV anastomoses (Figure 1 of Umur *et al.*[7]), implying that for single and unidirectional AV anastomoses, TTTS severity correlates with earlier gestational age at TTTS onset. However, single and unidirectional AV anastomoses are uncommon, occurring in only 5–20% of TTTS cases. In contrast, our model predicts that TTTS severity is not generally correlated with earlier gestational age at TTTS onset. For AV anastomoses accompanied by compensating anastomoses (VA, AA or VV), which occurs in 80–95% of TTTS placentas, anastomotic patterns and models demonstrate that severe TTTS may present later in gestation than mild TTTS (Figure 3.2). The underlying mechanism is that the initial appearance of TTTS develops owing to an AV feto-fetal transfusion, while the compensating effects of the other anastomoses may become effective subsequently, even after TTTS onset. For example, if an AA is the compensating anastomosis, onset of AA feto-fetal transfusion (recipient to donor) requires a higher recipient than donor arterial pressure. This pressure gradient has to be generated by the primary AV feto-fetal transfusion, which also causes the donor to develop oligohydramnios. Therefore, depending on AV capacity, donor oligohydramnios may present at earlier or later gestational ages. The capacity of compensating anastomoses compared with the AV capacity then determines whether compensation

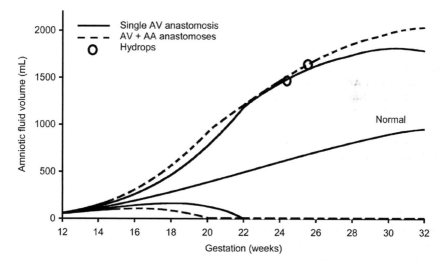

Figure 3.2. Numerical simulations of amniotic fluid volume of both donor (lower two curves) and recipient (upper two curves) twins for two anastomotic patterns; first, a serious TTTS case due to an uncompensated single AV anastomosis (AV resistance was 0.29 mmHg mL^{-1} 24 h at 40 weeks of gestation) (continuous lines) producing a stuck donor at 22 weeks and a hydropic recipient 2.4 weeks later, at 24.4 weeks; second, a milder TTTS case due to one much larger diameter (smaller resistance) AV anastomosis, inadequately compensated by one AA anastomosis (AV and AA resistances were 0.16 and 0.35 mmHg mL^{-1} 24 h at 40 weeks, respectively) (dashed lines), producing a stuck donor at 20 weeks, two weeks earlier than with the single AV, but hydrops in the recipient 1.2 weeks later than with the single AV, at 25.6 weeks

is inadequate (i.e. severe TTTS develops) or adequate (i.e. milder TTTS develops).

Placentas with TTTS include an AA anastomosis in only 20–30% of cases, compared with about 80% in non-TTTS placentas, which suggests that an AA anastomosis may be more protective than VA in compensating for the effects of the AV anastomosis. We incorporated the placental vascular tree by fractal geometry modelling, which allowed us to relate the anastomotic AV and VA resistances to their feeding arterial diameters, which were taken to be equal to the diameters of their draining vein.[11] In our model, AA anastomoses prevented TTTS over a large range of AA to AV diameter ratios, i.e. larger than about 0.65. In contrast, the VA to AV diameter ratios that prevented TTTS had a much more limited range: only between 0.8 and 1. The reason is that the resistance of a cotyledon is proportional to the resistance of its feeding artery, taken to be equal to the resistance of its draining vein. Therefore, a small decrease in the VA feeding/draining vessel diameter compared with the AV causes a significant increase in VA resistance. According to Poiseuille's law (Equation 2), an 84%, 76% or 71% decreased VA vessel diameter causes a two, three, or four times increased VA resistance, respectively (the inverse fourth power). An increase by a factor of two may still provide adequate compensation but not by a factor of four. In contrast, an AA anastomosis already has a 20–24 times lower resistance than an AV anastomosis with equal length and diameter of its feeding and draining vessels.[11] Consequently, a 20–24 times smaller pressure difference between recipient and donor arteries than between donor arteries and recipient veins already gives the same compensating AA and AV transfusions at equal vessel diameters. The conclusion was thus that for a monochorionic twin placenta containing multiple anastomoses, the probability that a VA anastomosis adequately compensates for the effects of the AV anastomosis is much smaller than the probability that an AA anastomosis of the same diameter compensates adequately. We proposed that this prediction explains the difference in AA anastomosis incidence in TTTS compared with non-TTTS placentas.

Figure 3.3 shows the predicted blood colloid concentrations, which are assumed to be representative of blood haemoglobin/haematocrit levels, for a single AV anastomosis versus a set of AV plus AA anastomoses. The single AV anastomosis generates large colloid discordances, even after a stuck donor develops at 22 weeks, in contrast to the AV plus AA combination which develops a much more reduced discordance in colloids despite an equally large initial discordance. We propose that these simulations reproduce the results reported above of strong haemoglobin discordance in bidirectional AV anastomoses, representative for single AV,[6] and much less discordance in AV plus AA patterns.

Discussion

Anastomoses are a significant cause of problems occurring in monochorionic but not in dichorionic twin pregnancies. Each anastomosis connects a part of the circulation of each twin, i.e. donor arterial–recipient venous (AV), donor venous–recipient arterial (VA), donor arterial–recipient arterial (AA) or donor venous–recipient venous (VV), allowing a feto-fetal transfusion of blood volume and constituents to develop between them. The combination of all the anastomoses can cause the feto-fetal transfusion to be chronically unbalanced, resulting in major clinical and pathological alterations in the fetal and placental development, frequently with serious adverse pregnancy outcomes. The clinical consequences of chronically unbalanced feto-fetal transfusion, such as abnormal development of amniotic fluid volume, estimated fetal dimensions, umbilical blood flow patterns, cardiac development and interstitial

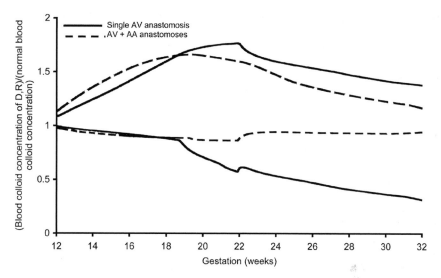

Figure 3.3.   Numerical simulations of blood colloid concentrations divided by the normal concentrations of both donor and recipient twins for an uncompensated single AV as in Figure 3.2 (continuous lines) and an AV plus AA anastomotic pattern (dashed lines) (AV and AA resistances were 0.16 and 0.13 mmHg mL⁻¹ 24 h at 40 weeks of gestation, respectively), which also produces a stuck donor at 22 weeks but hydrops in the recipient at 32.3 weeks; the difference between colloid concentrations is much smaller in the AV plus AA than the single AV case, reflecting a much smaller discordance in haematocrits.

volume overload, can be partly identified with ultrasonography. However, other important parameters of TTTS, such as blood pressures, the net feto-fetal transfusion along anastomoses, the transplacental and transvascular fluid flows, swallowing, lung secretion and the transmembranous fluid flow, cannot be studied. The impossibility of studying all mechanisms affecting TTTS onset is the main reason why computer modelling has become an important tool for identifying the importance and effects of these unmeasurable parameters, even though this approach is far from mainstream in obstetrics or physiological research. The systematic postnatal study of the pathology of monochorionic twin placentas is also uncommon. Our team has combined such modelling and placental studies since 1997, and this chapter has provided a brief summary of our results.

References

1.   Machin GA. Multiple pregnancies and conjoint twins. In: Gilbert-Barness E, editor. *Potter's Pathology of the Fetus and Infant,* vol. 1. London: Mosby; 1997. p. 281–321.
2.   Denbow ML, Cox P, Taylor M, Hammal DM, Fisk NM. Placental angioarchitecture in monochorionic twin pregnancies: relationship to fetal growth, fetofetal transfusion syndrome, and pregnancy outcome. *Am J Obstet Gynecol* 2000;182:417–26.
3.   van Gemert MJC, Umur A, Tijssen JGP, Ross MG. Twin–twin transfusion syndrome: etiology, severity and rational management. *Curr Opin Obstet Gynecol* 2001;13:193–206.

4.   Quintero RA, Morales WJ, Allen MH, Bornick PW, Johnson PK, Kruger M. Staging of twin–twin transfusion syndrome. *J Perinatol* 1999;19:550–5.
5.   Talbert DG, Bajoria R, Sepulveda W, Bower S, Fisk NM. Hydrostatic and osmotic pressure gradients produce manifestations of fetofetal transfusion syndrome in a computerized model of monochorial twin pregnancy. *Am J Obstet Gynecol* 1996;174:598–608.
6.   van Gemert MJC, Sterenborg HJCM. hemodynamic model of twin–twin transfusion syndrome in monochorionic twin pregnancies. *Placenta* 1998;19:195–208.
7.   Umur A, van Gemert MJC, Ross MG. Amniotic fluid and hemodynamic model in monochorionic twin pregnancies and twin–twin transfusion syndrome. *Am J Physiol Regul Integr Comp Physiol* 2001;280:R1499–509.
8.   van den Wijngaard JPHM, Umur A, Krediet RT, Ross MG, van Gemert MJC. Modeling a hydropic recipient twin in twin–twin transfusion syndrome. *Am J Physiol Regul Integr Comp Physiol* 2005;288:R799–814.
9.   Quintero RA, personal communication.
10. Van Gemert MJC, van den Wijngaard JPHM, de Vries HR, Nikkels PGJ. Invited comment on 'Taylor MJ, Talbert D, Fisk NM. Pseudo-arterio-arterial anastomoses in twin–twin transfusion syndrome. *Placenta* 2004;25:742–7.' *Placenta* 2004;25:748–51.
11. Umur A, van Gemert MJC, Nikkels PGJ, Ross MG. Monochorionic twins and twin–twin transfusion syndrome: the protective role of arterioarterial anastomoses. *Placenta* 2002;23:201–9.
12. Schaap AHP, van den Wijngaard JPHM, Nikkels PGJ, Suzuki S, van den Broek AJM, Snieders I, et al. Staging of twin–twin transfusion syndrome in monoamniotic twins. Unpublished data.
13. Hyrtl J. *Die Blutgefässe der menschlichen Nachgeburt in normalen und abnormalen Verhältnissen.* Vienna: Braumüller Verlag; 1870.
14. Ullberg U, Sandstedt B, Lingman G. Hyrtl's anastomosis, the only connection between the two umbilical arteries. A study in full term placentas from AGA infants with normal umbilical artery blood flow. *Acta Obstet Gynecol Scand* 2001;80:1–6.
15. Raio L, Ghezzi F, Di Naro E, Franchi M, Balestreri D, Dürig P, et al. In-utero characterization of the blood flow in the Hyrtl anastomosis. *Placenta* 2001;22:597–601.
16. Arts NFT. Investigations on the vascular system of the placenta. Part I. General introduction and the fetal vascular system. *Am J Obstet Gynecol* 1961;82:147–58.
17. Arts NFT, Lohman AHM. The vascular anatomy of monochorionic diamniotic twin placentas and the transfusion syndrome. *Eur J Obstet Gynecol* 1971;3:85–93.
18. Wee LY, Taylor M, Watkins N, Franke V, Parker K, Fisk NM. Characterisation of deep arteriovenous anastomoses within monochorionic placentae by vascular casting. *Placenta* 2005;26:19–24.
19. Lewi L, Cannie M, Jani J, Vandecaveye V, Dymarkowski S, Huber A, et al. Placental angiography of double survivors and double fetal deaths after laser for twin twin transfusion syndrome (TTTS). *Am J Obstet Gynecol* 2004;191 Suppl 1:s162.
20. Benirschke K, Kaufmann P. *Pathology of the Human Placenta*, 3rd edn. New York: Springer-Verlag; 1995.
21. van Gemert MJC, Umur A, van den Wijngaard JPHM, VanBavel E, Vandenbussche FPHA, Nikkels PGJ. Increasing cardiac output and decreasing oxygenation sequence in pump twins of acardiac twin pregnancies. *Phys Med Biol* 2005;50:N33–42.
22. Healey MG. Acardia: predictive risk factors for the co-twin's survival. *Teratology* 1994;50:205–13.
23. Umur A, van Gemert MJC, Nikkels PGJ. Monoamniotic versus diamniotic-monochorionic twin placentas: anastomoses and twin–twin transfusion syndrome. *Am J Obstet Gynecol* 2003;189:1314–19.
24. Nikkels PGJ, van Gemert MJC, Briët JW. Late onset of discordant growth in a monochorionic twin pregnancy: vascular anastomoses determine fetal growth pattern and not placental sharing. *Fetal Diagn Ther* 2001;16:23–5.
25. Nikkels PGJ, van Gemert MJC, Sollie-Szarynska KM, Molendijk H, Timmer B, Machin GA. Rapid onset of severe twin–twin transfusion syndrome caused by placental venous thrombosis. *Pediatr Develop Pathol* 2002;5:310–14.
26. Faber DJ, Aalders MCG, Mik EG, Hooper B, van Gemert MJC, van Leeuwen TG. Oxygen saturation-dependent absorption and scattering of blood. *Phys Rev Lett* 2004;93:028102(1–4).
27. Bermúdez C, Bercerra CH, Bornick PW, Allen MH, Arroyo J, Quintero RA. Placental types and twin–twin transfusion syndrome. *Am J Obstet Gynecol* 2002;187:489–94.
28. Murakoshi T, Quintero RA, Bornick PW, Allen MH. In vivo endoscopic assessment of arterioarterial anastomoses: insight into their hemodynamic function. *J Matern Fetal Neonatol Med* 2003;14:247–55.
29. de Vries HR, Aalders MC, Faber DJ, van den Wijngaard JP, Nikkels PG, van Gemert MJ. Colour oscillations in arterioarterial anastomoses reflect natural differences in donor and recipient

oxygenation and hematocrit. *Placenta* 2006. In press.

30. Tan TYT, Denbow ML, Cox PM, Talber D, Fisk NM. Occlusion of arterio-arterial anastomosis manifesting as acute twin–twin transfusion syndrome. *Placenta* 2004;25:238–42.

31. van Gemert MJC, van den Wijngaard JPHM, Umur A, Ross MG. Mathematical models of twin–twin transfusion syndrome pathophysiology. In: Quintero RA, editor. *Twin–Twin Transfusion Syndrome*. London: Taylor & Francis; in press.

32. van Gemert MJC, Vandenbussche FPHA, Schaap AHP, Zondervan HA, Nikkels PGJ, van Wijngaarden WJ, *et al.* Classification of discordant fetal growth may contribute to risk stratification in monochorial twin pregnancies. *Ultrasound Obstet Gynecol* 2000;16:237–44.

Chapter 4
Anomalous development in twins (including monozygotic duplication)

Neil J Sebire

Introduction

Twin pregnancy is a relatively common event, occurring in around 1–2% of all pregnancies worldwide (Table 4.1, Figure 4.1),[1–19] and the frequency has been increasing in recent years as a consequence of both increasing average maternal age and the use of fertility-enhancing treatments. There is some conflicting literature regarding the risk of congenital anomalies in twin compared with singleton pregnancies and, although there is general agreement that twins are more likely than singletons to be affected with a congenital malformation, the exact risks, associations with chorionicity and zygosity, and mechanisms remain largely unknown. This chapter will address these issues based on the currently available evidence.

Twin gestations represent about 1% of all pregnancies and approximately 80% are dichorionic.[20] However, there is a wide geographical variation in the prevalence of twinning, the lowest rates generally being reported in the Far East and the highest in Africa. These geographical variations are primarily because of differences in the rate of dizygotic twinning, monozygotic twinning being therefore of more relative importance in countries with lower overall twinning rates. The twinning rate in the USA has gradually increased from the 1960s to the 1990s, from 1 in 55 to 1 in 43 pregnancies, with a corresponding increase in the number of low birthweight infants and a disproportionate increase in the impact of multiple pregnancies on provision of perinatal care.[21] This change in rate is most marked for dizygotic twins but since 1975 there has also been a small but gradual increase in the monozygotic twinning rate, with their associated complications.[1,4,12,13,22–25] The rapid rise in multiple pregnancy rates since 1980, as a consequence of assisted reproduction techniques, has been reported worldwide.[26–31]

Perinatal mortality

The perinatal mortality rate in twins is about six-fold higher than in singletons (Figure 4.2).[1,4,10,12,16,32–34] About 40% of twin pregnancies spontaneously deliver prematurely,[35] and the overall excess in mortality in twins is primarily because of prematurity-related complications, whether this is examined using cause of death data[36] or by gestational age matching twins with singletons and comparing mortality

Table 4.1. Prevalence of twin pregnancies worldwide showing the twinning rate expressed as a percentage of all pregnancies

Study	Country	*n*	Twinning rate (%)
Botting *et al.* (1987)[1]	England	2 536 895	1.01
Kataki and Kouvatsi (1988)[2]	Greece	153 770	0.75
Bertranpetit and Marin (1988)[3]	Spain	498 586	0.76
Doherty (1988)[4]	Australia	1 832 414	0.99
Keith *et al.* (1988)[5]	USA	21 423	1.28
De Moraes *et al.* (1989)[6]	Brazil	26 520	0.81
Picard *et al.* (1989)[7]	Israel	19 207	1.20
Little and Nevin (1989)[8]	Northern Ireland	157 068	1.04
Ramos-Arroyo (1991)[9]	Spain	337 786	0.85
Kiely (1991)[10]	USA	349 188	1.05
Kato and Fujiki (1992)[11]	Japan	117 672	0.82
Chen *et al.* (1992)[12]	Taiwan	73 264	1.20
Goswami and Goswami (1993)[13]	India	13 887 943	1.37
Das Chaudhuri *et al.* (1993)[14]	West Bengal	119 107	1.06
Powers and Kiely (1994)[15]	USA	7 435 895	1.05
Pugliese *et al.* (1994)[16]	Italy	574 462	0.96
Zimon *et al.* (1998)[17]	Poland	28 051	1.10
Mastroiacovo *et al.* (1999)[18]	Worldwide	11 962 695	1.09
Sebire *et al.* (2001)[19]	England	423 107	1.28
Overall	**Worldwide**	**40 555 053**	**1.16**

rates.[37,38] Overall disability rates in twins are about 1.5-fold higher than in singletons, and for severe disability the increase is at least double.[39]

However, when perinatal mortality rates between twins and singletons matched for gestational age at delivery are considered, the results are dramatically different, with uncorrected perinatal mortality rates actually greater in singletons than twins at most gestational ages examined. After major congenital anomalies are excluded, gestational age corrected perinatal mortality remains significantly higher in singletons than in twins, further indicating preterm delivery as the major contributing factor to perinatal mortality in multiple pregnancies.[40,41] Overall, about 10–20% of all reported perinatal mortality may be associated with congenital anomaly but this is dependent on the extent of provision of prenatal diagnostic services. In twins, the relative contribution of congenital anomalies to perinatal mortality is much less, since the effect of prematurity is greater, and with increasing availability of prenatal diagnosis of fetal anomalies there has been a reduction in the contribution of congenital anomalies.[42]

The perinatal mortality rate for monozygotic twins is about 1.5-fold higher than for dizygotic twins[43] and in studies in which both chorionicity and zygosity were determined the perinatal mortality rate appears to be about 3–4 times greater for monochorionic than dichorionic twins regardless of their zygosity, indicating that chorionicity rather than zygosity is the main determinant of the additional adverse perinatal outcome.[44,45]

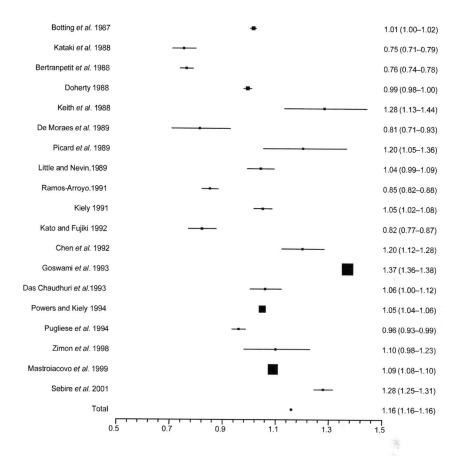

Botting *et al.* 1987	1.01 (1.00–1.02)
Kataki *et al.* 1988	0.75 (0.71–0.79)
Bertranpetit *et al.* 1988	0.76 (0.74–0.78)
Doherty 1988	0.99 (0.98–1.00)
Keith *et al.* 1988	1.28 (1.13–1.44)
De Moraes *et al.* 1989	0.81 (0.71–0.93)
Picard *et al.* 1989	1.20 (1.05–1.36)
Little and Nevin.1989	1.04 (0.99–1.09)
Ramos-Arroyo.1991	0.85 (0.82–0.88)
Kiely 1991	1.05 (1.02–1.08)
Kato and Fujiki 1992	0.82 (0.77–0.87)
Chen *et al.* 1992	1.20 (1.12–1.28)
Goswami *et al.* 1993	1.37 (1.36–1.38)
Das Chaudhuri *et al.*1993	1.06 (1.00–1.12)
Powers and Kiely 1994	1.05 (1.04–1.06)
Pugliese *et al.* 1994	0.96 (0.93–0.99)
Zimon *et al.* 1998	1.10 (0.98–1.23)
Mastroiacovo *et al.* 1999	1.09 (1.08–1.10)
Sebire *et al.* 2001	1.28 (1.25–1.31)
Total	1.16 (1.16–1.16)

Figure 4.1. Prevalence of twin pregnancies worldwide; there is variation in rates owing to differences in dizygotic twinning, with lower overall rates in Far Eastern countries and the highest rates in African and Indian countries; the overall twinning rate is around 1.2% of all pregnancies

Neurodevelopmental disability

Several studies have reported that the rate of permanent neurodisability, classified clinically as a cerebral palsy, is significantly higher among infants of multiple pregnancies compared with singletons,[46–48] and data from more recent studies ascertaining cerebral palsy rates in singleton and twin infants from the same populations, demonstrates the uncorrected odds ratio for cerebral palsy of about 4–6 for infants from multiple pregnancies compared with singletons (Figure 4.3).[49–53] These data are somewhat complicated by the finding that the risk is higher in monochorionic versus dichorionic twins and a proportion of such cases may also be associated with intrauterine death of the co-twin (see Chapter 16).[51,54,55] Nevertheless, regardless of the zygosity or chorionicity, twin pregnancy is associated with significant risk of severe

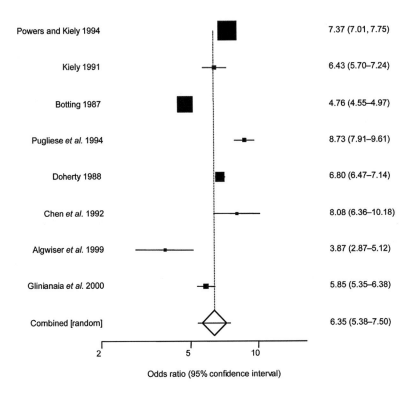

Odds ratio meta-analysis plot [random effects]

Powers and Kiely 1994	7.37 (7.01, 7.75)
Kiely 1991	6.43 (5.70–7.24)
Botting 1987	4.76 (4.55–4.97)
Pugliese et al. 1994	8.73 (7.91–9.61)
Doherty 1988	6.80 (6.47–7.14)
Chen et al. 1992	8.08 (6.36–10.18)
Algwiser et al. 1999	3.87 (2.87–5.12)
Glinianaia et al. 2000	5.85 (5.35–6.38)
Combined [random]	6.35 (5.38–7.50)

Odds ratio (95% confidence interval)

Figure 4.2. Perinatal mortality rates from studies reporting perinatal mortality data for singletons and twin infants from the same populations; there is some heterogeneity of magnitude of risk, but most studies report five- to ten-fold increases in uncorrected perinatal mortality rate, with a pooled odds ratio of around 6

preterm delivery, which represents the major contributor to the increased rate of neurodisability in twins, and such factors are even more important in higher order multiples.[54,55] Overall, infants from multiple gestations represent about 5–10% of the population affected by cerebral palsy.[56]

Since a significant proportion of twins arise as a consequence of assisted conception techniques, the effect has been examined using a national register-based cohort study including more than 18 000 singleton and twin pregnancies from assisted reproduction and natural conceptions with follow-up to age seven years. This study demonstrated that twins from assisted conception pregnancies have a similar risk of neurological sequelae as their naturally conceived controls.[52] Furthermore, in a similar manner to

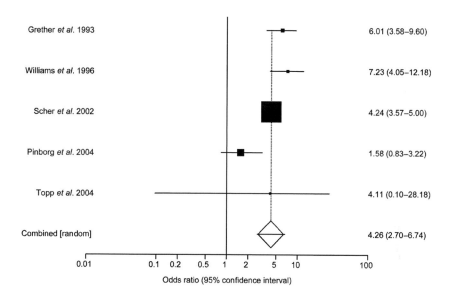

Figure 4.3.   Summary of odds ratios for uncorrected risk of cerebral palsy in twin versus singleton infants from the same populations

the effect on perinatal mortality, although twins are at increased risk of development of cerebral palsy overall compared with singletons, when matched for birthweight less than 2500 g, twin infants had lower cerebral palsy rates than singletons, although at greater birthweights the reported increased frequency in twins remained.[51,57] The greatest risk for cerebral palsy appears to be in surviving infants whose co-twin died *in utero* or is also affected by cerebral palsy.[51,57–59] Once correction for gestational age and birthweight is accounted for, the clinical type of cerebral palsy appears to be the same in multiples and singletons.[53] When birthweight-specific rates of cerebral palsy are examined, same-sex twins are at greater risk of cerebral palsy than opposite-sex twins and if both twins survive infancy the gestational age adjusted prevalence of cerebral palsy remains significantly less than when a co-twin has died *in utero*.[58–60] Although some studies report no difference in rates between monozygous and dizygous pairs, and in same-sex and opposite-sex pairs,[49,51,61,62] probably because the overriding risk factor overall is severe preterm delivery and most twins are dizygotic, others suggest monozygotic twins are at increased risk.[59,63] Indeed, using a multivariate technique to examine risk factors for cerebral palsy in infants less than 30 weeks of gestation, monochorionic twin placentation appears to be associated with a six-fold increase in risk.[64] Further detailed discussion of the issues surrounding cerebral palsy in twins is presented in Chapter 16.

Types of congenital anomalies in twin pregnancies

Some discussion of the terminology of congenital anomalies is required in order to understand the specific issues involved in the pathogenesis of these entities in twin pregnancies. A congenital anomaly is defined as any deviation from the expected structure, form or function that is interpreted as abnormal. Malformations are morphological abnormalities of organs or regions of the body resulting from an intrinsically abnormal developmental process. Disruptions are morphological defects of organs or regions of the body resulting from interference with an originally normal developmental process, such as a vascular event or infection; these are sometimes called secondary malformations. Deformations are abnormal forms, shapes or positions of part of the body caused by mechanical forces and a sequence is a pattern of multiple anomalies derived from a single presumed underlying defect.[65] It will become clear from the following data presentation and discussion that the range of congenital anomalies in twin pregnancies may result from any of these processes and the underlying mechanisms may be important in understanding the relative risks of congenital anomalies in twin versus singleton infants. Furthermore, although the conditions encompassed within the generic spectrum of congenital anomaly are wide (see below), for the purposes of the majority of this chapter congenital anomalies refer primarily to those structural malformations recognised prenatally or at birth and classified as such according to the International Classification of Disease (ICD) and World Health Organization (WHO) disease codes. Further details regarding other related conditions that may be associated with specific congenital anomalies, such as co-twin death-associated lesions and twin-to-twin transfusion syndrome (TTTS), are covered in detail in Chapters 10 and 12, respectively.

Congenital anomalies also found in singleton pregnancies

Congenital anomalies present in twin pregnancies of course include all anomalies that may also occur in singletons, including primary structural malformations, chromosomal defects and genetic syndromes; aspects of such abnormalities in twins in relation to genetic syndromes, penetrance and risk factors are discussed in detail in Chapter 5.

Structural malformations unique to the twinning process

Further to the abnormalities identical to those seen in singletons, there are additional anomalies unique to multiple pregnancies, which appear to be related to the underlying twinning process and aspects of placentation. Multiple pregnancies may be monozygotic ('identical') or polyzygotic ('non-identical' or 'fraternal'). The majority (about 70% in the UK) are polyzygotic, meaning each embryo is derived from a different ovum. Theoretically, these ova may arise from the same follicle, separate follicles maturing in the same cycle, or follicles maturing in sequential cycles (superfetation) and each ovum may be fertilised by sperm from the same source or from separate sources (superfecundation). However, in humans dizygotic twins result from polyovulation in the same cycle with fertilisation from the same source. In all cases of polyzygotic multiple pregnancy each zygote develops its own amnion, chorion and placental circulation, and hence will be polychorionic. Single-ovum multiple pregnancies result from a zygote being formed from the union of one ovum and one sperm which then undergoes a division to form two genetically identical individuals (monozygotic). The underlying mechanism has been suggested as either 'splitting' of the single cell mass ('splitting theory') or development of more than one organising axis ('co-dominant axis theory');[66,67] such underlying twinning processes are discussed in detail in Chapter 5. If these processes occur after several cell divisions have taken place, there is the potential for mis-segregation of genetic or cytoplasmic material, leading to two cell populations derived from the same underlying sperm and ovum but with subtly different characteristics owing to post-meiotic crossing over, post-zygotic non-disjunction, imprinting, discordant X-inactivation, anomalous homeobox gene expression, asymmetrical laterality and discordant cytoplasmic segregation.[68–73] The stimulus for monozygotic twinning remains unclear but this is most likely to be due to an environmental influence, perhaps with a possible susceptibility to development of co-dominant axes,[74] and influenced by sex chromosomal components, as evidenced by the increased prevalence of females in many monozygotic twinning disorders.[75] The impact of environmental influences can be highlighted by the increased rate of monozygotic twinning found in *in vitro* fertilisation (IVF) pregnancies and after ovulation induction,[76–79] and it has been suggested that this may be a result of changes in the zona pellucida brought about by the culture medium.[80] Potential complications of the twinning process are discussed below.

Anomalies of monozygotic duplication

The pattern of placentation in monozygotic twins depends primarily upon the timing of the underlying twinning process. Early division, within the first three days post-fertilisation, results in dichorionic placentation; twinning at approximately three to nine days post-fertilisation results in monochorionic twin placentation; and splitting after around nine days post-fertilisation results in monoamniotic twins.[81–83] Since it is not usual for the single early embryonic cell mass to form two fetuses, many consider that monozygotic twinning is itself a congenital abnormality and also within the spectrum of abnormalities of monozygotic duplication are the entities of 'symmetrical' conjoined twins and asymmetrical duplications. Such asymmetrical duplications are usually divided into those with an external twin entity present (such as acardiac or acephalic twinning, twin reversed arterial perfusion (TRAP) sequence, or chorioangiopagus parasiticus), those associated with bizarre structural external defects of an otherwise normal fetus, known as ectoparasitic twin, and a final group of internal asymmetrical duplications termed endoparasitic twin or fetus in fetu, which usually present as an amorphous mass within the retroperitoneal region of an otherwise normal fetus. Differentiation of endoparasitic twinning from teratoma may be difficult but is traditionally performed on the basis of the presence of an organised spinal column in the endoparasitic twin.[84] Further discussion of ectoparasitic and endoparasitic asymmetrical duplication will not be included here, since, although the underlying pathophysiology is believed to be related to the twinning process, these are rare entities that present as abnormal apparent singleton infants, for which the diagnosis and management falls outside of the scope of management of twin pregnancy. Various other aspects of monozygotic duplications are detailed below.

Monochorionic twin pregnancies demonstrate varying degrees of unequal placental share and the vast majority of monochorionic twin pregnancies are characterised by the presence of inter-twin placental vascular anastomoses resulting in communication between the two feto-placental circulations (see Chapter 11). In about 15–25% of cases, imbalance in the net flow of blood across such vessels results in haemodynamic consequences and development of the clinical features of

TTTS.[85–90] The precise underlying mechanisms by which a select population of monochorionic pregnancies with vascular communications develops TTTS is not fully understood but the donor fetus suffers from hypovolaemia and hypoxia, while the recipient fetus becomes hypervolaemic, polyuric and hyperosmolar with high cardiac output state and polyhydramnios.[91–93] Several secondary congenital abnormalities have been recorded in infants suffering from TTTS, including hypertrophic, dilated and dyskinetic heart with pulmonary stenosis in the recipient fetus and cardiac dilation, hyperechogenic bowel and ventriculomegaly/microcephaly in the donor (see Chapter 12), in addition to other intrauterine disruptive lesions (see below). Postnatally, infants from pregnancies with TTTS demonstrate a three-fold increase in the frequency of congenital heart disease, often discordant, and predominantly affecting the recipient twin.[94] Full details of the pathophysiology, pathology and management of TTTS are discussed in Chapters 11 and 12.

Monoamniotic twinning is a rare variant of monozygotic monochorionic twinning in which the twinning process is thought to occur after approximately nine days post-fertilisation. Monoamniotic twins represent only approximately 1% of twins and fetal anomaly rates in such cases are reported to be around 20–25%, even when conjoined twins (which are monoamniotic) are excluded.[95] A full discussion of the issues surrounding monoamniotic twinning can be found later in the chapter.

Conjoined twins represent a rare form of monoamniotic twinning with specific and complex issues regarding their management, which are discussed later in the chapter.

Acardiac twinning, or TRAP sequence, is a specific type of abnormal external duplication affecting monochorionic twins.[84] Its pathogenesis, pathology and management are discussed in detail in Chapter 13.

Consequences of intrauterine death of a co-twin

Intrauterine death of a fetus in a monochorionic twin pregnancy may be associated with death or disability of the co-twin owing to hypotensive episodes secondary to the presence of the inter-fetal placental vascular communications in around 20–40% of cases, depending on the gestation of co-twin death.[96] Neurologically damaged twin infants, when compared with normal twin infants, are associated with co-twin death later in gestation, a shorter interval between co-twin death and delivery, and delivery earlier in gestation.[97] A full discussion of the risks and mechanisms of co-twin death is provided in Chapter 10.

Intrauterine disruptions

Disruptions represent secondary anomalous development of structures which originally began developing normally, and are therefore due to 'environmental' agents, with the most common aetiologies being infective and vascular. In addition to those disruptions occurring owing to the same agents as in singletons, such as infection or teratogenic drugs, many disruptions occur in monochorionic twins that appear to be a consequence of abnormalities in fetal and placental haemodynamics secondary to the presence of placental vascular communications between the circulations. Although many such disruptions have been reported following death of the co-twin (see above and Chapter 10), they have also been described in monochorionic twins with two surviving infants. Many organ systems may be affected, the most common and most serious being those leading to secondary hypoxic–ischaemic brain disruptions such as microcephaly, hydrocephaly, porencephalic cysts and hydranencephaly, but other organ systems commonly involved include gastrointestinal (intestinal atresia) and skin (aplasia cutis congenita).[84,98] Further support for the secondary vascular hypothesis is provided by a study reporting on small intestinal atresias in which the rate was higher among twins than singletons, but affecting same-sex twins and in relation to jejunoileal atresia rather than duodenal atresia, which is usually a malformation.[99] Further discussion of specific types of abnormalities associated with vascular events in twins is provided below.

Frequency of congenital anomalies in twins compared with singletons

Several historical studies based on obstetric or pathological data have suggested that the overall rate of congenital anomalies per infant is greater in twin compared with singleton pregnancies, both for anomalies in general and specific structural malformations.[84,100–112] However, to quantify accurately the relative increase in anomaly rate between twin and singleton infants it is necessary to examine those studies in which identical criteria were used in both groups for the definition of congenital anomaly and those in which twin and singleton subjects were recruited from the same overall population. Furthermore, since many congenital anomalies are individually rare, studies recruiting large numbers of cases are required in order to investigate the significance of any apparent differences in frequencies. Therefore, much of the best currently available data is provided from large national or international registries.

The combined data from eight major studies comparing congenital anomaly rates in singletons and twin infants from the same populations, including more than 17 million singleton births and more than 380 000 twin births (2.2% of infants), demonstrate that the overall odds ratio for congenital anomaly in twins is about 1.3 (Table 4.2, Figure 4.4).[11,12,17,18,113–116] The figure demonstrates that the majority of

Table 4.2. Studies reporting the rate of congenital abnormalities in twins compared with singletons from the same population using identical criteria for the definition of congenital anomaly

Study	Congenital abnormality rate		Odds ratio (95% CI)
	Singletons	Twins	
Windham and Bjerkedal (1984)[113]	23 141 of 766 000	426 of 15 320	0.92 (0.83–1.38)
Doyle et al. (1991)[114]	95 510 of 3 700 000	1925 of 76 000	0.98 (0.94–1.03)
Chen et al. (1992)[12]	27 of 4573	31 of 1468	3.63 (2.09–6.35)
Kato and Fujiki (1992)[11]	1721 of 116 686	42 of 1936	1.48 (–)
Zimon et al. (1998)[17]	725 of 27 741	23 of 620	1.44 (–)
Mastroiacovo et al. (1999)[18]	202 423 of 11 818	354 5572 of 260 856	1.25 (1.22–1.29)
Jacquemyn et al. (2003)[115]	162 of 4384	110 of 4384	0.67 (0.52–0.86)
Li et al. (2003)[116]	44 505 of 922 791	2127 of 23 069	2.00 (1.02–1.64)
Total	**368 214 of 17 360 529**	**10 256 of 383 683**	**1.30 (1.02–1.64)**

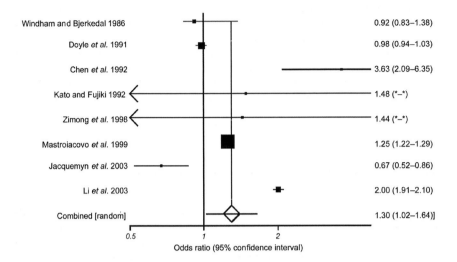

Windham and Bjerkedal 1986	0.92 (0.83–1.38)
Doyle et al. 1991	0.98 (0.94–1.03)
Chen et al. 1992	3.63 (2.09–6.35)
Kato and Fujiki 1992	1.48 (*–*)
Zimong et al. 1998	1.44 (*–*)
Mastroiacovo et al. 1999	1.25 (1.22–1.29)
Jacquemyn et al. 2003	0.67 (0.52–0.86)
Li et al. 2003	2.00 (1.91–2.10)
Combined [random]	1.30 (1.02–1.64)]

Odds ratio (95% confidence interval)

Figure 4.4. Congenital anomaly rates in twins and singleton infants derived from the same populations using identical criteria for definition of congenital anomaly; the larger series derive from regional, national or international registries; the majority of studies demonstrate an increased frequency of congenital anomalies in twin infants but since the prevalence of anomalies is relatively low, the smaller studies demonstrate wide confidence intervals; the overall pooled odds ratio for anomalies in twins, using a random effects model, is 1.3 times the rate in singletons (there is heterogeneity of results which is not easily explained by the populations or methodologies used, but no significant publication bias of studies is apparent; $P = 0.96$)

studies show consistent effects of increased anomaly rates in twins but some have large confidence intervals owing to their relatively small size. In addition, there is heterogeneity of results, with some studies apparently demonstrating no difference in rates, which cannot readily be explained on the basis of methodological features. Nevertheless, the two more recent, larger and most detailed, studies[18,116] show consistent effects and weighted meta-analysis using a random effects model suggests an overall increase in anomaly rate in twins of 1.3 compared with singletons. This estimate is also entirely consistent with the expected effect based on malformations in specific twinning subtypes (see later section). Although this represents the best available evidence it should be noted that there are potential problems with the use of registry data since ascertainment of anomalies is not known and there may be variability in definition of congenital anomalies for inclusion across different studies. Since many twin pregnancies may be the result of assisted conception techniques it should be noted that there does not appear to be any significant increase in malformation rate following intracytoplasmic sperm injection (ICSI) or IVF compared with naturally conceived pregnancies, so this in itself should not be a significant factor.[117–119]

Malformation rates in monozygotic versus dizygotic twins

Data from the above large registry studies include sufficient numbers of cases to provide a best estimate of the overall increased anomaly rate in twins of about 1.3

compared with singletons. However, in order to examine this finding further, in particular the possible relationship between zygosity or chorionicity and anomaly rates, data are required detailing congenital anomaly rates by fetal sex, formal genetic zygosity testing or chorionicity rates in twins. Unfortunately, no such data are available from any of the large registries. Indeed, only one study is available providing direct data on congenital anomaly rates in singleton and twin infants from the same population in whom zygosity determination has been performed.[12] In this study, of 73 264 deliveries in Taipei, including 1688 twin infants, zygosity was determined by infant sex, placentation and analysis of red blood cell antigens in 1468 cases, comprising 964 monozygotic and 504 dizygotic twin infants. Although the overall frequency of malformations in twin infants was greater than singletons (see Figure 4.4), subgroup analysis revealed that the prevalence of malformations was actually not significantly different between singletons and dizygotic twin infants, whereas the rate for monozygotic twins was about five-fold greater than singletons. Several other small studies, while not providing such quantitative estimates, do, however, provide further supportive evidence that the prevalence of congenital malformations in twin infants appears to be greater in same-sex twins with little or no increased frequency of malformations among opposite-sex, therefore proven dizygotic dichorionic, twin pairs. In particular, defects of the central nervous system, cardiovascular system and genitourinary systems appear to be significantly more frequent in same-sex twins (see below).[84,103,104,111,120-125]

Concordance rates for fetal malformations in twins

Monozygotic twins will, of course, be concordant for chromosomal or genetic defects in most circumstances, but the majority of twin pregnancies are discordant for fetal malformations regardless of type of anomaly. Data from the largest available series report 81% discordance for any type of anomaly,[116] which is consistent with similar rates reported in several smaller reports.[84,126] However, no large studies are available that provide information on zygosity, chorionicity or fetal sex in relation to concordance rates. In the only study of malformations in twins and singletons in which zygosity data were provided, the concordance rate of major congenital malformations was 18% for monozygotic twins; no dizygotic twin pair was concordant for any malformation, although the number of affected dizygotic twins was too small for adequate analysis.[12] This is consistent with the hypothesis that malformations in dizygotic twins occur at a similar rate to singletons, making the probability of two affected dizygotic co-twins very small, and that the majority of anomalies in monozygotic twins are either the result of the anomalous twinning process itself or complications of inter-fetal haemodynamics, both of which would affect the two fetuses unequally.

Specific malformation types in twins

The spectrum of potential congenital anomalies affecting twin infants and their proposed pathophysiological mechanisms are discussed above. Further examination of specific anomaly rates in twins versus singletons allows more rational comment regarding prenatal counselling. Since many individual anomalies are very rare, such data are available only from large, population-based registry studies, of which two provide detailed description of specific anomalies with their relative risks (Figures 4.5 and 4.6).[18,116] Unfortunately, no such detailed data are available regarding specific anomaly rates by zygosity or chorionicity. A further detailed description of anomalies

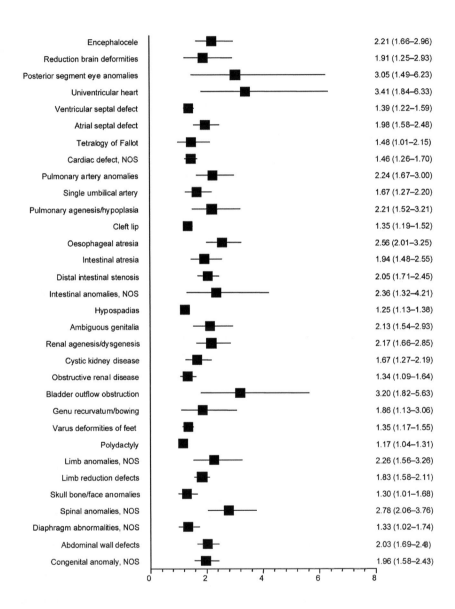

Figure 4.5. Specific malformation types at significantly increased risk in in twin compared with singleton infants with calculated odds ratios and 95% confidence intervals; NOS = not otherwise specified; adapted from Mastroiacovo et al. (1999)[18]

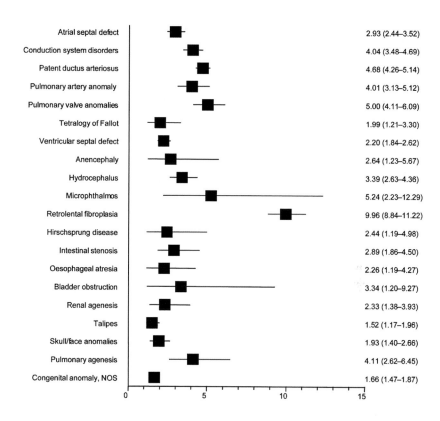

Atrial septal defect	2.93 (2.44–3.52)
Conduction system disorders	4.04 (3.48–4.69)
Patent ductus arteriosus	4.68 (4.26–5.14)
Pulmonary artery anomaly	4.01 (3.13–5.12)
Pulmonary valve anomalies	5.00 (4.11–6.09)
Tetralogy of Fallot	1.99 (1.21–3.30)
Ventricular septal defect	2.20 (1.84–2.62)
Anencephaly	2.64 (1.23–5.67)
Hydrocephalus	3.39 (2.63–4.36)
Microphthalmos	5.24 (2.23–12.29)
Retrolental fibroplasia	9.96 (8.84–11.22)
Hirschsprung disease	2.44 (1.19–4.98)
Intestinal stenosis	2.89 (1.86–4.50)
Oesophageal atresia	2.26 (1.19–4.27)
Bladder obstruction	3.34 (1.20–9.27)
Renal agenesis	2.33 (1.38–3.93)
Talipes	1.52 (1.17–1.96)
Skull/face anomalies	1.93 (1.40–2.66)
Pulmonary agenesis	4.11 (2.62–6.45)
Congenital anomaly, NOS	1.66 (1.47–1.87)

Figure 4.6. Specific malformation types at significantly increased risk in twin compared with singleton infants with calculated odds ratios and 95% confidence intervals; NOS = not otherwise specified; adapted from Li *et al.* (2003)[116]

found in a large autopsy series of twins is also available,[84] the findings being consistent with those presented in Figures 4.5 and 4.6. The reported anomalies may affect all organ systems but the most common are cardiovascular, nervous system, ophthalmic and gastrointestinal abnormalities, with the findings broadly consistent across studies. It should be noted, however, that those anomalies reported with significantly increased prevalence in twin infants can be divided into several groups. Firstly, those presumed primary malformations that may be related to midline formation and/or dependent on laterality, such as neural tube defects and some of the cardiac defects. Secondly, those anomalies that have a presumed disruptive aetiology, usually a consequence of haemodynamic abnormalities, such as encephaloclastic brain lesions, limb reduction defects, some cardiac defects, renal agenesis, aplasia cutis and intestinal atresias. Indeed, one study specifically examined small intestinal atresias and reported that the rate was three-fold greater in twin infants, predominantly in same-sex twins, and predominantly associated with jejunoileal atresia.[99] Thirdly, those anomalies associated with prematurity, including patent ductus arteriosus and retrolental fibroplasia, and finally, those not fitting any of the above categories.

It is interesting to note that monozygotic twinning has also been reported to occur with increased frequency in Beckwith–Wiedemann syndrome (BWS). In one study, 12 sets of monozygotic twins with BWS were reported, of which 11 were female, and in all cases but one, the infants were discordant for the BWS phenotype despite being monozygotic. Since BWS is essentially a defect of imprinting, such findings suggest that monozygotic twinning may be associated with intrinsically anomalous imprinting, although the mechanism remains uncertain.[127] Furthermore, an increased twinning rate has been reported in families with a history of singleton neural tube defects, suggesting a possible role of either a genetic predisposition to both abnormalities or a metabolic defect which predisposes to both conditions.[128]

Summary of congenital anomalies in twins

Despite the limitations of the available data, best estimates suggest that the overall rate of congenital anomalies in twin infants is about 1.3 times higher than in singletons. Since such calculations are based primarily on infant registry data, which often include such entities as retrolental fibroplasia, a proportion of this increased risk may be directly attributable to the higher frequency of prematurity-related complications in multiple pregnancies, which will affect twin infants regardless of zygosity or chorionicity. The limited data available suggest that once prematurity-related complications are excluded, the congenital anomaly rate in dizygotic twins is not significantly greater than for singletons. Since the overall anomaly rate in twins is increased 1.3-fold, this suggests that the congenital anomaly rate in monozygotic twin infants (based on the assumption that monozygotic twin pregnancies account for about one-third of all twin pregnancies) must be at least double that in dizygotic twins or singletons. This is in accordance with data from the limited studies that have provided such information and is also compatible with data examining specific malformation types. This suggests that the majority of anomalies seen with increased frequencies in twin infants could be associated with defects in laterality or secondary to vascular disruptions, both of which mechanisms would preferentially affect only monozygotic, and predominantly monochorionic, twins. By inference, since monochorionic twins account for about two-thirds of monozygotic twins, it is likely that, in reality, the congenital anomaly rate in monochorionic twins is three- to four-fold greater than for dichorionic twins or singletons.

Chromosomal abnormalities in twin pregnancies

In singleton pregnancies the risks of many chromosomal abnormalities, such as autosomal trisomy, increase with maternal age. Since on average the maternal age of multiple pregnancies is higher than that for singletons, a corresponding greater absolute risk for trisomy might be expected in this population. However, several studies have reported on the frequency of chromosomal abnormalities in twin pregnancies which demonstrate that risk for fetal aneuploidy is the same or lower than for singleton pregnancies from the same population.[9,105,114,116,129,130] Therefore, it is reasonable on the basis of the data currently available to suggest that the risk for chromosomal abnormality is probably the same per fetus in twin as in singleton pregnancies but obviously in monozygotic twin pregnancies both fetuses will be affected (although there are occasional case reports of monozygotic twins who are apparently discordant for chromosomal abnormalities, usually sex chromosome anomalies, presumably as a consequence of defective post-fertilisation divisions).[84] In dizygotic pregnancies the risk for chromosomal abnormalities for each twin is probably the same as for singletons but, because two fetuses are present, the risk that at least one fetus would be affected in that pregnancy is at least twice as high as for singletons, which may have implications for counselling.

In singleton pregnancies screening for trisomy 21 by a combination of maternal age and second-trimester maternal serum biochemistry can detect about 50–60% of cases for a 5% false positive rate.[131] In twin pregnancies the median value for maternal serum markers, such as α-fetoprotein (AFP), human chorionic gonadotrophin (hCG), unconjugated oestriol (uE3), free α hCG, free β hCG and inhibin A,[132–136] are about twice those for singleton pregnancies. When this is taken into account in the mathematical modelling for calculation of risks, it was estimated that serum screening in twins may be associated with a similar overall detection rate as in singletons.[133,137,138] However, there are several additional issues to be addressed regarding aneuploidy screening in multiple pregnancies. Firstly, the detection rate must be associated with an acceptably low false positive rate since invasive testing in multiple pregnancies is technically more demanding. Secondly, in the presence of a 'screen positive' result the test should indicate which fetus is affected; and thirdly, if the pregnancy is discordant for aneuploidy further management by way of selective termination carries lower loss rates when carried out in the first trimester. Therefore, the most appropriate methodology for screening in twin pregnancies may be a combination of maternal serum biochemistry and nuchal translucency measurement at 11–14 weeks of gestation, in which a detection rate of 75% for trisomy 21 has been reported for a 6–7% false positive rate.[139]

Fetal karyotyping currently requires invasive testing by amniocentesis or chorionic villus sampling (CVS) and in singleton pregnancies the procedure-related risks of both techniques appear similar. In twin pregnancies the relative safety of the procedures, certainty of sampling both fetuses and the likely subsequent management affect the choice of appropriate technique. Both amniocentesis and CVS have now been well described in twin pregnancies using one or two separate uterine insertions of the needle.[140] Invasive testing in twin pregnancies should always be performed in a specialist centre where selective feticide can be undertaken because, to avoid the potential disaster of feticide of the wrong fetus, it is vital that at the time of the amniocentesis a careful ultrasound examination is performed to classify the fetuses as twin I and II. Amniocentesis and CVS in twin pregnancies appear to have similar procedure-related loss rates to singletons when performed by experienced operators. CVS has the potential advantage of providing cytogenetic results in the first trimester allowing earlier, and hence safer, selective termination if required. However, with CVS there is a potential small risk of sampling error (about 1–5% of cases),[141] and CVS in twins requires a high degree of expertise in ultrasonography and invasive procedures. Therefore, CVS may be the preferred option for pregnancies at high risk of chromosomal defects, whereas amniocentesis may be preferable if the risk is low; however, decisions must ultimately be taken on a case-by-case basis and according to operator expertise in invasive testing techniques.

Management of twin pregnancies discordant for fetal abnormality

In twin, compared with singleton, pregnancies affected by a prenatally detected fetal abnormality, the main additional factor to be considered in their management is the potential impact of the malformation on the structurally normal co-twin. As such, any potential intrauterine procedure for the malformed fetus needs to be weighed against the potential risk of pregnancy loss of the structurally normal co-twin, and the issue of the multiple pregnancy resulting in a disabled twin must also be considered. Essentially, there are two options for the management of multiple pregnancies discordant for structural fetal abnormalities: they can be managed either expectantly or by selective termination of the abnormal twin. In cases where the abnormality is non-lethal but may result in disability the parents must decide whether the risk of loss of the normal co-twin from feticide-related complications outweighs that of the risk of a disabled child. In cases where the abnormality is lethal, in some circumstances it may be best to avoid the risk of feticide-associated loss unless the malformation itself threatens the survival of the normal twin, an example of which is discordant anencephaly, which although lethal may be associated with a 50% risk of development of severe polyhydramnios which places the normal co-twin at risk of severe preterm delivery related complications.[142] Regardless of management, compared with normal twin pregnancies, those discordant for fetal abnormality appear to be associated with a significantly increased preterm delivery rate.[143] The issues regarding techniques, rationale, timing and risks of selective termination are discussed in Chapter 6.

Twin pregnancies with complete hydatidiform mole

There is a very specific scenario in which obstetric management differs from that of other twin pregnancies discordant for anomaly, namely that of a dizygotic twin pregnancy in which one fetus appears structurally normal, associated with a complete hydatidiform mole, which occurs in about 1/20 000 to 1/100 000 gestations. In such cases there is a 50% risk of spontaneous pregnancy loss or severe pre-eclampsia requiring termination of pregnancy before 24 weeks of gestation, and, of those reaching potential viability, a further 25% will result in fetal death. The overall probability of delivering a live infant is therefore about 35–40%. The risk of developing persistent gestational trophoblastic disease (pGTD) appears similar to singleton pregnancies with complete mole (about 15–20%), and the risk of pGTD is not different in early termination of pregnancy compared with continuation to delivery or spontaneous loss.[144]

Monoamniotic twinning

Monoamniotic twins represent about 1–2% of twin gestations, occurring in around one in 3000 to one in 6000 pregnancies,[145–149] and are at increased risk for a number of antenatal complications. Some of these appear to be as a result of the twinning process itself, with high fetal structural anomaly rates recorded. It should be noted that since conjoined twins are also monoamniotic, these are often included in the literature regarding anomalous monoamniotic twins. However, this section refers only to non-conjoined monoamniotic twins, which appear to be associated with a significant risk of structural anomalies of around 20–25%.[84] In addition to direct complications of the twinning process, monoamniotic twins are at increased risk of intrauterine death and other obstetric complications because of umbilical cord entanglement or major haemodynamic alterations via the large chorionic vascular connections between the two fetal circulations in proximity to the closely inserted umbilical cords, which are present in most cases.[150]

Early pathological studies often attributed complications such as fetal death to the presence of umbilical cord entanglement in monoamniotic twins. With the introduction of routine sonographic evaluation of such pregnancies from the first trimester it has become apparent that cord entanglement is a very common finding, being reported in 20–100% of monoamniotic twin pregnancies depending on the gestational age at recruitment and methodologies used; however, the majority (80–100%) of cases examined in the first and second trimesters in more recent studies appear to be associated with sonographic evidence of cord entanglement.[148,151,152] Nevertheless, the significance of such cord entanglement remains unclear, since it does occur very commonly and most monoamniotic twins do not succumb to cord accidents. It has also been reported unequivocally in pregnancies with two surviving infants in addition to those resulting in intrauterine deaths.[150,153–163] Furthermore, although TTTS (see Chapter 11) can theoretically occur in monoamniotic twin pregnancies, and has been reported,[164] classical chronic TTTS is rare owing to the differences in cord proximity and anastomosis patterns between monoamniotic and diamniotic monochorionic twin pregnancies. Monoamniotic placentas usually have large arterio-arterial anastomoses, fewer arteriovenous anastomoses and shorter intercord distances. The vascular pattern described predicts that classical TTTS would be expected to occur in only about 5% of monoamniotic monochorionic twin pregnancies although acute haemodynamic changes via arterio-arterial anastomoses remain a significant risk.[150,165]

The available evidence regarding outcome and anomaly rates in monoamniotic twins is suboptimal since data are essentially derived from either small case series or recruitment of larger retrospective series ascertained primarily from obstetric or neonatal databases in which early deaths may not be included, and which therefore preferentially include those surviving beyond 24 weeks of gestation. Furthermore, in some larger series it is unclear whether anomalous infants are included in the calculation of survival data. Nevertheless, the best currently available evidence, based on the combined data from ten series including more than 250 monoamniotic twin pregnancies in total, suggests an overall livebirth rate of 82% and a congenital anomaly rate of 21%.[145,148,151,152,166–171] However, because of the retrospective and potentially biased nature of ascertainment in some series and the variable, and often unknown, gestational age at recruitment, for antenatal counselling purposes the best estimate of intrauterine survival is probably 40–80% for structurally normal fetuses, the lower value being derived from a small series recruiting all cases in the first trimester, in which survival was much lower than reported in the registry-derived series.[148] Further multicentre studies of outcome of monoamniotic twin pregnancies following ascertainment in the first trimester are required in order to provide counselling information, understand the timing of fetal demise and investigate surveillance strategies. However, the congenital anomaly data are more consistent with a rate of 20–25% of infants in almost all studies (Figure 4.7) with a wide range of anomalies reported in monoamniotic twins, most discordant, including several cases of discordant severe renal tract anomalies, such as bilateral renal agenesis, in which the monoamniotic nature of the pregnancy prevented the Potter phenotype and pulmonary complications from developing in the affected infant.[84,172–176]

Since few data are available regarding antenatal outcome, timing and mechanisms of fetal loss in monoamniotic twins, it is not surprising that the optimal management and surveillance of such pregnancies is also undetermined. Several studies have reported on the use of pulsed and colour Doppler assessment of umbilical blood flow to detect and evaluate the presence of umbilical cord entanglement, but with no evidence supporting its interpretation and usefulness in preventing fetal complications in this clinical setting.[177–187] Furthermore, opinions in the existing literature also vary

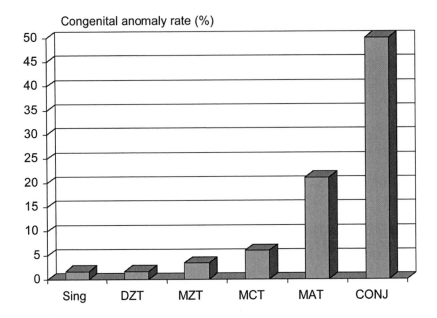

Congenital anomaly rate (%)

Figure 4.7. Summary of best estimates of fetal/infant congenital anomaly rates in singletons (Sing) and twins: dizygotic (DZT), monozygotic (MZT), monochorionic (MCT), monoamniotic (MAT) and conjoined (CONJ), based on appropriate published studies (see text); the rate of congenital anomalies of conjoined twins not directly related to the conjoined region is difficult to determine but appears to be at least 50% and up to 80% in some studies

regarding the methods of antepartum monitoring, timing and mode of delivery in such cases. Generally, it is agreed that there should be regular antepartum fetal heart rate monitoring and serial sonograms with umbilical artery Doppler flow study, although the evidence for their effectiveness is limited. Many studies also advocate delivery at 32 weeks to reduce the risk of late intrauterine deaths, although it remains uncertain whether such a strategy is beneficial. Caesarean section is generally the preferred mode of delivery although successful vaginal delivery has been reported.[188]

Since cord entanglement is a common complication of monoamniotic twins which it is assumed may be the cause of fetal mortality, it has been hypothesised that reducing amniotic fluid volume could stabilise fetal lie and reduce the risk of cord complications. In a pilot study of three cases of monoamniotic twin pregnancies with cord entanglement, sulindac, a nonsteroidal anti-inflammatory drug (NSAID), was administered to the mothers and was associated with a reduction in amniotic fluid index, with all six infants liveborn.[189] However, there was no control group and similar reported use of sulindac in other studies has been reported in association with a fetal loss rate of up to 75%.[148] Currently, the evidence does not suggest that such NSAID use is effective in this clinical group to reduce morbidity or mortality.

Conjoined twinning

Given their rarity and clinical importance, there is a disproportionately large body of literature regarding various aspects of conjoined twins, including extensive teratological, moral and ethical issues, in addition to numerous single case reports. However, this section will focus purely on aspects directly relevant to clinical care in the obstetric setting.

The frequency of conjoined twinning is obviously related to the underlying frequency of monozygotic twinning in general, such that the reported prevalence of conjoined twinning is only one in 200 000 in Africa, one in 97 000 in the USA, and as high as one in 6000 pregnancies in Taipei. However, worldwide, conjoined twins account for around one in 90 000 to one in 100 000 gestations based on analysis of data from 28 million births from international registry data and several other smaller national studies.[190–194] There does not appear to be any influence of maternal age, parity or family history on the likelihood of conjoined twinning. However, there is a clear female preponderance in the majority of cases of conjoined twins in almost all studies reported, with the largest registry data set recording 61% as female.[84,190] The underlying pathogenic mechanism of conjoined twinning remains uncertain, with numerous studies hypothesising on this matter. Theories include incomplete separation of the developing embryo, development of co-dominant axes with abnormalities due to organising regions located too close and exerting an abnormal effect, and embryonic fusion. It has been suggested that all types of conjoined twins (see below) could be explained by several possible sites of union in the early embryo, including fusion of parallel notochords, cranial and caudal neuropores, pharyngeal and cloacal membranes, cardiac anlage, umbilicus and edges of the two embryonic discs.[195,196]

There is also a large body of literature that classifies anatomical types of conjoined twinning. This appears to be largely an academic exercise but there clearly are some fairly regular forms, which may simplify understanding of the condition. For example, in general, only similar body parts are joined; junction of limbs alone does not seem to occur and conjoined twins are usually approximately symmetrical, being joined laterally or face-to face. Detailed descriptions of the anatomical classifications of conjoined twins are available for the interested reader,[84] but the classifications can be simplified into three conjoined regions: upper body, lower body or midzone regions; further complicating this matter, multiple terminologies are used with often little consistency.[197] Conjoining of the central, thoracic region is the most common group (thoracopagus), often with associated abdominal conjoining (thoraco-omphalopagus), pure abdominal conjoining (omphalopagus) and, less commonly, lower body/pelvic conjoining (ischiopagus) or cranial conjoining (craniopagus).[84,193] These patterns suggest that most conjoined twins appear to have two notochordal axes with the ventral organs severely disorientated, malformed, or aplastic owing to secondary disorganisation, with some organs and tissues probably failing to develop because of abnormal morphogenic gradients.[198] The vast majority of placentas of conjoined twins are monochorionic monoamniotic, with either a single umbilical cord appearing to originate from the placenta (usually with multiple apparent vessels demonstrable with prenatal imaging),[199] which then divides, or two long umbilical cords apparently originating separately. However, there are now two reports of conjoined twins with pathologically confirmed diamniotic monochorionic placentas, the theoretical explanation being early duplication of the primitive streak during gastrulation.[200,201]

By definition, conjoined twinning is itself a malformation and is associated with both secondary changes of the abnormal conjoined organs with probable superimposed effects of abnormal haemodynamics, and other congenital anomalies not apparently directly related to the conjoined components in up to 80% of cases.[202] In general, the degree of cardiovascular anomaly in conjoined twins is the main limiting factor to consideration of separation procedures, and therefore long-term survival. Several studies have provided detailed descriptions of such cardiovascular anomalies, ranging from a single conventional heart with isomerism, two conventional hearts with abnormal laterality, to complex compound hearts with fusions of venous sinuses, atria, or atria and ventricles. Cardiac morphogenesis in conjoined twins is highly complex and appears to depend on both the site of the fusion and the effects of secondary temporal and spatial influences.[203–205]

The best estimate of overall intrauterine lethality of conjoined twins, based on more than 300 cases derived from historical pooled registry data, is 47%.[190] However, accurate recent counselling data are difficult to obtain since prognosis is strongly related to the type of conjoining in each individual case and many parents opt for termination of pregnancy following early prenatal diagnosis.[148] Nevertheless, in one recent series of 14 cases of prenatally diagnosed conjoined twins at a single referral centre, 20% opted for termination of pregnancy, 10% died *in utero* and the overall individual survival rate to discharge of those attempting pregnancy continuation was about 25%.[206] Most cases are now prenatally diagnosed and delivered by elective caesarean section, but vaginal deliveries of conjoined twins are well reported.[207–210] However, risk of dystocia and uterine rupture has been reported in association with prenatally undiagnosed cases.[211,212]

Prenatal diagnosis of conjoined twins is now well reported from the mid first-trimester, using B-mode ultrasound, Doppler, colour Doppler and three-dimensional imaging techniques, with detailed assessment of cardiovascular anatomy important for determining prognosis and planning management.[213–237] Further antenatal management is usually termination of pregnancy or conservative management with planned delivery, although *in utero* therapy in a set of omphalopagus-conjoined twins has been reported using thermocoagulation in the early second trimester with the live birth of one twin.[238]

Successful surgical separation of conjoined twins has been described for many years, with the success rate essentially dependent on the extent of organ sharing and anatomical features. Therefore, planning of each case must be individualised, with overall success rates of 25–70% reported.[239–254] Nevertheless, several general factors associated with successful separation procedures may be identified. In a review of 47 reported pairs of surgically separated thoracopagus-conjoined twins, in patients with completely separate hearts, 70% survived, in those with only atrial connections 10% survived, while none of the patients with atrial and ventricular interconnections survived. The overall survival rate of surgically separated thoracopagus-conjoined twins in this series was 48%.[250] In another series from a single centre, 10 separations were attempted from 13 sets of conjoined twins, with 16 operative survivors (61% survival); however, this study included long-term follow-up and significantly, up to ten years after surgery, there were a further six deaths (40% of initial operative survivors) because of complications of serious associated congenital anomalies, predominantly cardiac.[246] More recently, in a review of 17 sets managed at a single tertiary centre, five (29%) had non-operable anatomy and all died. In seven (41%), separation was attempted as an emergency procedure because of the presence of a life-threatening anomaly, of which 29% of infants survived, while in five cases (30%) elective separation was carried out and 80% of infants survived. The overall survival of those with attempted separation was 50% of infants.[255] It is therefore reasonable to suggest from the available data that at least 30% of conjoined twins will be associated with non-operable anatomy and will die, of those operable cases around 50% of infants will survive the procedure, with significantly greater survival for cases operated electively and with non-shared cardiac anatomy, and there is a further long-term mortality rate of up to 40% of immediate survivors.

In addition to mortality, it should be noted that conjoined twins may be associated with significant morbidities both before and after separation. For example, to enable adequate coverage following separation, extensive use of skin expanders may be required,[256] and there may be significant long-term orthopaedic, neurological and spinal problems,[257-260] gastrointestinal complications requiring stomas,[261] and urogenital complications requiring complex genital reconstructions and urinary drainage procedures.[262-265] In one series, complex urological problems were present in all twins with omphalo-ischiopagus, including crossed, fused renal ectopias, common bladders, common genitalia, partial urethral duplications and hypospadias.[264]

References

1. Botting BJ, Macdonald Davies I, Macfarlane AJ. Recent trends in the incidence of multiple births and associated mortality. *Arch Dis Child* 1987;62:941–50.

2. Kataki A, Kouvatsi A. Twinning in Greece. *Acta Genet Med Gemellol (Roma)* 1988;37:147–50.

3. Bertranpetit J, Marin A. Demographic parameters and twinning: a study in Catalonia, Spain. *Acta Genet Med Gemellol (Roma)* 1988;37:127–35.

4. Doherty JDH. Perinatal mortality in twins, Australia, 1973–1980. *Acta Genet Med Gemellol (Roma)* 1988;37:313–19.

5. Keith LG, Depp R, Method MW, Wittman R, Lopez-Zeno J, Minoque J, *et al.* The Northwestern University twin study. V: twin deliveries at Prentice Womens Hospital and Maternity Center, 1978–83. *Acta Genet Med Gemellol (Roma)* 1988;37:1–10.

6. De Moraes MHB, Beiguelman B, Krieger H. Decline of the twinning rate in Brazil. *Acta Genet Med Gemellol (Roma)* 1989;38:57–63.

7. Picard R, Fraser D, Hagay ZJ, Leiberman JR. Twinning in southern Israel: secular trends, ethnic variation and effects of maternal age and parity. *Eur J Obstet Gynecol Reprod Biol* 1989;33:131–39.

8. Little J, Nevin NC. Congenital anomalies in twins in Northern Ireland. I: Anomalies in general and specific anomalies other than neural tube defects and of the cardiovascular system, 1974–1979. *Acta Genet Med Gemellol (Roma)* 1989;38:1–16.

9. Ramos-Arroyo MA. Birth defects in twins: study in a Spanish population. *Acta Genet Med Gemellol (Roma)* 1991;40:337–44.

10. Kiely JL. Time trends and neonatal mortality among twins and singletons in New York City, 1968–1986. *Acta Genet Med Gemellol (Roma)* 1991;40:303–9.

11. Kato K, Fujiki K. Multiple births and congenital anomalies in Tokyo Metropolitan Hospitals, 1979–1990. *Acta Genet Med Gemellol (Roma)*. 1992;41:253–9.

12. Chen CJ, Wang CJ, Yu MW, Lee TK. Perinatal mortality and prevalence of major congenital malformations of twins in Taipei City. *Acta Genet Med Gemellol (Roma)* 1992;41:197–203.

13. Goswami R, Goswami HK. Changing trends in twinning. *Acta Genet Med Gemellol (Roma)* 1993;42:289–94.

14. Das Chaudhuri AB, Basu S, Chakraborty S. Twinning rate in the Muslim population of West Bengal. *Acta Genet Med Gemellol (Roma)* 1993;42:35–9.

15. Powers WF, Kiely JL. The risks confronting twins: a national perspective. *Am J Obstet Gynecol* 1994;170:456–61.

16. Pugliese A, Arsieri R, Patriarca V, Spagnolo A. Incidence and neonatal mortality of twins: Italy 1981–90. *Acta Genet Med Gemellol (Roma)* 1994;43:139–44.

17. Zimon T, Walczak M, Fydryk J, Materna-Kiryluk A, Mejnartowicz J, Latos-Bielenska A, *et al.* Prevalence and forms of congenital anomalies in twins born in Pomeranian District during the period from 1.07.1997 to 31.12.1998. Polish Register of Congenital Anomalies. *Acta Genet Med Gemellol (Roma)* 1998;47:255–9.

18. Mastroiacovo P, Castilla EE, Arpino C, Botting B, Cocchi G, Goujard J, *et al.* Congenital malformations in twins: an international study. *Am J Med Genet* 1999;83:117–24.

19. Sebire NJ, Jolly M, Harris J, Nicolaides KH, Regan L. Risks of obstetric complications in

multiple pregnancies: an analysis of more than 400,000 pregnancies in the UK. *Prenat Neonat Med* 2001;6:89–94.

20. Cameron AH, Edwards JH, Derom R, Thiery M, Boelaert R. The value of twin surveys in the study of malformations. *Eur J Obstet Gynecol Reprod Biol* 1983;14:347–56.

21. Luke B. The changing pattern of multiple births in the United States: maternal and infant characteristics, 1973–1990. *Obstet Gynecol* 1994;84:101–6.

22. Bressers WMA, Eriksson AW, Kostense PJ, Parisi P. Increasing trend in the monozygotic twinning rate. *Acta Genet Med Gemellol (Roma)* 1987;36:397–408.

23. Allen G, Parisi P. Trends in monozygotic and dizygotic twinning rates by maternal age and parity. Further analysis of Italian data, 1949–1985, and rediscussion of US data, 1964–1985. *Acta Genet Med Gemellol (Roma)* 1990;39:317–28.

24. Orlebeke JF, Eriksaw AW, Boomsma DI, Vlietinck R, Tas FJ, De Geus EC. Changes in the DZ unlike/like sex ratio in the Netherlands. *Acta Genet Med Gemellol (Roma)* 1991;40:319–23.

25. Imaizumi Y. Twinning rates in Japan, 1951–1990. *Acta Genet Med Gemellol (Roma)* 1992;41:165–75.

26. Vaksmann S, Bouchart P, Patey-Savatier P, Maunoury-Lefebvre C, Vinatier D, Monnier JC. Multiple pregnancies. II. Epidemiology, clinical aspects. *J Gynecol Obstet Biol Reprod Paris* 1990;19:383–94.

27. Parazzini F, Tozzi L, Mezzanotte G, Bocciolone L, La Vecchia C, Fedele L, *et al.* Trends in multiple births in Italy: 1955–1983. *Br J Obstet Gynaecol* 1991;98:535–9.

28. Millar WJ, Wadhera S, Nimrod C. Multiple births: trends and patterns in Canada, 1974–1990. *Health Rep* 1992;4:223–50.

29. Parazzini F, Villa A, Moroni S, Tozzi L, Restelli S. The epidemiology of multiple pregnancies. *Acta Genet Med Gemellol (Roma)* 1994;43:17–23.

30. Mushinski M. Trends in multiple births. *Stat Bull Metrop Insur Co* 1994;75: 28–35.

31. Luke B, Keith LG. The contribution of singletons, twins and triplets to low birth weight, infant mortality and handicap in the United States. *J Reprod Med* 1992;37:661–6.

32. Powers WF, Kiely JL. The risks confronting twins: a national perspective. *Am J Obstet Gynecol* 1994;170:456–61.

33. Algwiser A, Al Sultan S, Mesleh RA, Ayoub H. Twin pregnancies: incidence and outcome – Riyadh Armed Forces Hospital experience. *J Obstet Gynaecol* 1999;19:587–93.

34. Glinianaia SV, Pharoah P, Sturgiss SN. Comparative trends in cause-specific fetal and neonatal mortality in twin and singleton births in the North of England, 1982–1994. *BJOG* 2000;107:452–60.

35. US Department of Health. *Department of Health Statistics and Research (SR28) Annual Summaries of LHS 27/1 Returns.* United States Annual Vital Statistics Reports. Vol I. Natality. 1989. Washington: Department of Health; 1993.

36. Fowler MGF, Kleinman JC, Kiely JL, Kessel SS. Double jeopardy: twin infant mortality in the United States, 1983–1984. *Am J Obstet Gynecol* 1991;165:15–22.

37. Fleming AD, Rayburn WF, Mandsager NT, Hill WC, Levine MG, Lawler R. Perinatal outcomes of twin pregnancies at term. *J Reprod Med* 1990;35:881–5.

38. Buekens P, Wilcox A. Why do small twins have a lower mortality rate than small singletons? *Am J Obstet Gynecol* 1993;168:937–41.

39. Hecht BR. The impact of assisted reproduction technologies on the incidence of multiple gestation. In: Keith DM, Luke B, editors. *Multiple Pregnancy. Epidemiology, Gestation and Perinatal Outcome.* London: The Parthenon Publishing Group; 1995. p. 175–90.

40. Kilpatrick SJ, Jackson R, Croughan-Minihane MS. Perinatal mortality in twins and singletons matched for gestational age at delivery at > or = 30 weeks. *Am J Obstet Gynecol* 1996;174:66–71.

41. Hedriana HL, Eby-Wilkens EM, Gilbert WM. Perinatal mortality and morbidity rates among singleton, twin, and triplet gestations. *Prim Care Update Ob Gyns* 1998;5:184–5.

42. Glinianaia SV, Pharoah P, Sturgiss SN. Comparative trends in cause-specific fetal and neonatal mortality in twin and singleton births in the North of England, 1982–1994. *BJOG* 2000;107:452–60.

43. Rydhstrom H. The effects of maternal age, parity and sex of the twins on twin perinatal mortality. A population based study. *Acta Genet Med Gemellol (Roma)* 1990;39:401–8.

44. Derom R, Derom C, Vlietinck R. Placentation. In: Keith LG, Papiernik E, Keith DM, Luke B, editors. *Multiple Pregnancy.* London: Parthenon Press; 1995. p. 113–28.

45. Machin G, Bamforth F, Innes M, Minichul K. Some perinatal characteristics of monozygotic twins who are dichorionic. *Am J Med Genet* 1995;55:71–6.

46. Ward RH, Whittle M, editors. *Multiple Pregnancy.* London: RCOG; 1995.

47. MacGillivray I, Campbell DM. The changing pattern of cerebral palsy in Avon. *Paediatr Perinat Epidemiol* 1995;9:146–55.

48. Touyama M, Ochiai Y, Touyama J. Cerebral palsy in twins in Okinawa. *No To Hattatsu* 2000;32:35–8.

49. Grether JK, Nelson KB, Cummins SK. Twinning and cerebral palsy: experience in four northern California counties, births 1983 through 1985. *Pediatrics* 1993;92:854–8.

50. Williams K, Hennessy E, Alberman E. Cerebral palsy: effects of twinning, birthweight, and gestational age. *Arch Dis Child Fetal Neonatal Ed* 1996;75: F178–82.

51. Scher AI, Petterson B, Blair E, Ellenberg JH, Grether JK, Haan E, *et al.* The risk of mortality or cerebral palsy in twins: a collaborative population-based study. *Pediatr Res* 2002;52:671–81.

52. Pinborg A, Loft A, Schmidt L, Greisen G, Rasmussen S, Andersen AN. Neurological sequelae in twins born after assisted conception: controlled national cohort study. *BMJ* 2004;329:311.

53. Topp M, Huusom LD, Langhoff-Roos J, Delhumeau C, Hutton JL, Dolk H; SCPE Collaborative Group. Multiple birth and cerebral palsy in Europe: a multicenter study. *Acta Obstet Gynecol Scand* 2004;83:548–53.

54. Blickstein I. Do multiple gestations raise the risk of cerebral palsy? *Clin Perinatol* 2004;31:395–408.

55. Pharoah PO. Risk of cerebral palsy in multiple pregnancies. *Obstet Gynecol Clin North Am* 2005;32:55–67.

56. Topp M, Huusom LD, Langhoff-Roos J, Delhumeau C, Hutton JL, Dolk H; SCPE Collaborative Group. Multiple birth and cerebral palsy in Europe: a multicenter study. *Acta Obstet Gynecol Scand* 2004;83:548–53.

57. Pharoah PO, Cooke T. Cerebral palsy and multiple births. *Arch Dis Child Fetal Neonatal Ed* 1996;75:F174–7.

58. Pharoah PO, Adi Y. Consequences of in-utero death in a twin pregnancy. *Lancet* 2000;355:1597–602.

59. Pharoah PO. Twins and cerebral palsy. *Acta Paediatr Suppl* 2001;90:6–10.

60. Pharoah PO, Price TS, Plomin R. Cerebral palsy in twins: a national study. *Arch Dis Child Fetal Neonatal Ed* 2002;87:F122–4.

61. Petterson B, Nelson KB, Watson L, Stanley F. Twins, triplets, and cerebral palsy in births in Western Australia in the 1980s. *Br Med J* 1993;307:1239–43.

62. Nelson KB, Ellenberg JH. Childhood neurological disorders in twins. *Paediatr Perinat Epidemiol* 1995;9:135–45.

63. Koterazawa K, Shimogaki K, Nabetani M, Miyata H, Kodama S, Nakamura H. A study on the incidence of cerebral palsy among twins in Himeji City. *No To Hattatsu* 1998;30:20–3.

64. Burguet A, Monnet E, Pauchard JY, Roth P, Fromentin C, Dalphin ML, *et al.* Some risk factors for cerebral palsy in very premature infants: importance of premature rupture of membranes and monochorionic twin placentation. *Biol Neonate* 1999;75:177–86.

65. Gilbert-Barness E, editor. *Potter's Pathology of the Fetus and Infant.* St Louis: Mosby; 1997.

66. Hall JG. Twinning: mechanisms and genetic implications. *Curr Opin Genet Dev* 1996;6:343–7.

67. Boklage CE. On the timing of monozygotic twinning events. *Prog Clin Biol Res* 1981;69:155–65.

68. Storrs EE, Williams RJ. A study of monozygous quadruplet armadillos in relation to mammalian inheritance. *Proc Natl Acad Sci USA* 1968;60:910–14.

69. Solter D. Differential imprinting and expression of maternal and paternal genomes. *Annu Rev Genet* 1988;22:127–64.

70. Hall JG. Genomic imprinting: review and relevance to human diseases. *Am J Hum Genet* 1990;46:857–73.

71. De Robertis EM, Oliver G, Wright CV. Homeobox genes and the vertebrate body plan. *Sci Am* 1990;263:46–52.

72. Cote GB, Gyftodimou J. Twinning and mitotic crossing over: some possibilities and their implications. *Am J Hum Genet* 1991;49:120–30.

73. Winchester B, Young E, Geddes S, Genet S, Hurst J, Middleton-Price H, *et al.* Female twin with Hunter disease due to non-random inactivation of the X-chromosome: a consequence of twinning. *Am J Med Genet* 1992;4:834–8.

74. Segreti WO, Winter PM, Nance WE. Familial studies in monozygotic twinning. *Prog Clin Biol Res* 1978;24 Pt B:55–60.

75. Burn J, Corney G. Zygosity determination and the types of twinning. In: MacGillivray I, Campbell DM, Thompson B, editors. *Twinning and Twins.* Chichester: John Wiley; 1988. p. 7–25.

76. Mettler L, Riedel HH, Grillo M, Michelmann HW, Baukloh V, Weisner D, *et al.* Pregnancy and birth of monozygous female twins following *in vitro* fertilization and embryo transfer. *Geburtshilfe Frauenheilkd* 1984;44:670–6.

77. Edwards RG, Mettler L, Walters DE. Identical twins and *in vitro* fertilization. *J In Vitro Fert Embryo Transf* 1986;3:114–17.

78. Derom C, Vlietinck R, Derom R, Van Den Berghe H, Thiery M. Increased monozygotic twinning rate after ovulation induction. *Lancet* 1987;1:1236–8.

79. Murphy M, Seagroatt V. Twin peaks, extramarital conceptions, and virgin births: is there a connection? *Arch Dis Child* 1992;67:189–91.

80. Alikani M, Noyes N, Cohen J, Rosenwaks Z. Monozygotic twinning in the human is associated with the zona pellucida architecture. *Hum Reprod* 1994;9:1318–21.

81. Benirschke K, Kim CK. Multiple pregnancy. *N Eng J Med* 1973;288:1276–84.

82. Hrubec Z, Robinette D. The study of human twins in medical research *N Engl J Med* 1984;310:435–41.

83. Derom R, Orlebeke J, Eriksson A, Thiery M. The epidemiology of multiple births in Europe. In: Keith LG, Papiernik E, Keith DM, Luke B, editors. *Multiple Pregnancy*. London: Parthenon Press; 1995. p. 129–38.

84. Baldwin VJ. *Pathology of Multiple Pregnancy*. New York: Springer-Verlag; 1994.

85. Benirschke K. Twin placenta in perinatal mortality. *N Y St J Med* 1961;61:1499–508.

86. Arts NFT, Lohman AHM. The vascular anatomy of monochorionic diamniotic twin placentas and the transfusion syndrome. *Eur J Obstet Gynecol* 1971;3:85–93.

87. Sekiya S, Hafez ESE. Physiomorphology of twin transfusion syndrome. A study of 86 twin gestations. *Obstet Gynecol* 1977;50:288–92.

88. Galea P, Scott JM, Goel KM. Feto-fetal transfusion syndrome. *Arch Dis Child* 1982;57:781–94.

89. Machin GA, Still K. The twin–twin transfusion syndrome: vascular anatomy of monochorionic placentas and their clinical outcomes. In: Keith LG, Papiernik E, Keith M, Luke B, editors. *Multiple Pregnancy*. London: Parthenon Press; 1995. p. 367–93.

90. Sebire NJ, Souka A, Skentou H, Geerts L, Nicolaides KH. Early prediction of severe twin-to-twin transfusion syndrome. *Hum Reprod* 2000;15:2008–10.

91. Saunders NJ, Snijders RJM, Nicolaides KH. Therapeutic amniocentesis in twin–twin transfusion syndrome appearing in the second trimester of pregnancy. *Am J Obstet Gynecol* 1992;166:820–4.

92. Saunders NJ, Snijders RJM, Nicolaides KH. Twin–twin transfusion syndrome in the second trimester is associated with small inter-twin hemoglobin differences. *Fetal Diagn Ther* 1991;6:34–6.

93. Rosen D, Rabinowitz R, Beyth Y, Feijgin MD, Nicolaides KH. Fetal urine production in normal twins and in twins with acute polyhydramnios. *Fetal Diagn Ther* 1990;5:57–60.

94. Karatza AA, Wolfenden JL, Taylor MJ, Wee L, Fisk NM, Gardiner HM. Influence of twin–twin transfusion syndrome on fetal cardiovascular structure and function: prospective case–control study of 136 monochorionic twin pregnancies. *Heart* 2002;88:271–7.

95. Baldwin VJ. Anomalies of monozygotic duplication. In: Baldwin VJ, editor. *Pathology of Multiple Pregnancy*. New York: Springer-Verlag; 1994. p. 277–348.

96. Murphy KW. Intrauterine death in a twin: implications for the survivor. In: Ward RH, Whittle M, editors. *Multiple Pregnancy*. London: RCOG; 1995. p. 218–30.

97. Liu S, Benirschke K, Scioscia AL, Mannino FL. Intrauterine death in multiple gestation. *Acta Genet Med Gemellol (Roma)* 1992;41:5–26.

98. Jung JH, Graham JM Jr, Schultz N, Smith DW. Congenital hydranencephaly/porencephaly due to vascular disruption in monozygotic twins. *Pediatrics* 1984;73:467–9.

99. Cragan JD, Martin ML, Waters GD, Khoury MJ. Increased risk of small intestinal atresia among twins in the United States. *Arch Pediatr Adolesc Med* 1994;148:733–9.

100. Ferguson WF. Perinatal mortality in multiple gestations. A review of perinatal deaths from 1,609 multiple gestations. *Obstet Gynecol* 1964;23:861–70.

101. Hay S, Wehrung DA. Congenital malformations in twins. *Am J Hum Genet* 1970;22:662–78.

102. Onyskowova Z, Dolezal A, Jedlicka V. The frequency and the character of malformations in multiple births. *Acta Univ Carol* 1970;16:333–76.

103. Myrianthopoulos NC. Congenital malformations in twins: epidemiologic survey. *Birth Defects* 1975;11:1–39.

104. Cameron AH, Edwards JH, Derom R, Thiery M, Boelaert R. The value of twin surveys in the study of malformations. *Eur J Obstet Gynecol Reprod Biol* 1983;14:347–56.

105. Kallen B. Congenital malformations in twins: a population study. *Acta Genet Med Gemellol (Roma)* 1986;35:167–78.

106. Little J, Nevin NC. Congenital abnormalities in twins in Northern Ireland. II: Neural tube defects, 1974–79. *Acta Genet Med Gemellol (Roma)* 1989;38:17–25.

107. Little J, Nevin NC. Congenital abnormalities in twins in Northern Ireland. III: Anomalies of the cardiovascular system, 1974–78. *Acta Genet Med Gemellol (Roma)* 1989;38:27–35.

108. Little J, Nevin NC. Congenital abnormalities in twins in Northern Ireland. I: Anomalies in general and specific anomalies other than neural tube defects, 1974–79. *Acta Genet Med Gemellol (Roma)* 1989;38:1–16.

109. Fowler MGF, Kleinman JC, Kiely JL, Kessel SS. Double jeopardy: twin infant mortality in the United States, 1983–1984. *Am J Obstet Gynecol* 1991;165:15–22.

110. Imaizumi Y, Yamamura H, Nishikawa M, Matsuoka M, Moriyama I. The prevalence at birth of congenital malformations at a maternity hospital in Osaka City, 1948–1990. *Jinrui Idengaku Zasshi* 1991;36:275–87.

111. Ramos-Arroyo MA. Birth defects in twins: study in a Spanish population. *Acta Genet Med Gemellol (Roma)* 1991;40:337–44.

112. Kleinman JC, Fowler MG, Kessel SS. Comparison of infant mortality among twins and singletons: United States 1960 and 1983. *Am J Epidemiol* 1991;133:133–43.

113. Windham GC, Bjerkedal T. Malformations in twins and their siblings, Norway, 1967–79. *Acta Genet Med Gemellol (Roma)* 1984;33:87–95.

114. Doyle PE, Beral V, Botting B, Wale CJ. Congenital malformations in twins in England and Wales. *J Epidemiol Comm Health* 1991;45:43–8.

115. Jacquemyn Y, Martens G, Ruyssinck G, Michiels I, Van Overmeire B. A matched cohort comparison of the outcome of twin versus singleton pregnancies in Flanders, Belgium. *Twin Res* 2003;6:7–11.

116. Li SJ, Ford N, Meister K, Bodurtha J. Increased risk of birth defects among children from multiple births. *Birth Defects Res A Clin Mol Teratol* 2003;67:879–85.

117. Rizk B, Doyle P, Tan SL, Rainsbury P, Betts J, Brinsden P, et al. Perinatal outcome and congenital malformations in in-vitro fertilization babies. *Hum Reprod* 1991;6:1259–64.

118. Wennerholm UB, Bergh C, Hamberger L, Lundin K, Nilsson L, Wikland M, et al. Incidence of congenital malformations in children born after ICSI. *Hum Reprod* 2000;15:944–8.

119. Pinborg A, Loft A, Rasmussen S, Schmidt L, Langhoff-Roos J, Greisen G, Andersen AN. Neonatal outcome in a Danish national cohort of 3438 IVF/ICSI and 10,362 non-IVF/ICSI twins born between 1995 and 2000. *Hum Reprod* 2004;19:435–41.

120. Layde PM, Erickson JD, Falek A, McCarthy BJ. Congenital malformation in twins. *Am J Hum Genet* 1980;32:69–78.

121. Windham GC, Bjerkedal T. Malformations in twins and their siblings, Norway, 1967–79. *Acta Genet Med Gemellol (Roma)* 1984;33:87–95.

122. Campana MA, Roubicek MM. Maternal and neonatal variables in twins: an epidemiological approach. *Acta Genet Med Gemellol (Roma)* 1996;45:461–9.

123. Corney G, MacGillivray I, Campbell DM, Thompson B, Little J. Congenital anomalies in twins in Aberdeen and Northeast Scotland. *Acta Genet Med Gemellol (Roma)* 1983;32:31–5.

124. Hay S, Wehrung DA. Congenital malformations in twins. *Am J Hum Genet* 1970;22:662–78.

125. Onyskowova Z, Dolezal A, Jedlicka V. The frequency and the character of malformations in multiple births. *Acta Univ Carol* 1970;16:333–76.

126. Malone FD, Craigo SD, Chelmow D, D'Alton ME. Outcome of twin gestations complicated by a single anomalous fetus. *Obstet Gynecol* 1996;88:1–5.

127. Clayton-Smith J, Read AP, Donnai D. Monozygotic twinning and Wiedemann–Beckwith syndrome. *Am J Med Genet* 1992;42:633–7.

128. Garabedian BH, Fraser FC. A familial association between twinning and upper neural tube defects. *Am J Hum Genet* 1994;55:1050–3.

129. Hay S, Wehrung DA. Congenital malformations in twins. *Am J Hum Genet* 1970;22:662–78.

130. Jamar M, Lemarchal C, Lemaire V, Koulischer L, Bours V. A low rate of trisomy 21 in twin-pregnancies: a cytogenetics retrospective study of 278 cases. *Genet Couns* 2003;14:395–400.

131. Snijders RJ, Noble P, Sebire N, Souka A, Nicolaides KH. UK multicentre project on assessment of risk of trisomy 21 by maternal age and fetal nuchal-translucency thickness at 10–14 weeks of gestation. Fetal Medicine Foundation First Trimester Screening Group. *Lancet* 1998;352:343–6.

132. Nebiolo LM, Adams WB, Miller SL, Milunsky A. Maternal serum human chorionic gonadotropin levels in twin pregnancies. *Prenat Diagn* 1991;11:463–6.

133. Wald N, Cuckle H, Wu TS, George L. Maternal serum unconjugated oestriol and human chorionic gonadotrophin levels in twin pregnancies: implications for screening for Down's syndrome. *Br J Obstet Gynaecol* 1991;98:905–8.

134. Wald NJ, Densem JW. Maternal serum free beta-human chorionic gonadotrophin levels in twin pregnancies: implications for screening for Down's syndrome. *Prenat Diagn* 1994;14:319–20.

135. Wald NJ, Densem JW. Maternal serum free alpha-human chorionic gonadotrophin levels in twin pregnancies: implications for screening for Down's syndrome. *Prenat Diagn* 1994;14:717–9.

136. Watt HC, Wald NJ, George L. Maternal serum inhibin-A levels in twin pregnancies: implications for screening for Down's syndrome. *Prenat Diagn* 1996;16:927–9.

137. Spencer K, Salonen R, Muller F. Down's syndrome screening in multiple pregnancies using alpha-fetoprotein and free beta hCG. *Prenat Diagn* 1994;14:537–42.

138. Neveux LM, Palomaki GE, Knight GJ, Haddow JE. Multiple marker screening for Down syndrome in twin pregnancies. *Prenat Diagn* 1996;16:29–34.

139. Spencer K, Nicolaides KH. Screening for trisomy 21 in twins using first trimester ultrasound and maternal serum biochemistry in a one-stop clinic: a review of three years experience. *BJOG* 2003;110:276–80.

140. Sebire NJ, Noble PL, Odibo A, Malligiannis P, Nicolaides KH. Single uterine entry for genetic amniocentesis in twin pregnancies. *Ultrasound Obstet Gynecol* 1996;7:26–31.

141. Brambati B, Tului L, Baldi M, Guercilena S. Genetic analysis prior to selective fetal reduction in multiple pregnancies: technical aspects and clinical outcome. *Hum Reprod* 1995;10:818–25.

142. Sebire NJ, Sepulveda W, Hughes KS, Noble P, Nicolaides KH. Management of twin pregnancies discordant for anencephaly. *Br J Obstet Gynaecol* 1997;104:216–19.

143. Nassar AH, Adra AM, Gomez-Marin O, O'Sullivan MJ. Perinatal outcome of twin pregnancies with one structurally affected fetus: a case–control study. *J Perinatol* 2000;20:82–6.

144. Sebire NJ, Foskett M, Paradinas FJ, Fisher RA, Francis RJ, Short D, *et al.* Outcome of twin pregnancies with complete hydatidiform mole and healthy co-twin. *Lancet* 2002; 359: 2165–6.

145. Lumme RH, Saarikoski SV. Monoamniotic twin pregnancy. *Acta Genet Med Gemellol(Roma)* 1986;35:99–105.

146. Blane CE, Dipietro MA, Johnson MZ, White SJ, Louwsma GI, Hamman JE. Sonographic detection of monoamniotic twins. *J Clin Ultrasound* 1987;15:394–6.

147. Carr SR, Aronson MP, Coustan DR. Survival rates of monoamniotic twins do not decrease after 30 weeks' gestation. *Am J Obstet Gynecol* 1990;163:719–22.

148. Sebire NJ, Souka A, Skentou H, Geerts L, Nicolaides KH. First trimester diagnosis of monoamniotic twin pregnancies. *Ultrasound Obstet Gynecol* 2000;16:223–5.

149. Demaria F, Goffinet F, Kayem G, Tsatsaris V, Hessabi M, Cabrol D. Monoamniotic twin pregnancies: antenatal management and perinatal results of 19 consecutive cases. *BJOG* 2004;111:22–6.

150. Bajoria R. Abundant vascular anastomoses in monoamniotic versus diamniotic monochorionic placentas. *Am J Obstet Gynecol* 1998;179:788–93.

151. Rodis JF, McIlveen PF, Egan JF, Borgida AF, Turner GW, Campbell WA. Monoamniotic twins: improved perinatal survival with accurate prenatal diagnosis and antenatal fetal surveillance. *Am J Obstet Gynecol* 1997;177:1046–9.

152. Townsend RR, Filly RA. Sonography of nonconjoined monoamniotic twin pregnancies. *J Ultrasound Med* 1988;7:665–70.

153. Swain FM. A case of knotted cords in a monoamniotic twin pregnancy. *Am J Obstet Gynecol* 1954;68:720–1.

154. Librach S, Terrin AJ. Monoamniotic twin pregnancy with report of three cases of double survival, one of them with knotted cords. *Am J Obstet Gynecol* 1957;74:440–3.

155. Nyberg DA, Filly RA, Golbus MS, Stephens JD. Entangled umbilical cords: a sign of monoamniotic twins. *J Ultrasound Med* 1984;3:29–32.

156. Bhakthavathsalan A, Heinz L, Wafalosky J, Armstrong CL, Kirkhope TG. Ultrasound diagnosis of monoamniotic twins with cord entanglement: case report with double survival. *J Clin Ultrasound* 1985;13:137–40.

157. Lyndrup J, Schouenborg L. Cord entanglement in monoamniotic twin pregnancies. *Eur J Obstet Gynecol Reprod Biol* 1987;26:275–8.

158. Hod M, Merlob P, Friedman S, Ovadia J. Single intrauterine fetal death in monoamniotic twins due to cord entanglement. *Clin Exp Obstet Gynecol* 1988;15:63–5.

159. Annan B, Hutson RC. Double survival despite cord entwinement in monoamniotic twins. Case report. *Br J Obstet Gynaecol* 1990;97:950–1.

160. Ritossa M, O'Loughlin J. Monoamniotic twin pregnancy and cord entanglement: a clinical dilemma. *Aust N Z J Obstet Gynaecol* 1996;36:309–12.

161. Bhattacharyya A, Jones AB. Spontaneous vaginal delivery of monoamniotic twin pregnancy despite extensive cord entanglement. *J Obstet Gynaecol* 1998;18:283.

162. Sau AK, Neales K. Double survival despite cord intertwining in monoamniotic twins. *Acta Obstet Gynecol Scand* 2001;80:974–5.

163. Kantanka KS, Buchmann EJ. Vaginal delivery of monoamniotic twins with umbilical cord entanglement. A case report. *J Reprod Med* 2001;46:275–7.

164. Suzuki S, Kaneko K, Shin S, Araki T. Incidence of intrauterine complications in monoamniotic twin gestation. *Arch Gynecol Obstet* 2001;265:57–9.

165. Umur A, van Gemert MJ, Nikkels PG. Monoamniotic- versus diamniotic-monochorionic twin placentas: anastomoses and twin–twin transfusion syndrome. *Am J Obstet Gynecol* 2003;189:1325–9.

166. Aisenbrey GA, Catanzarite VA, Hurley TJ, Spiegel JH, Schrimmer DB, Mendoza A. Monoamniotic and pseudomonoamniotic twins: sonographic diagnosis, detection of cord entanglement, and obstetric management. *Obstet Gynecol* 1995;86:218–22.

167. Beasley E, Megerian G, Gerson A, Roberts NS. Monoamniotic twins: case series and proposal for antenatal management. *Obstet Gynecol* 1999;93:130–4.

168. Allen VM, Windrim R, Barrett J, Ohlsson A. Management of monoamniotic twin pregnancies: a case series and systematic review of the literature. *BJOG* 2001;108:931–6.

169. Sau AK, Langford K, Elliott C, Su LL, Maxwell DJ. Monoamniotic twins: what should be the optimal antenatal management? *Twin Res* 2003;6:270–4.

170. Roque H, Gillen-Goldstein J, Funai E, Young BK, Lockwood CJ. Perinatal outcomes in monoamniotic gestations. *J Matern Fetal Neonatal Med* 2003;13:414–21.

171. Heyborne KD, Porreco RP, Garite TJ, Phair K, Abril D. Improved perinatal survival of monoamniotic twins with intensive inpatient monitoring. *Am J Obstet Gynecol* 2005;192:96–101.

172. Mauer SM, Dobrin RS, Vernier RL. Unilateral and bilateral renal agenesis in monoamniotic twins. *J Pediatr* 1974;84:236–8.

173. McNamara MF, McCurdy CM, Reed KL, Philipps AF, Seeds JW. The relation between pulmonary hypoplasia and amniotic fluid volume: lessons learned from discordant urinary tract anomalies in monoamniotic twins. *Obstet Gynecol* 1995;85:867–9.

174. Cilento BG Jr, Benacerraf BR, Mandell J. Prenatal and postnatal findings in monochorionic, monoamniotic twins discordant for bilateral renal agenesis–dysgenesis (perinatal lethal renal disease). *J Urol* 1994;151:1034–5.

175. Klinger G, Merlob P, Aloni D, Maayan A, Sirota L. Normal pulmonary function in a monoamniotic twin discordant for bilateral renal agenesis: report and review. *Am J Med Genet* 1997;73:76–9.

176. Perez-Brayfield MR, Kirsch AJ, Smith EA. Monoamniotic twin discordant for bilateral renal agenesis with normal pulmonary function. *Urology* 2004;64:589.

177. Belfort MA, Moise KJ Jr, Kirshon B, Saade G. The use of color flow Doppler ultrasonography to diagnose umbilical cord entanglement in monoamniotic twin gestations. *Am J Obstet Gynecol* 1993;168:601–4.

178. Abuhamad AZ, Mari G, Copel JA, Cantwell CJ, Evans AT. Umbilical artery flow velocity waveforms in monoamniotic twins with cord entanglement. *Obstet Gynecol* 1995;86:674–7.

179. Shahabi S, Donner C, Wallond J, Schlikker I, Avni EF, Rodesch F. Monoamniotic twin cord entanglement. A case report with color flow Doppler ultrasonography for antenatal diagnosis. *J Reprod Med* 1997;42:740–2.

180. Arabin B, Laurini RN, van Eyck J. Early prenatal diagnosis of cord entanglement in monoamniotic multiple pregnancies. *Ultrasound Obstet Gynecol* 1999;13:181–6.

181. Overton TG, Denbow ML, Duncan KR, Fisk NM. First-trimester cord entanglement in monoamniotic twins. *Ultrasound Obstet Gynecol* 1999;13:140–2.

182. Rosemond RL, Hinds NE. Persistent abnormal umbilical cord Doppler velocimetry in a monoamniotic twin with cord entanglement. *J Ultrasound Med* 1998;17:337–8.

183. Suzuki S, Ishikawa G, Sawa R, Yoneyama Y, Asakura H, Araki T. Umbilical venous pulsation indicating tight cord entanglement in monoamniotic twin pregnancy. *J Ultrasound Med* 1999;18:425–7.

184. Tongsong T, Chanprapaph P. Picture of the month. Evolution of umbilical cord entanglement in monoamniotic twins. *Ultrasound Obstet Gynecol* 1999;14:75–7.

185. Sherer DM, Sokolovski M, Haratz-Rubinstein N. Diagnosis of umbilical cord entanglement of monoamniotic twins by first-trimester color Doppler imaging. *J Ultrasound Med* 2002;21:1307–9.

186. Vayssiere C, Plumere C, Gasser B, Neumann M, Favre R, Nisand I. Diagnosing umbilical cord entanglement in monoamniotic twins: becoming easier and probably essential. *Ultrasound Obstet Gynecol* 2004;24:587–9.

187. Faber R, Stepan H. Umbilical cord entanglement in monoamniotic twins. *Ultrasound Obstet Gynecol* 2004;24:592–3.

188. Su LL. Monoamniotic twins: diagnosis and management. *Acta Obstet Gynecol Scand* 2002;81:995–1000.

189. Peek MJ, McCarthy A, Kyle P, Sepulveda W, Fisk NM. Medical amnioreduction with sulindac to reduce cord complications in monoamniotic twins. *Am J Obstet Gynecol* 1997;176:334–6.

190. The International Clearinghouse for Birth Defects Monitoring Systems. Conjoined twins – an epidemiological study based on 312 cases. The International Clearinghouse for Birth Defects Monitoring Systems. *Acta Genet Med Gemellol (Roma)* 1991;40:325–35.

191. Castilla EE, Lopez-Camelo JS, Orioli IM, Sanchez O, Paz JE. The epidemiology of conjoined twins in Latin America. *Acta Genet Med Gemellol (Roma)* 1988;37:111–18.

192. Imaizumi Y. Conjoined twins in Japan, 1979–1985. *Acta Genet Med Gemellol (Roma)* 1988;37:339–45.

193. Edmonds LD, Layde PM. Conjoined twins in the United States, 1970–1977. *Teratology* 1982;25:301–8.

194. Kallen B, Rybo G. Conjoined twinning in Sweden. *Acta Obstet Gynecol Scand* 1978;57:257–9.

195. Spencer R. Conjoined twins: theoretical embryologic basis. *Teratology* 1992;45:591–602.

196. Spencer R. Theoretical and analytical embryology of conjoined twins. Part I. Embryogenesis. *Clin Anat* 2000;13:36–53.

197. Spencer R. Anatomic description of conjoined twins: a plea for standardized terminology. *J Pediatr Surg* 1996;31:941–4.

198. Machin GA. Conjoined twins: implications for blastogenesis. *Birth Defects Orig Artic Ser* 1993;29:141–79.

199. Cohen HL, Shapiro ML, Haller JO, Schwartz D. The multivessel umbilical cord: an antenatal indicator of possible conjoined twinning. *J Clin Ultrasound* 1992;20:278–82.

200. Weston PJ, Ives EJ, Honore RL, Lees GM, Sinclair DB, Schiff D. Monochorionic diamniotic minimally conjoined twins: a case report. *Am J Med Genet* 1990;37:558–61.

201. Kapur RP, Jack RM, Siebert JR. Diamniotic placentation associated with omphalopagus conjoined twins: implications for a contemporary model of conjoined twinning. *Am J Med Genet* 1994;52:188–95.

202. Metneki J, Czeizel A. Conjoined twins in Hungary, 1970–1986. *Acta Genet Med Gemellol (Roma)* 1989;38:285–99.

203. Seo JW, Shin SS, Chi JG. Cardiovascular system in conjoined twins: an analysis of 14 Korean cases. *Teratology* 1985;32:151–61.

204. Gerlis LM, Seo JW, Ho SY, Chi JG. Morphology of the cardiovascular system in conjoined twins: spatial and sequential segmental arrangements in 36 cases. *Teratology* 1993;47:91–108.

205. Gilbert-Barness E, Debich-Spicer D, Opitz JM. Conjoined twins: morphogenesis of the heart and a review. *Am J Med Genet* 2003;120:568–82.

206. Mackenzie TC, Crombleholme TM, Johnson MP, Schnaufer L, Flake AW, Hedrick HL, *et al.* The natural history of prenatally diagnosed conjoined twins. *J Pediatr Surg* 2002;37:303–9.

207. Greening DG. Vaginal delivery of conjoined twins. *Med J Aust* 1981;2:356–60.

208. Sakala EP. Obstetric management of conjoined twins. *Obstet Gynecol* 1986;67:21S–5S.

209. Agarwal U, Dahiya P, Khosla A. Vaginal birth of conjoined thoracopagus – a rare event. *Arch Gynecol Obstet* 2003;269:66–7.

210. Harma M, Harma M, Mil Z, Oksuzler C. Vaginal delivery of dicephalic parapagus conjoined twins: case report and literature review. *Tohoku J Exp Med* 2005;205:179–85.

211. Harper RG, Kenigsberg K, Sia CG, Horn D, Stern D, Bongiovi V. Xiphopagus conjoined twins: a 300-year review of the obstetric, morphopathologic, neonatal, and surgical parameters. *Am J Obstet Gynecol* 1980;137:617–29.

212. Aiyedun TA. The conjoined twins of Gusau, Nigeria. *West Afr J Med* 2002;21:256–7.

213. Gore RM, Filly RA, Parer JT. Sonographic antepartum diagnosis of conjoined twins. Its impact on obstetric management. *JAMA* 1982;247:3351–3.

214. Chatterjee MS, Weiss RR, Verma UL, Tejani NA, Macri J. Prenatal diagnosis of conjoined twins. *Prenat Diagn* 1983;3:357–61.

215. Chen HY, Hsieh FJ, Huang LH. Prenatal diagnosis of conjoined twins by real-time sonography: a case report. *J Clin Ultrasound* 1983;11:94–6.

216. Koontz WL, Herbert WN, Seeds JW, Cefalo RC. Ultrasonography in the antepartum diagnosis of conjoined twins. A report of two cases. *J Reprod Med* 1983;28:627–30.

217. Siegfried MS, Koptik GF. Prenatal sonographic diagnosis of conjoined twins. *Postgrad Med* 1983;73:317–19.

218. Fitzgerald EJ, Toi A, Cochlin DL. Conjoined twins. Antenatal ultrasound diagnosis and a review of the literature. *Br J Radiol* 1985;58:1053–6.

219. Maggio M, Callan NA, Hamod KA, Sanders RC. The first-trimester ultrasonographic diagnosis of conjoined twins. *Am J Obstet Gynecol* 1985;152:833.

220. Kalchbrenner M, Weiner S, Templeton J, Losure TA. Prenatal ultrasound diagnosis of thoracopagus conjoined twins. *J Clin Ultrasound* 1987;15:59–63.

221. Quiroz VH, Sepulveda WH, Mercado M, Bermudez R, Fernandez R, Varela J. Prenatal ultrasonographic diagnosis of thoracopagus conjoined twins. *J Perinat Med* 1989;17:297–303.

222. Dev V, Pothineni RB, Rohatgi M, Shrivastava S. Echo-Doppler assessment of cardiac status in conjoined (thoraco-omphalopagus) twins. *Pediatr Cardiol* 1990;11:91–2.

223. Barth RA, Filly RA, Goldberg JD, Moore P, Silverman NH. Conjoined twins: prenatal diagnosis and assessment of associated malformations. *Radiology* 1990;177:201–7.

224. Karsdorp VH, van der Linden JC, Sobotka-Plojhar MA, Prins H, van der Harten JJ, van Vugt JM. Ultrasonographic prenatal diagnosis of conjoined thoracopagus twins: a case report. *Eur J Obstet Gynecol Reprod Biol* 1991;39:157–61.

225. Monni G, Useli C, Ibba RM, Lai R, Olla G, Cao A. Early antenatal sonographic diagnosis of conjoined syncephalus–craniothoraco–omphalopagus twins. Case report. *J Perinat Med* 1991;19:489–92.

226. Hubinont C, Kollmann P, Malvaux V, Donnez J, Bernard P. First-trimester diagnosis of conjoined twins. *Fetal Diagn Ther* 1997;12:185–7.

227. Hill LM. The sonographic detection of early first-trimester conjoined twins. *Prenat Diagn* 1997;17:961–3.

228. Bonilla-Musoles F, Raga F, Bonilla F Jr, Blanes J, Osborne NG. Early diagnosis of conjoined twins using two-dimensional color Doppler and three-dimensional ultrasound. *J Natl Med Assoc* 1998;90:552–6.

229. Lam YH, Sin SY, Lam C, Lee CP, Tang MH, Tse HY. Prenatal sonographic diagnosis of conjoined twins in the first trimester: two case reports. *Ultrasound Obstet Gynecol* 1998;11:289–91.

230. Maymon R, Halperin R, Weinraub Z, Herman A, Schneider D. Three-dimensional transvaginal sonography of conjoined twins at 10 weeks: a case report. *Ultrasound Obstet Gynecol* 1998;11:292–4.

231. Bega G, Wapner R, Lev-Toaff A, Kuhlman K. Diagnosis of conjoined twins at 10 weeks using three-dimensional ultrasound: a case report. *Ultrasound Obstet Gynecol* 2000;16:388–90.

232. Kuroda K, Kamei Y, Kozuma S, Kikuchi A, Fujii T, Unno N, *et al*. Prenatal evaluation of cephalopagus conjoined twins by means of three-dimensional ultrasound at 13 weeks of pregnancy. *Ultrasound Obstet Gynecol* 2000;16:264–6.

233. Sen C, Celik E, Vural A, Kepkep K. Antenatal diagnosis and prognosis of conjoined twins – a case report. *J Perinat Med* 2003;31:427–30.

234. Daskalakis G, Pilalis A, Tourikis I, Moulopoulos G, Karamoutzos I, Antsaklis A. First trimester diagnosis of dicephalus conjoined twins. *Eur J Obstet Gynecol Reprod Biol* 2004;112:110–13.

235. MacKenzie AP, Stephenson CD, Funai EF, Lee MJ, Timor-Tritsch I. Three-dimensional ultrasound to differentiate epigastric heteropagus conjoined twins from a TRAP sequence. *Am J Obstet Gynecol* 2004;191:1736–9.

236. Shimizu Y, Fukuda J, Sato W, Kumagai J, Hirano H, Tanaka T. First-trimester diagnosis of conjoined twins after in-vitro fertilization-embryo transfer (IVF-ET) at blastocyst stage. *Ultrasound Obstet Gynecol* 2004;24:208–9.

237. Fang KH, Wu JL, Yeh GP, Chou PH, Hsu JC, Hsieh CT. Ischiopagus conjoined twins at 9 weeks of gestation: three-dimensional ultrasound and power Doppler findings. *Ultrasound Obstet Gynecol*;2005:309–10.

238. Lam YH, Lee CP, Tang MH, Lau E. Thermocoagulation for selective reduction of conjoined twins at 12 weeks of gestation. *Ultrasound Obstet Gynecol* 2000;16:267–70.

239. Gans SL, Morgenstern L, Gettelman E, Zukow AH, Cooperman H. Separation of conjoined twins in the newborn period. *J Pediatr Surg* 1968;3:565–74.

240. Mestel AL, Golinko RJ, Wax SH, Steiger B, Kenin A, Filler R, *et al*. Ischiopagus tripus conjoined twins: case report of a successful separation. *Surgery* 1971;69:75–83.

241. Kling S, Johnston RJ, Michalyshyn B, Turner FW, Brownlee RT. Successful separation of xiphopagus-conjoined twins. *J Pediatr Surg* 1975;10:267–71.

242. Boles ET Jr, Vassy LE. Thoraco–omphalopagus conjoined twins: successful surgical separation. *Surgery* 1979;86:485–92.

243. Messmer BJ, Hornchen H, Kosters C. Surgical separation of conjoined (Siamese) xiphopagus twins. *Surgery* 1981;89:622–5.

244. Golladay ES, Williams GD, Seibert JJ, Dungan WT, Shenefelt R. Dicephalus dipus conjoined twins: a surgical separation and review of previously reported cases. *J Pediatr Surg* 1982;17:259–64.

245. Hung WT, Chen WJ, Chen HT, Hsu TC, Chao CC, Wu TT. Successful separation of ischiopagus tripus conjoined twins. *J Pediatr Surg* 1986;21:920–3.

246. O'Neill JA Jr, Holcomb GW III, Schnaufer L, Templeton JM Jr, Bishop HC, Ross AJ, *et al*. Surgical experience with thirteen conjoined twins. *Ann Surg* 1988;208:299–312.

247. Campbell GD, Brown SW, Anderson M, Anderson PG. Separation of conjoined twins. *Aust NZ J Surg* 1990;60:59–61.

248. Fowler CL, Pulito AR, Warf BC, Vandenbrink KD. Separation of complex pygopagus conjoined twins. *J Pediatr Surg* 1999;34:619–22.

249. Chen WJ, Lai HS, Chu SH, Lee PH, Chen MT, Chen SC, Huang SC. Separation of ischiopagus tripus conjoined twins. *J Pediatr Surg* 1994;29:1417–20.

250. Chiu CT, Hou SH, Lai HS, Lee PH, Lin FY, Chen WJ, *et al*. Separation of thoracopagus conjoined twins. A case report. *J Cardiovasc Surg* 1994;35:459–62.

251. Wirt SW, Algren CL, Wallace VR, Glass N. Separation of conjoined twins. *AORN J* 1995;62:527–5.

252. Doski JJ, Heiman HS, Solenberger RI, Stefko RM, Kuivila T, Rozanski TA, *et al*. Successful separation of ischiopagus tripus conjoined twins with comparative analysis of methods for abdominal wall closure and use of the tripus limb. *J Pediatr Surg* 1997;32:1761–6.

253. Hilfiker ML, Hart M, Holmes R, Cooper M, Kriett J, Collins D, *et al*. Expansion and division of conjoined twins. *J Pediatr Surg* 1998;33:768–70.

254. McDowell BC, Morton BE, Janik JS, Gerow RK, Handler MH, Lowenstein AD, *et al*. Separation of conjoined pygopagus twins. *Plast Reconstr Surg* 2003;111:1998–2002.

255. Spitz L, Kiely EM. Experience in the management of conjoined twins. *Br J Surg* 2002;89:1188–92.

256. Zuker RM, Filler RM, Lalla R. Intra-abdominal tissue expansion: an adjunct in the separation of conjoined twins. *J Pediatr Surg* 1986;21:1198–200.

257. Albert MC, Drummond DS, O'Neill J, Watts H. The orthopedic management of conjoined twins: a review of 13 cases and report of 4 cases. *J Pediatr Orthop* 1992;12:300–7.

258. Fieggen AG, Dunn RN, Pitcher RD, Millar AJ, Rode H, Peter JC. Ischiopagus and pygopagus conjoined twins: neurosurgical considerations. *Childs Nerv Syst* 2004;20:640–51.

259. Fieggen G, Millar A, Rode H, Ngiloi P, Andronikou S, Peter J. Spinal cord involvement in pygopagus conjoined twins: case report and review of the literature. *Childs Nerv Syst* 2003;19:183–7.

260. Hockley AD, Gornall P, Walsh R, Nishikawa H, Lam H, MacPherson L, *et al*. Management of pyopagus conjoined twins. *Childs Nerv Syst* 2004;20:635–9.

261. Hoyle RM, Thomas CG Jr. Twenty-three-year follow-up of separated ischiopagus tetrapus conjoined twins. *Ann Surg* 1989;210:673–9.

262. Holcomb GW III, Keating MA, Hollowell JG, Murphy JP, Duckett JW. Continent urinary reconstruction in ischiopagus tripus conjoined twins. *J Urol* 1989;141:100–2.

263. Hsu HS, Duckett JW, Templeton JM Jr, O'Neill JA Jr. Experience with urogenital reconstruction of ischiopagus conjoined twins. *J Urol* 1995;154:563–7.

264. Wilcox DT, Quinn FM, Spitz L, Kiely EM, Ransley PG. Urological problems in conjoined twins. *Br J Urol* 1998;81:905–10.

265. Kim SS, Waldhausen JH, Weidner BC, Grady R, Mitchell M, Sawin R. Perineal reconstruction of female conjoined twins. *J Pediatr Surg* 2002;37:1740–3.

Chapter 5
Genetic aspects of twinning

David Chitayat and Judith G Hall

Introduction

Twinning has captured our imagination for centuries and has been the source of many tales that have shaped religions and cultures.

The Bible described the twins Jacob and Esau, who were probably dizygotic (DZ) as Esau was large, had red hair and was hirsute while Jacob was smaller and with unremarkable hair colour. Their membranes ruptured at about the same time and Jacob was born clinging to his brother's heel. He was thus called Jacob, which means a follower. This story also shows that DZ twins are not only different in their genetic makeup but also in their environmental exposure. Their mother Rebekah preferred Jacob to Esau, which caused the latter to be angry and depressed.

Greek mythology used the two bright stars of Gemini to feed their imagination about the DZ twins Castor and Pollux, who were conceived by different fathers and went together to heaven. The Romans created the legend of the twins Romulus and Remus to decorate the origins of Rome.

Advances in technology have made it possible to detect twins early in gestation, including identifying the zygosity and determining complications associated with twinning early in pregnancy. Furthermore, techniques have been developed to treat, both pre- and postnatally, the malformations, disruptions and deformations associated with twinning. During the last few decades, expertise has been developed to artificially induce ovulation and fertilise eggs by intrauterine insemination (IUI), *in vitro* fertilization (IVF) and intracytoplasmic sperm injection (ICSI). This has resulted in an increased incidence of both monozygotic (MZ) and DZ twins and has opened a Pandora's box of complications, such as prematurity, associated with these fertility methods.

Most of the current health issues are complex. Chronic disorders such as diabetes mellitus, autoimmune disorders and autism appear to be caused by the interaction of genes and environment[1] and can be effectively studied by comparing DZ and MZ twins. Changes in environment during the last two centuries have apparently led to the development of disorders with an underlying genetic predisposition, and twin studies can help in detecting the genetic versus environmental origins of many of these types of disorder.[2]

Definition

In 1874, Camille Dareste was the first to report, to the Société d'Anthropologie, that there are two types of twins: monozygotic and dizygotic. MZ twins result from a zygote that splits into two separate individuals and such twins have thus been called natural clones, but this is of course not biologically accurate.

DZ twins result from two different eggs each fertilised by a different sperm derived from the same or different individuals at the same or at different times. Almost all DZ twins have the same father and thus are not different from any of their siblings. They share on average 50% of their genes, and thus can be expected to be identical at 25% of their loci.[3,4]

Incidence

Fluctuations in the incidence of twins are mainly due to variations in the incidence of DZ twins as the incidence of MZ twins has been fairly constant around the world. The incidence of MZ twins is about 1/300 and the incidence of DZ twins ranges from 1/11 in the Yoruba tribe in Nigeria, through 1/100 among Caucasians, to 1/250 in Orientals. In the 20th century there was initially a gradual decrease in the incidence of twins, associated first with urbanisation and later also with the use of oral contraceptives. In the last few decades, however, an increase in the incidence of twins has been observed and this has mainly been due to improved nutrition (including folic acid supplementation) and health, increasing maternal age and the use of assisted reproductive technology (ART) (see Chapter 1).

The incidence of DZ twinning appears to change as a result of interaction between genetic and environmental factors, while MZ twinning is an anomaly and the result of postzygotic changes in the developing embryo.

To obtain a rough population incidence of MZ versus DZ twins, Weinberg[5] proposed that since all MZ twins are of the same sex and one-half of DZ twins are also of the same sex, the number of DZ twins equals the number of non-same-sex twins multiplied by two. Thus, the number of MZ twins is the total number of twins minus the calculated number of DZ twins. However, more recently, some exceptions to this rule have been found, such as MZ twins that differ in their sex owing to sex chromosome mosaicism, e.g. 45,X/46,XY. These are rare, however, and Weinberg's theory in general holds true.

Zygosity, chorionicity and amnionicity

Zygosity refers to the type of conception, chorionicity refers to the type of placentation and amnionicity refers to the number of amniotic cavities in which the twins reside.

To define the zygosity in a specific case, researchers use the same techniques used for paternity testing. Initially, apart from the chorionicity, the only tool available was physical examination and dermatoglyphics. In the 1940s determination of the ABO blood group and serological testing for Rh, Kell and Duffy were added. In the 1970s HLA typing was added to the arsenal and in the last two decades DNA fingerprinting has been used. Chorionicity is still the most important way to determine zygosity and by definition monochorionic twins are MZ. However, several exceptions to even this rule have recently been found.

In MZ twins, approximately one-third are dichorionic-diamniotic and cannot be distinguished from DZ twins by chorionicity. These MZ twins are thought to represent division of the embryo into the two twins by day 3 (i.e. after conception but before the chorion and amnion have differentiated). In 25% of dichorionic-diamniotic MZ twins the placentas are fused and in 10% there appears to be only one placenta.[2]

Most MZ twins (70–80%) will have monochorionic placentas, which are thought to be associated with division of the embryo between days 3 and 7. About 1–2% of MZ twins will have monochorionic-monoamniotic placentas where there is no intervening membrane. In this situation, the fetuses and cords can freely intermingle and entwine. This type of MZ twins is thought to be the result of division between days 7 and 11 after conception.

Conjoined twins are believed to be the result of division of the embryo after day 14, after the primitive streak has begun to differentiate. However, how long after day 14 and by what mechanism is not clear.

Chorionicity and amnionicity can be determined by early vaginal ultrasound with an accuracy of almost 100%.[6]

Since 70–80% of MZ twins are monochorionic and have placental vascular connections, the DNA in their blood cells is likely to appear to be identical even when the twin pair is genetically or epigenetically discordant. Furthermore, several examples of DZ twins with vascular connections between their placentas are now being recognised and in at least one case the bone marrow of one twin filled the marrow of the other.[7] Thus, to determine zygosity using DNA fingerprinting, a tissue sample such as cord or skin should be obtained, rather than a blood or bone marrow sample.

Dizygotic twins

Aetiology

DZ twinning is the result of natural or artificial (via ART) hyperovulation (more than one dominant ovarian follicle maturing during the same menstrual cycle). A number of factors are known to influence the incidence of natural DZ twinning:

- **Maternal age:** The incidence of DZ twins increases with maternal age, with an annual increase of about 2.4%, and reaches a maximum at the age of 35–39 years.

- **Fecundity:** There is a higher incidence in women with higher probability of conceiving a child per cohabitation. (An increased number of children leads to increased occurrence of DZ twins.)

- **Nutrition:** Starvation decreases the incidence of DZ twins whereas improved nutrition increases the incidence. Folic acid supplementation may result in an increased incidence of DZ twins and/or their survival to birth.

- **Ethnicity:** African and African-American women have a higher incidence of DZ twins while Oriental women have a low incidence. This increased incidence in African women correlates with the levels of follicle-stimulating hormone (FSH) in the maternal blood. Thus, the high incidence of DZ twins among women from the Yoruba tribe in Nigeria (1/11) is associated with higher blood FSH levels and these women have also been found to have larger pituitary glands.

- **ART:** Increases in the incidence of DZ twins have been seen in association with the increased use of ART. However, the recent trend towards increased regulation of the number of fertilised eggs being transferred to the uterus will probably result in a decrease in the number of DZ twins associated with ART.

DZ twinning has a multifactorial mode of inheritance with an empirical recurrence, for the mothers, of four times the general population incidence. Males who are DZ twins or who fathered DZ twins do not result in an increased incidence.[8]

Abnormalities associated with DZ twinning

The incidence of congenital abnormalities in DZ twins (one or both) is twice the baseline risk for singletons and is thus 6%. The crowding associated with DZ twins, by virtue of having two babies in a space usually occupied by one, results in a slight increase in deformations (abnormal form, shape or position of part of the body caused by mechanical forces) such as head moulding, club foot, bowing of legs and dislocated hips.

Monozygotic twins

Aetiology

MZ twinning is an anomaly caused by a split of the zygote into two separate embryos. The aetiology is probably heterogeneous and is currently unknown.

Since MZ twinning is a postzygotic event, it is most probably the result of one or more postzygotic mutations in a gene and/or an abnormality in cell surface proteins, or related to the formation of the zona pellucida, which subsequently leads to the separation of two distinct cell masses. Discordance for physical findings, karyotype or single-gene disorders supports this hypothesis:

- **Single-gene disorders:** MZ twins discordant for single-gene disorders have been reported, including discordance for growth hormone deficiency, Noonan syndrome, cystic fibrosis and Van der Woude syndrome.

- **X-inactivation:** Discordance for X-linked conditions such as colour-blindness, haemophilia A and B and Lesch–Nyhan syndrome has been reported in female MZ twins. This discordance can be the result of a skewed X-inactivation for a gene inherited from the father or the mother or a new condition caused by postzygotic mutation in an X-linked gene in the sperm or egg that conceived the twins. The finding that the majority of monoamniotic MZ twins and conjoined twins are female further supports this theory.

- **Imprinting:** a defect in imprinting can result in MZ twinning. Many cases of MZ twins discordant for Beckwith–Wiedemann syndrome have been reported, particularly among females.

- **Chromosome abnormalities:** discordance for chromosome abnormalities such as 45, X, trisomy 21 trisomy 1p has been reported and may be the reason for the MZ twinning.

- **Malformations:** 10–15% of all liveborn MZ twins have abnormalities and in most of them the aetiology is not known. Most of these abnormalities are malformations (a defect in the embryological development) and may be the reason for the twinning. Furthermore, some abnormalities are more common in MZ twins (e.g. sirenomelia and cloacal anomalies). Thus, the genes or processes causing these anomalies may also be involved in the process of MZ twinning.

There is a 2–5 times increase in the incidence of MZ liveborn twins in pregnancies conceived by IVF. This could be the result of breaks in the zona pellucida caused by handling, the media used, use of ICSI, zona hardening related to ageing, the drugs used or the underlying cause of infertility.

Conjoined twins

Conjoined twins are always MZ and are the result of an incomplete twinning event. They develop past 14 days of embryonic development, since at approximately day 14 the primitive streak sets up lateralisation (assuming MZ twins follow the 'normal' human developmental schedule). They occur in about 1 in 100 000 births and, as indicated above, there is an excess of females. They are classified by the site of attachment. Many do not fit the expected attachment sites of 'normal' separation. In 10% of conjoined twins the second fetus arises from and is attached to the initial one (fetus in fetu).

Abnormalities associated with MZ twinning: disruptions, malformations and deformations

Abnormalities are detected in 10–15% of MZ twins. Some of these abnormalities are the result of disruptions (a morphological defect of an organ, part of an organ or a larger region of the body resulting from an extrinsic breakdown of, or an interference with, an initially normal developmental process). The shared chorion, in these MZ twins, contains numerous vascular interconnections that can lead to complications such as twin reversed arterial perfusion (TRAP) (see Chapter 13), twin-to-twin transfusion syndrome (TTTS) (see Chapters 11 and 12) and disruptive congenital anomalies.

Disruptions in MZ twins are likely to be caused by hypotension and decreased perfusion. Disruptions known to be associated with MZ twins include hydranencephaly, porencephaly, limb reduction defect, gastroschisis, amyoplasia and intestinal atresia.

MZ twins also have an increased incidence of malformations (a morphological defect of an organ, part of an organ or larger region of the body resulting from an intrinsically abnormal developmental process), including holoprosencephaly, cardiac abnormalities, cloacal anomalies, neural tube defects and sirenomelia.

MZ twins are also prone to deformations such as club foot, dislocated hips and cranial synostosis due to crowding, as is the case with DZ twins.

As mentioned above, it has become clear that most, if not all, MZ twins are discordant in some aspect in spite of the fact that most are very similar in appearance. In the future, we may be able to identify in MZ twins discordance for genes that express early in embryogenesis but do not cause phenotypic abnormalities.

Twin studies

Comparisons of MZ and DZ twins are often used to estimate the environmental (nurture) and heritable (nature) factors contributing to complex diseases. These studies assume that MZ twins are genetically identical and thus that any phenotypic differences between MZ twins must be caused by environmental influence. Discordance between DZ twins, on the other hand, may be caused by both genetic and environmental changes.

However, as indicated above, MZ twins can be discordant for chromosome abnormalities and single-gene disorders, as well as for imprinting disorders. They have a higher incidence of intrauterine growth restriction (IUGR), which is known to be associated with late-onset diseases such as hypertension, cardiovascular disease and diabetes mellitus in singletons. Furthermore, an increased incidence of breast cancer and testicular cancer as well as autism, has been reported in both MZ and DZ twins. Twin studies can thus produce ambiguous results.

Conclusion

In summary, human twinning, and MZ twinning in particular, is a fascinating experiment of nature that can provide important information regarding the genes involved in early embryogenesis and the intrauterine factors that affect pre- and postnatal growth and development. Documentation of zygosity pre- and postnatally is of the utmost importance in order to identify twins prone to develop complications and abnormalities. Since one-third of MZ twins are dichorionic-diamniotic and cannot be distinguished from DZ twins, DNA fingerprinting may be indicated in all same-sex apparently DZ twins. To avoid confusion caused by placental vascular connections, the DNA should be extracted from a tissue such as umbilical cord.

References

1. Mayeux R. Mapping the new frontier: complex genetic disorders. *J Clin Invest* 2005;115:1404–7.
2. Phelan M. Twins. In: Stevenson R, Hall JG, Goodman R, editors. *Human Malformations and Associated Anomalies*. Oxford: Oxford University Press; 1993. p. 1047–79.
3. Benirschke K, Kim CK. Multiple pregnancy 1. *N Engl J Med* 1973;288:1276–84.
4. Benirschke K, Kim CK. Multiple pregnancy 2. *N Engl J Med* 1973;288:1329–36.
5. Weinberg W. Beiträge zur Physiologie und der Pathologie der Mehrlingsgeburten beim Menschen. *Arch Physiol* 1902;88:346.
6. Tong S, Vollenhoven B, Meagher S. Determining zygosity in early pregnancy by ultrasound. *Ultrasound Obstet Gynecol* 2004;23:36–7.
7. Rubocki RJ, McCue BJ, Duffy KJ, Shepard KL, Shepard SJ, Wisecarver JL. Natural DNA mixtures generated in fraternal twins *in utero. J Forensic Sci* 2001;46:120–5.
8. Hall JG. Twinning. *Lancet* 2003;362:735–43.

Chapter 6

Selective reduction and termination of multiple pregnancies

Ruwan C Wimalasundera

Introduction

The incidence of multiple births in developed countries has increased dramatically since the early 1970s, with an approximate doubling of twin births and a trebling of triplet births.[1] Although the incidence of spontaneous multiple pregnancies has increased slightly,[1-3] the overall rise in multiple births is primarily due to the increasing use of assisted reproductive technologies (ART). Bergh *et al*.[4] attributed a third of the increase in multiple pregnancies in Sweden to *in vitro* fertilisation (IVF), a third to ovulation induction and a third to advancing maternal age. In the UK 46% of babies born after IVF are now from a multiple pregnancy.[5] However, many parents and physicians underestimate the negative consequences of multiple pregnancy. A triplet pregnancy has a 9.7% chance of perinatal mortality for each triplet[6] and a 7–8% chance of one or more of the triplets developing cerebral palsy.[7] There are further significant adverse obstetric, neonatal, financial, emotional and social consequences of multiple pregnancies. Although triplet pregnancies are increasingly acknowledged as a failing of ART, most iatrogenic morbidity and mortality currently result from twin pregnancies.

Management of multiple pregnancies is now a common problem for all obstetricians in their day-to-day practice. Prevention of higher order multiple pregnancies has to be the primary objective. Approaches such as ultrasound monitoring of ovulation induction and superovulation intrauterine insemination (IUI) cycles with cancellation or transfer to IVF if excessive ovulation is predicted, as well as the relatively recent restrictions on embryo transfer in IVF and intracytoplasmic sperm injection (ICSI) cycles,[8] have been shown to dramatically reduce the high order multiple birth rate without significantly reducing the pregnancy rate. However, once a high order multiple pregnancy has occurred or indeed a discordant severe fetal anomaly has been diagnosed in a fetus of a multiple pregnancy then the option of multifetal pregnancy reduction (MFPR) or selective fetal termination needs to be considered.

Multifetal pregnancy reduction

MFPR has been used over the last 15–20 years to reduce high order multiple pregnancies to twins in the late first trimester. The perinatal outcome of reduced twins has approached but not quite reached that of spontaneous twins.[9] A final number of two has become standard practice, as the perinatal outcome of twin pregnancies is considered acceptable and as two fetuses still leaves an option of selective feticide if discordant fetal abnormalities manifest later on ultrasound scans. Most groups regard MFPR as a necessary, but unpalatable, option for treating the complications of aggressive fertility therapy, rather than a humanistic approach to maximising pregnancy rates and perinatal outcome.

Expansion of the technique has been associated with a progressive fall in miscarriage rates, owing to a combination of improved ultrasound resolution and the increasing experience of the fetal medicine specialists performing the technique.[10] The procedure is performed by an intracardiac injection of strong potassium chloride solution (1.5 g in 10 mL) into the targeted fetus under ultrasound guidance using a 20 gauge needle. Because of a lower miscarriage rate (5.4% versus 12%), the transabdominal approach has almost entirely replaced the transvaginal technique.[10,11]

MFPR is performed most commonly between 11 and 14 weeks of gestation for three reasons:

- the risk of spontaneous reduction or 'vanishing twin' has by then passed[12]
- limited anomaly scans can be performed to detect gross structural anomalies and features of aneuploidy to guide selection of the fetus(es) for reduction[13]
- screening for aneuploidy using nuchal translucency (NT) can also be performed prior to MFPR, again to guide selection if the NT measurements are discordant.

Pregnancy outcome appears to be similar whether or not invasive prenatal diagnosis by chorionic villus sampling (CVS) is performed prior to fetal reduction.[14] However, CVS is considered by many to be a relative contraindication in polychorionic multiple pregnancies because of the risk of contamination. The availability of NT screening, together with the recognition that Down syndrome is comparatively rare in twins,[15] means that CVS is now rarely performed prior to MFPR.

To minimise the risk of ascending infection, if there are no structural anomalies and the NT risk of aneuploidy is low, the fetus furthest away from the cervix is normally selected for reduction.

Results of MFPR

In the most recent international registry analysis of 3513 patients undergoing MFPR prior to 24 weeks of gestation in 11 centres, the overall pregnancy loss rate was 9.6%, with 3.7% of deliveries occurring at between 25 and 28 weeks,[10] both of which are substantially better than the published outcomes for unreduced multiple pregnancies.[16–19] The likelihood of poor pregnancy outcome strongly correlated with both the starting number of fetuses and the final number after MFPR. For starting numbers of four to six fetuses, the loss rate was 12–22%, with a severe prematurity rate of 4–11%. The rates for triplets were 6% and 3%, respectively, and for twins they were 6% and 1.3%, respectively. The risk of pregnancy loss and prematurity decreased sequentially from a final number of three fetuses (20% loss, 6.5% severe prematurity), through two (9% and 4%) and one (9% and 1.6%).

Reduction of triplets to twins

Although the evidence of improved perinatal and obstetric outcomes after reduction of four or more fetuses is undisputed, whether triplets reduced to twins fare better than unreduced triplets has been somewhat controversial, with many viewing this instead as a social rather than a medical issue.

It is worth noting at this stage that the published literature on the comparison between MFPR and conservative management of triplet pregnancies is limited and that the evidence is not based on randomised studies. At best, it is based on systematic reviews and meta-analyses of smaller comparative studies of reduced and unreduced triplets and at worst on small case series. Indeed, as the decision to opt for MFPR is based on individuals' moral and religious beliefs, many would argue that it would not be ethically justified to perform a randomised study in this situation. Therefore, the recommendations on MFPR in triplets need to be considered within the context of the limited evidence on which they are based.

The literature is relatively evenly divided as to whether MFPR in triplets improves outcome compared with unreduced triplets. Evans et al.[10] maintain that triplets reduced to twins perform essentially as if they started as twins, with pregnancy loss rates (4.5%) lower than that of unreduced triplets (8.3%). In contrast, Papageorgiou et al.[20] reported a meta-analysis of studies of reduced versus unreduced triplets. In this paper they presented data suggesting that the rate of pregnancy loss prior to 24 weeks of gestation was significantly lower in unreduced triplets (3.7%) than in reduced triplets (7.8%, $P = 0.03$). However, on careful reanalysis of their data it was apparent that an error had been made in the meta-analysis of unreduced triplets. A study by Check et al.[21] that was included in the meta-analysis was reported to have had no miscarriages in 23 triplets managed expectantly. However, a review of that study showed that it had actually reported that in 6 out of 24 unreduced triplet pregnancies the whole pregnancy was lost (it is unclear whether all were before 24 weeks). If this figure is used and the meta-analysis is reanalysed, the pregnancy loss rate in the unreduced group is 5.6%, and is not significantly different from the reduced group ($P = 0.38$).

It is clear from the international registry of MFPR[10] that there is a learning curve with MFPR and that the risk of pregnancy loss falls with experience. We undertook a meta-analysis of all studies listed on Medline between 1984 and 2005 with more than 20 patients that included data on triplets reduced to twins, in order to exclude small studies with higher pregnancy loss rates related to inexperience. This was compared with comparable studies of unreduced triplets published during the same period, again with more than 20 patients, as this would suggest greater experience in managing triplets expectantly (Table 6.1). Outcome measures investigated were the pregnancy loss before 24 weeks of gestation, delivery between 24 and 28 weeks, delivery before 32 weeks, perinatal mortality rate and take-home-baby rate. Overall there were 14 studies of MFPR comprising a total of 2641 cases in which any of the above outcome measure could be derived and 17 studies of unreduced triplets comprising 1041 cases. The raw data are presented in the table and the summary data illustrated in Figure 6.1.

The pregnancy loss rate before 24 weeks of gestation for triplets reduced to twins appeared to be lower than that of unreduced triplets but was not statistically significant (5.7% versus 7.5%, odds ratio (OR) 0.74, 95% CI 0.54–1.03, $P = 0.09$). It would therefore appear that the increase in risk of miscarriage inherent in any invasive procedure is in this instance offset by the reduction in risk of miscarriage of the reduced fetal number. However, the extreme preterm delivery rate before 28 weeks was significantly lower for the reduced group (4% versus 10%, OR 0.37, 95% CI 0.24–0.57, $P < 0.0001$), as was the rate of preterm delivery before 32 weeks (9% versus 25.1%; OR 0.32, 95% CI 0.25–0.42, $P < 0.0001$) and the perinatal mortality

Table 6.1. Meta-analysis of studies listed on Medline from 1984 to 2005 with outcome measures (miscarriage before 24 weeks of gestation, delivery before 28 weeks and delivery before 32 weeks, perinatal mortality rate (PNMR) and take-home-baby rate per pregnancy (THBR)) of multifetal pregnancy reduction of triplets to twins compared with conservatively managed triplets; the data were analysed using χ^2 and are presented as odds ratios with 95% confidence intervals; $P<0.05$ was accepted as significant

	n	Miscarriage	Delivery <28 weeks	Delivery <32 weeks	PNMR[a]	THBR
Reduced triplet pregnancies						
Evans et al. (2001)[10]	1318	63				
Sebire et al. (1997)[18]	66	5		5		
Lipitz et al. (1996)[9]	43		1	8	2	
Torok et al. (1998)[47]	233		7	21		
Lipitz et al. (1994)[17]	34	3		3	0	30/34
Boulot et al. (2000)[48]	65	2	2	7	1 (7 IUD)	
Lipitz et al. (2001)[13]	95	4	1	7	1 (1 IUD)	90/95
Berkowitz et al (1996)[26]	179		4	10		
Geva et al. (2000)[49]	47	5			2 (IUD)	
Yaron et al. (1999)[16]	143	9	7			
Papageorghiou et al. (2002)[20]	133	12	13	12	26	121/133
Geipel et al. (2004)[28]	54	1	1	2		
Antsaklis et al. (2004)[23]	185	15	19	22		
Leondires et al. (2000)[58]	46	6				
Total	**2641**	**125/2186**	**36/908**	**92/982**	**56/1285**	**241/262**
Rate		**5.7%**	**4%**	**9%**	**43/1000**	**92%**
Unreduced triplet pregnancies						
Sebire et al. (1997)[18]	47	1		11		
Lipitz et al. (1994)[17]	106	22		20	11	79/106
Boulot et al. (2000)[48]	83	5	5	21	4 (11 IUD)	
Smith-Levitin et al. (1996)[50]	54		1	13		
Kadhel et al. (1998)[51]	24		1	0	3 (SB)	
Skrablin et al. (2000)[52]	52		7	7	21 (16 SB)	
Ziadeh et al. (2000)[19]	41				2 (30 SB)	
Pons et al. (1998)[53]	91		8	11	12 (9)	
Kaufman et al. (1998)[54]	55	4	5	17	4 (4 SB)	
Roest et al. (1997)[56]	19	2		1	2 (9 SB)	
Melgar et al. (1991)[11]	20				2 (5)	20/20
Leondires et al. (2000)[58]	125	4		28		
Geipel et al. (2005)[22]	51	5	9	22	30	
Abu-Heija (2003)[55]	21	15				
Barkehall-Thomas et al. (2004)[57]	57	3	8	23	13	
Papageorghiou et al. (2002)[20]	125	4	13	28	31	119/125
Antsaklis et al. (2004)[23]	70	2	25			
Total	**1041**	**56/743**	**57/571**	**228/908**	**227/2065**	**218/251**
Rate		**7.5%**	**10%**	**25.1%**	**110/1000**	**87%**
Comparison		OR 0.74 (0.54–1.03)	OR 0.37 (0.24–0.57)	OR 0.32 (0.25–0.42)	OR 0.30 (0.23–0.40)	OR 0.69 (0.39–1.20)
Reduced vs unreduced		$P=0.09$	$P<0.0001$	$P<0.0001$	$P<0.0001$	$P=0.23$

[a] The number of intrauterine deaths (IUD) or stillbirths (SB) is given in brackets; where it was not clear which, only the number is given

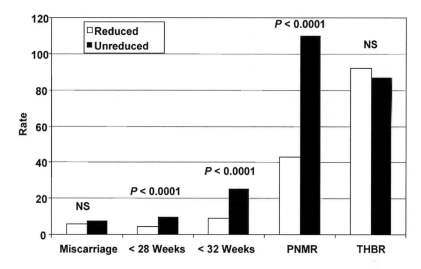

Figure 6.1. Meta-analysis of studies listed on Medline between 1984 and 2005 with outcome measures (miscarriage before 24 weeks of gestation, delivery before 28 weeks and before 32 weeks, perinatal mortality rate (PNMR) and take-home-baby rate per pregnancy (THBR)) of multifetal pregnancy reduction of triplets to twins compared with expectantly managed triplets; the data are presented as percentages (except PNMR, which is per 1000 live births) and the statistical significance of the difference in proportions between the groups was analysed using the χ^2 test, with significance being $P<0.05$

rate (43/1000 live births versus 110/1000, OR 0.30, 95% CI 0.23–0.40 $P<0.0001$) compared with unreduced triplets, although there was no significant difference in the take-home-baby rate (92% versus 87%, OR 0.69, 95% CI 0.39–1.20, $P=0.23$).

As mentioned earlier, some caution is needed given the lack of randomised studies and the retrospective nature of the mainly small series conducted in different centres over different time periods – it is clear that a randomised controlled trial could never be considered. Based on the evidence available it would appear that a reduction of triplets to twins significantly improves the perinatal outcome.

A major flaw with the published data on unreduced triplets is that many of the studies do not differentiate between trichorionic triplets and non-trichorionic (dichorionic or monochorionic) triplets where the triplet pregnancy includes a set of monochorionic (MC) twins. Whereas in the MFPR studies, triplets with an MC twin set would have been excluded as reduction to dichorionic twins using intracardiac potassium would not have been possible. It is clear that dichorionic (DC) or indeed MC triplet pregnancies are at considerably greater risk of poor outcome than trichorionic triplets. Geipel *et al.*[22] reported on 176 expectantly managed triplet pregnancies where outcome was expressed in relation to chorionicity. In this study 18.1% ($n=32$) of triplets referred to two tertiary centres in Germany were MC or DC, with 81.8% being trichorionic ($n=144$). The miscarriage rate in the non-trichorionic group (8.8%) was significantly higher than in the trichorionic group (1.5%, $P<0.01$). The premature delivery rate before 32 weeks of gestation was higher (47.4% versus 32.2%) and the overall survival was lower (84.2% versus 91.7%) in the non-trichorionic group, although these did not reach significance. It is therefore possible that the higher miscarriage rate, premature delivery rate and overall perinatal mortality rate in the unreduced triplet group in our meta-analysis is falsely high because it does not differentiate trichorionic from non-trichorionic triplets.

Despite the flaws in the meta-analysis in the report by Papageorghiou et al.,[20] it is by far the most robust analysis and presents the largest single-centre series comparing reduced with unreduced trichorionic triplets. Data are presented on 133 trichorionic triplets reduced to DC twins and compared with 125 trichorionic triplets managed expectantly in the same centre over the same time period. The data demonstrate that although the risk of miscarriage was lower in the unreduced group (3.2% versus 8.3%) it was not a significant difference ($P = 0.09$). However, the rate of preterm delivery before 32 weeks of gestation was significantly lower in the reduced group (9.0% versus 22.4%, $P = 0.005$). This is supported by a similar study by Antsaklis et al.[23] who compared 185 trichorionic triplets reduced to twins with 70 expectantly managed trichorionic pregnancies. They also demonstrated a higher miscarriage rate in the reduced group (8.1% versus 2.9%), which was again not significant, but there was a significantly lower risk of preterm delivery before 32 weeks (11% versus 37%) and low birthweight babies under 1500 g (11% versus 28%) in the reduced group compared with the unreduced group. Both these studies are consistent with our meta-analysis.

There are few data on neurological outcomes after MFPR from triplets to twins. However, if postnatal outcomes in the group reduced from triplets to twins were similar to those of unreduced twins,[9] it would suggest that MFPR to twins substantially reduces the rate of cerebral palsy. This is supported by the fact that MFPR to twins reduces the preterm delivery rate and it is established that the incidence of cerebral palsy in multiple pregnancies is primarily related to gestation at delivery.[24] Although few studies have investigated the true incidence of cerebral palsy in triplets with or without reduction, a questionnaire survey by Dimitriou et al.[25] of general practitioners of women who had delivered trichorionic triplets following expectant management or after reduction to twins suggested that there was no difference in the incidence of cerebral palsy between the two groups despite a significantly later gestation at delivery in the reduced group. This was, however, a retrospective GP survey with a response rate of less than 40% that was not powered adequately to detect a significant difference between the two groups and that did not involve any standardised neurological follow-up of the cases to confirm the diagnosis of cerebral palsy. It is clear that there is a great need for further follow-up studies to adequately ascertain whether reduction to twins has any effect on the rates of cerebral palsy as this evidence would dramatically affect any recommendations on MFPR.

It does, however, appear that even when chorionicity is taken into consideration, reducing triplets to twins does reduce the rate of preterm delivery and low birthweight babies, with probably no significant increase in the risk of miscarriage. Nevertheless, it is clear that expectant management of trichorionic triplets does still have a reasonably good perinatal outcome. It is also clear that there is a far stronger argument for MFPR in non-trichorionic triplets, although newer more advanced vascular occlusive techniques may need to be used and there is little in the way of published data on the potentially higher risks of miscarriage with these techniques.

MFPR has a significant psychological impact on the parents. Bergh et al.[4] suggested that parents' recall of events surrounding the MFPR was of 'chaos and emotional disturbance' and in one of 13 cases the mother 'regretted the decision'. In a retrospective telephone survey, Berkowitz et al.[26] found that 65% of parents recalled acute emotional pain, stress and fear, with 18% reporting feelings of guilt and anger.

There is also the ethical issue of terminating the lives of otherwise healthy fetuses in order to increase the potential for the others. Infertile couples who conceive after ART are often nulliparous and invariably anxious to have children and the ethical dilemma of a decision to undergo MFPR is thus acute, especially against the background of the emotional effort and expense of their IVF treatment. Parents therefore need to be counselled not just about the effects on perinatal outcome but also about their ethical and religious beliefs. If all life is sacred to the couple, then they should be supported in any decision to continue the triplet pregnancy. If, however, their primary concern is to reduce the complications of a triplet pregnancy, they should be counselled towards MFPR.

Reduction to singleton

A number of studies have reported on the outcomes of triplet and higher order pregnancies reduced to singleton. Papageorghiou et al.[20] suggested that, in a series of 22 trichorionic triplets reduced to a singleton, the risk of miscarriage before 24 weeks of gestation (13.6%) was higher than when trichorionic triplets were reduced to twins (8.3%) or, indeed, expectantly managed triplets, although this did not reach significance because of the power of the study. However, the risk of preterm delivery was lower when the triplets were reduced to a singleton (4.5%) then when they were reduced to twins (9%) or were expectantly managed (22.4%), and the gestation at delivery was greater (median gestation and range: singleton 38 weeks (24–40); twins 36 weeks (25–41); triplets 34 weeks (24–39)). Again, this did not reach significance. Antsaklis et al.[27] reported a smaller series ($n = 7$) but again showed a higher rate of miscarriage (one of seven, 14.3%) with a later median age at delivery (38 weeks) compared with reduction to twins (miscarriage 2.7%, median gestation at delivery 36 weeks).

The argument for reduction to a singleton in DC triplet pregnancies where there is an MC twin component, by using a simple intracardiac potassium chloride injection into the MC twins, would appear to be clearer when compared with the significantly increased risk of expectant management of DC triplets. Geipel et al.[28] reported nine cases of DC triplets where the MC twin set was reduced to a singleton. One of the nine miscarried before 24 weeks (11%), with the remaining eight singletons delivering at a mean gestation of 39 ± 1 weeks and no preterm deliveries. This compares favourably with their published data[22] on conservatively managed non-trichorionic triplets where the miscarriage rate was 10% but the preterm delivery (< 32 weeks) rate was 63%. It would therefore appear reasonable to offer women with non-trichorionic triplet pregnancies the option of reduction to a singleton using a simple technique.

Selective feticide for fetal anomaly

Selective termination for fetal anomalies, whether chromosomal or structural, differs from MFPR in terms of the usually later gestation at which anomalies are detected. In view of the increased risk of miscarriage following karyotyping in multiple pregnancies, most anomalies in multiple pregnancies are diagnosed following nuchal translucency screening at 11–13 weeks of gestation or a detailed anomaly scan at 20–22 weeks. Evans et al.[29] published the largest series from the international registry on selective termination in multiple pregnancies for structural or chromosomal anomalies. They reported that the miscarriage rate before 24 weeks was 7.1% when twins were reduced to a singleton but was as high as 13% when triplets or higher order pregnancies were reduced to twins. There also appeared to be a slight increase in the miscarriage rate with the gestation at the time of the procedure, with rates of 5.4% at 9–12 weeks, 8.7% at 13–18 weeks and 9.1% at more than 25 weeks, although these did not reach significance. The mean gestation at delivery was 35.7 weeks, with a liveborn infant in over 90% of cases.

Eddleman *et al.*[30] reported 200 cases of selective feticide from a single centre. The median gestation at procedure was 19.6 weeks. They also showed a low risk of miscarriage before 24 weeks in twins reduced to a singleton (2.4%), but a significantly higher rate (12.5%) in triplets reduced to twins. The median gestation at delivery was 37.1 weeks. These studies demonstrate that selective termination for fetal anomalies is a feasible option in any trimester.

Selective feticide/MFPR in monochorionic pregnancies

Selective feticide using intracardiac strong potassium chloride as a management option has historically not been considered feasible in MC twins because of the risk of transplacental passage of the lethal agent, as well as the high risk of agonal inter-twin transfusion at the time of fetal demise and its co-twin sequelae.

It has only been since the development of vascular occlusive techniques, which completely occlude flow through the targeted fetus's umbilical cord in order to prevent feto-fetal haemorrhage through placental anastomoses, that selective feticide has become a feasible management option in MC twin pregnancies discordant for fetal abnormalities.

A variety of techniques has been tried for occlusive feticide, with the literature supporting bipolar cord occlusion as the procedure of choice in mid-pregnancy, with the option of interstitial laser coagulation in early pregnancy, and ultrasound-guided cord ligation in the third trimester if needed.

Elective delayed feticide at, for example, 32 weeks of gestation is a recognised strategy in DC twins to avoid procedure-related loss of the healthy co-twin but it is inappropriate in MC twins. Indeed, in MC twin pregnancies it is probably preferable to perform selective feticide soon after diagnosis of the indication as this will obviate subsequent transfusional risks of the MC placentation.

Early gestation

Fetoscopically guided neodymium-doped yttrium aluminium garnet (Nd:YAG) laser coagulation of the cord or the vessels at the insertion of the cord has been used successfully in MC pregnancies between 16 and 20 weeks of gestation. A double needle loaded with a 1 mm fetoscope is inserted into the sac of the affected fetus. A 400 μm laser fibre is used to coagulate the umbilical cord under direct vision.[31] This technique has a high failure rate above 20–22 weeks of gestation, when the vessels may be too large or the cord too hydropic to allow successful coagulation.[32,33] The procedure can also be limited by poor visibility from blood-stained liquor if one of the vessels ruptures intraamniotically.

Ultrasound-guided interstitial laser can be used up to 20 weeks of gestation and overcomes the complications associated with fetoscopic laser coagulation. Our group described the technique of interstitial laser in the treatment of acardiac twins.[34] This involves a 17 gauge needle that is introduced into the fetal abdomen under continuous ultrasound guidance. Colour/power Doppler is then used to direct the

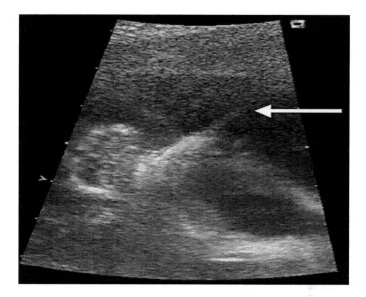

Figure 6.2.   Interstitial laser coagulation procedure in an acardiac twin; the arrow shows a 17 gauge needle inserted percutaneously through the maternal abdomen into the fetal abdomen with the laser fibre protruding just beyond the needle tip adjacent to the intrahepatic vessels

needle to the intrahepatic vein and the distal fetal aorta or intraabdominal umbilical vessels. A 400 or 600 μm laser fibre is then passed down the lumen of the needle until it is seen protruding approximately 4 mm beyond the needle tip on scan (Figure 6.2). Laser coagulation is commenced at 20 W with 10 W increments as necessary up to a maximum of 50 W. The vessels are coagulated until blood flow in the vitelline artery and intrahepatic vein is seen to stop. This technique, which has now also been used successfully by several other groups, avoids accidental cord rupture. However, it is limited by the size of the fetal vessels to be coagulated and thus the volume of flow to be stopped; its use is not recommended in appropriately sized twins after 16 weeks, although we have applied it successfully in smaller acardiac acephalic twins as late as 20 weeks of gestation.

Mid-gestation (17–25 weeks)

As laser coagulation techniques cannot be used at later gestations, bipolar energy has been used to occlude the cord.[35] This procedure is used for cord occlusion between 17 and 25 weeks of gestation, where the maximum diameter of the cord is less than 15 mm. The technique involves inserting a 3 mm port into the sac of the affected fetus under continuous ultrasound guidance and passing 2.7 mm bipolar coagulation forceps that have a maximum blade opening width of 15 mm (Everest Medical, Minneapolis, USA). The bipolar forceps are then used to grasp the cord of the affected fetus under ultrasound guidance. Once complete cord occlusion is demonstrated by closing the forceps and observing cessation of flow using colour/power Doppler of the cord, the cord is then coagulated using bipolar energy between 20 and 50 W. Each point of the cord is coagulated three times for approximately 60 seconds and three separate areas of cord are coagulated to ensure complete occlusion. This technique has the advantage of simultaneously obliterating the umbilical arteries and vein causing immediate cessation of flow and thus preventing agonal inter-fetal haemorrhage. A definite advantage of such bipolar cord occlusion over the older fetoscopic ligation techniques is that it can be can be done through a single port under ultrasound guidance. This allows the procedure to be performed under conditions in which fetoscopy would be difficult, such as blood-stained amniotic fluid. Compared with cord ligation, the duration of the procedure is also markedly shorter. Notwithstanding this, bipolar cord occlusion is complicated by an approximately 20% incidence of iatrogenic amniorrhexis, although liquor leakage in these circumstances is not usually associated with severe oligohydramnios or short procedure-to-delivery intervals.[36]

Late gestation (after 26 weeks)

After 26 weeks of gestation, the cord is considered to be too large for the bipolar forceps to grasp, so the technique of choice is cord ligation. This causes complete and permanent arterial and venous occlusion, and has survival rates of about 70%.[37] The older fetoscopic procedure carries a substantial risk of premature rupture of the membranes of 30% before 32 weeks and, even in experienced hands, fails in about 10% of cases.[32,38] It has been speculated that a higher risk for rupture of membranes after fetoscopic cord ligation is related to the complexity of the procedure, the higher number of ports and longer operating times.[39] This technique can also be used earlier in gestation when other techniques have failed or are not technically possible, for example when the cord is too oedematous.

Lemery et al.[37] reported an ultrasound-guided technique of cord ligation, which we have used successfully for selective feticide in an MC pregnancy referred at 32 weeks of gestation that was discordant for severe ventriculomegaly. The procedure can be performed under epidural anaesthesia with continuous ultrasound monitoring. A free loop of cord of the affected fetus is identified by ultrasound scan and a 3 mm port (Karl Stortz, Germany, no. 30114G) is inserted percutaneously into the uterine cavity. One end of a 1-Vicryl® (polyglactin) suture is tied in a loop to aid ultrasound visualisation. The looped end of the Vicryl suture is then introduced through the 3 mm port using a 2 mm knot tier (Karl Stortz, Germany, no. 30200FNS), with the other end of the suture securely held outside the maternal abdomen. The Vicryl suture is then guided past one side of the free loop of cord and released behind the cord. The grasper is then withdrawn to above the cord and directed down the other side of the cord to grasp the loop of Vicryl behind the cord. The loop end of the suture is then withdrawn through the 3 mm port using the grasping forceps. An extracorporeal knot is then tied and the knot pushed through the port using a knot pusher (Karl Stortz, Germany, no. 26167DS). The knot is tightened around the cord until pulse wave Doppler confirms no flow in the cord. Care must to be taken to avoid pulling on the cord itself as this may cause it to rupture with the consequent exsanguination of both twins. A second knot is tied extracorporeally and pushed down to secure the first knot. The procedure is then repeated in a second position along the cord to avoid any risk of incomplete occlusion from the first ligation. Although this procedure involves a single portal entry with a likely lower risk of iatrogenic amniorrhexis, it can still be a difficult procedure because of the difficulties of grasping the suture material in the uterine cavity and the risk of cord rupture.[40]

Other techniques

Embolisation of the fetal cord with various thrombogenic substances such as alcohol, coils or enbucrilate gel have been described, but is now contraindicated because of a too high incidence of intrauterine death of both twins, probably caused by incomplete obliteration of the umbilical cord vessels.[41,42] Denbow *et al.*[41] reported 12 cases in which embolisation with alcohol or enbucrilate gel was attempted, with the co-twin being lost in 66% of cases owing to agonal transfusion from incomplete occlusion.[43]

Rodeck[44] reported monopolar thermocoagulation of the fetal aorta, successfully arresting flow in acardiac twins. However, it remains to be determined whether arresting flow in the aorta precludes feto-fetal haemorrhage in other situations with normal haemodynamic flow in the affected fetus. For example, the technique does not work in twin-to-twin transfusion syndrome, suggesting that occlusion, if there are high-flow vessels, is not ensured. Monopolar thermocoagulation also has the added risk of coagulation occurring throughout the length of the needle with resultant risk of maternal injury and fistula formation. Sepulveda *et al.*[45] reported a simple device for monopolar diathermy that avoids the need for specialised equipment. It consists of a 1 mm insulated semi-rigid solid wire obtained from a six-wire phone cable, which can be housed in an 18 gauge disposable Echotip® needle and used in a similar manner to that described for interstitial laser coagulation.

A more recently described minimally invasive technique, which has been developed in animal models and applied in humans with a high success rate, is radiofrequency ablation (RFA).[46] RFA is a technique that uses high-energy radio waves to cause coagulation. The coagulative damage can be restricted by deploying the RFA device through a 14 gauge needle in direct contact with the target tissue such as the umbilical cord or intra-fetal vessels and thereby avoiding injury to the co-twin.[47] The technique can be performed under ultrasound guidance. A 3 mm (14 gauge) RFA needle is introduced into the fetal abdomen at the level of the cord insertion. The RFA device is passed down the needle so that it is adjacent to the vessels and energy is then applied, starting at 10 W and increasing by 10 W every two minutes, up to 80 W, until colour/power Doppler observation indicates termination of blood flow.[46] This has been used as late as 23 weeks of gestation, but does require specialised equipment. Tsao *et al.*[46] reported 13 acardiac twin pregnancies where selective reduction of the abnormal twin using RFA was used. Twelve of 13 normal (pump) twins survived, with one, delivered at 24 weeks, dying in the neonatal period because of complications of prematurity.

An anecdotally reported alternative to selective feticide is sectio parvae, where one fetus is delivered by hysterotomy. This approach is likely to be associated with significant maternal morbidity, risk of placental abruption and preterm rupture of membranes, and a low chance of long-term retention of the healthy twin *in utero*.[34]

All these procedures for selective feticide are associated with some risk of complications and death in the normal twin. Specific criteria for selecting patients and the optimal timing of the procedure have not been definitively established. As the balance between the risks and benefits is unclear, the decision is usually based on parental wishes and local experience. Generally, prior to 16 weeks of gestation, ultrasound-guided interstitial laser coagulation is the preferred technique. After 18 weeks, bipolar cord coagulation is the method of choice. Beyond 25 or 26 weeks of gestation, selective feticide is rarely indicated, but ultrasound-guided cord ligation may be used.

Summary

The dramatic increase in higher order multiple pregnancies as a result of ART has necessitated the development of MFPR as a mechanism for improving perinatal outcome. There is now no doubt that in pregnancies with starting numbers greater than three MFPR to twins significantly improves outcome.

The issue of MFPR in triplets remains somewhat contentious. It is apparent that expectant management of trichorionic triplets has improved significantly in the last two decades and now has reasonably good outcomes. However, the evidence, although limited, suggests that reduction to dichorionic twins significantly reduces the risk of preterm delivery and low birthweight babies without a significant increase in the risk of miscarriage. Therefore, parents of trichorionic triplets need balanced counselling early in pregnancy where clear facts are presented and time is provided to enable them to make an informed decision based on their individual moral and religious values. It is also very clear that follow-up data of neurological outcome in reduced and unreduced triplets are essential if we are to get a true picture of the risks or MFPR compared with conservative management.

MFPR of non-trichorionic triplets and selective termination for anomalies in monochorionic pregnancies has advanced significantly in recent years with the development of vascular occlusive techniques. However, clinicians need to be aware of the differences in the management of these pregnancies compared with polychorionic multiple pregnancies. This applies particularly to the need to avoid delays before referral to specialist centres, as the techniques and risks involved vary depending on gestation.

References

1. Wood R. Trends in multiple births: 1938–1995 *Popul Trends* 1997;87: 29–35.
2. James WH. Are 'natural' twinning rates continuing to decline? *Hum Reprod* 1995;10:3042–4.
3. Bortolus R, Parazzini F, Chatenoud L, Benzi G, Bianchi MM, Marini A. Epidemiology of multiple births. *Hum Reprod Update* 1999;5:179–87.
4. Bergh T, Ericson A, Hillensjo T, Nygren KG, Wennerholm UB. Deliveries and children born after in-vitro fertilisation in Sweden: 1982–95: a retrospective cohort study. *Lancet* 1999;354:1579–85.
5. Human Fertilisation and Embryology Authority. *Annual Report and Accounts*. London: *Stationery Office*; 2000.
6. Devine PC, Malone FD, Athanassiou A, Harvey-Wilkes K, D'Alton ME. Maternal and neonatal outcome of 100 consecutive triplet pregnancies. *Am J Perinatol* 2001;18:225–35.
7. Petterson B, Nelson KB, Watson L, Stanley F. Twins, triplets, and cerebral palsy in births in Western Australia in the 1980s. *BMJ* 1993;307:1239–43.
8. Human Fertilisation & Embryology Authority. *Code of Practice 6th Edition*. London: HFEA; 2003 [www.hfea.gov.uk/HFEAPublications/CodeofPractice].
9. Lipitz S, Uval J, Achiron R, Schiff E, Lusky A, Reichman B. Outcome of twin pregnancies reduced from triplets compared with nonreduced twin gestations. *Obstet Gynecol* 1996;87:511–14.
10. Evans MI, Berkowitz RL, Wapner RJ, Carpenter RJ, Goldberg JD, Ayoub MA, et al. Improvement in outcomes of multifetal pregnancy reduction with increased experience. *Am J Obstet Gynecol* 2001;184:97–103.
11. Melgar CA, Rosenfeld DL, Rawlinson K, Greenberg M. Perinatal outcome after multifetal reduction to twins compared with nonreduced multiple gestations. *Obstet Gynecol* 1991;78(5 Pt 1):763–7.
12. Landy HJ, Keith LG. The vanishing twin: a review. *Hum Reprod Update* 1998;4:177–83.
13. Lipitz S, Shulman A, Achiron R, Zalel Y, Seidman DS. A comparative study of multifetal pregnancy reduction from triplets to twins in the first versus early second trimesters after detailed fetal screening. *Ultrasound Obstet Gynecol* 2001;18:35–8.
14. Brambati B, Tului L. First trimester fetal reduction: its role in the management of twin and higher order multiple pregnancies. *Hum Reprod Update* 1995;1:397–408.

15. Cuckle H. Down's syndrome screening in twins. *J Med Screen* 1998;5:3–4.
16. Yaron Y, Bryant-Greenwood PK, Dave N, Moldenhauer JS, Kramer RL, Johnson MP, *et al.* Multifetal pregnancy reductions of triplets to twins: comparison with nonreduced triplets and twins. *Am J Obstet Gynecol* 1999;180:1268–71.
17. Lipitz S, Reichman B, Uval J, Shalev J, Achiron R, Barkai G, *et al.* A prospective comparison of the outcome of triplet pregnancies managed expectantly or by multifetal reduction to twins. *Am J Obstet Gynecol* 1994;170:874–9.
18. Sebire NJ, D'Ercole C, Sepulveda W, Hughes K, Nicolaides KH. Effects of embryo reduction from trichorionic triplets to twins. *Br J Obstet Gynaecol* 1997;104:1201–3.
19. Ziadeh SM. Perinatal outcome in 41 sets of triplets in Jordan. *Birth* 2000;27:185–8.
20. Papageorghiou AT, Liao AW, Skentou C, Sebire NJ, Nicolaides KH. Trichorionic triplet pregnancies at 10–14 weeks: outcome after embryo reduction compared to expectant management. *J Matern Fetal Neonatal Med* 2002;11:307–12.
21. Check JH, Nowroozi K, Vetter B, Rankin A, Dietterich C, Schubert B. Effects of multiple gestation and selective reduction on fetal outcome. *J Perinat Med* 1993;21:299–302.
22. Geipel A, Berg C, Katalinic A, Plath H, Hansmann M, Germer U, *et al.* Prenatal diagnosis and obstetric outcomes in triplet pregnancies in relation to chorionicity. *BJOG* 2005;112:554–8.
23. Antsaklis A, Souka AP, Daskalakis G, Papantoniou N, Koutra P, Kavalakis Y, *et al.* Embryo reduction versus expectant management in triplet pregnancies. *J Matern Fetal Neonatal Med* 2004;16:219–22.
24. Pharoah PO, Cooke T. Cerebral palsy and multiple births. *Arch Dis Child Fetal Neonatal Ed* 1996;75:F174–7.
25. Dimitriou G, Pharoah PO, Nicolaides KH, Greenough A. Cerebral palsy in triplet pregnancies with and without iatrogenic reduction. *Eur J Pediatr* 2004;163:449–51.
26. Berkowitz RL, Lynch L, Stone J, Alvarez M. The current status of multifetal pregnancy reduction. *Am J Obstet Gynecol* 1996;174:1265–72.
27. Antsaklis A, Souka AP, Daskalakis G, Papantoniou N, Koutra P, Kavalakis Y, *et al.* Pregnancy outcome after multifetal pregnancy reduction. *J Matern Fetal Neonatal Med* 2004;16:27–31.
28. Geipel A, Berg C, Katalinic A, Plath H, Hansmann M, Smrcek J, *et al.* Targeted first-trimester prenatal diagnosis before fetal reduction in triplet gestations and subsequent outcome. *Ultrasound Obstet Gynecol* 2004;24:724–9.
29. Evans MI, Goldberg JD, Horenstein J, Wapner RJ, Ayoub MA, Stone J, *et al.* Selective termination for structural, chromosomal, and Mendelian anomalies: international experience. *Am J Obstet Gynecol* 1999;181:893–7.
30. Eddleman KA, Stone JL, Lynch L, Berkowitz RL. Selective termination of anomalous fetuses in multifetal pregnancies: two hundred cases at a single center. *Am J Obstet Gynecol* 2002;187:1168–72.
31. Lewi L, Van SD, Gratacos E, Witters I, Timmerman D, Deprest J. Monochorionic diamniotic twins: complications and management options. *Curr Opin Obstet Gynecol* 2003;15:177–94.
32. Deprest JA, Van Ballaer PP, Evrard VA, Peers KH, Spitz B, Steegers EA, *et al.* Experience with fetoscopic cord ligation. *Eur J Obstet Gynecol Reprod Biol* 1998;81:157–64.
33. Ville Y, Hyett JA, Vandenbussche FP, Nicolaides KH. Endoscopic laser coagulation of umbilical cord vessels in twin reversed arterial perfusion sequence. *Ultrasound Obstet Gynecol* 1994;4:396–8.
34. Jolly M, Taylor M, Rose G, Govender L, Fisk NM. Interstitial laser: a new surgical technique for twin reversed arterial perfusion sequence in early pregnancy. *BJOG* 2001;108:1098–102.
35. Deprest JA, Audibert F, Van SD, Hecher K, Mahieu-Caputo D. Bipolar coagulation of the umbilical cord in complicated monochorionic twin pregnancy. *Am J Obstet Gynecol* 2000;182:340–5.
36. Taylor MJ, Shalev E, Tanawattanacharoen S, Jolly M, Kumar S, Weiner E, *et al.* Ultrasound-guided umbilical cord occlusion using bipolar diathermy for Stage III/IV twin–twin transfusion syndrome. *Prenat Diagn* 2002;22:70–6.
37. Lemery DJ, Vanlieferinghen P, Gasq M, Finkeltin F, Beaufrere AM, Beytout M. Fetal umbilical cord ligation under ultrasound guidance. *Ultrasound Obstet Gynecol* 1994;4:399–401.
38. Quintero RA, Romero R, Reich H, Goncalves L, Johnson MP, Carreno C, *et al. In utero* percutaneous umbilical cord ligation in the management of complicated monochorionic multiple gestations. *Ultrasound Obstet Gynecol* 1996;8:16–22.
39. Deprest JA, Lerut TE, Vandenberghe K. Operative fetoscopy: new perspective in fetal therapy? *Prenat Diagn* 1997;17:1247–60.
40. Gallot D, Laurichesse H, Lemery D. Selective feticide in monochorionic twin pregnancies by ultrasound-guided umbilical cord occlusion. *Ultrasound Obstet Gynecol* 2003;22:484–8.
41. Denbow ML, Overton TG, Duncan KR, Cox PM, Fisk NM. High failure rate of umbilical vessel

occlusion by ultrasound-guided injection of absolute alcohol or enbucrilate gel. *Prenat Diagn* 1999;19:527–32.

42. Porreco RP, Barton SM, Haverkamp AD. Occlusion of umbilical artery in acardiac, acephalic twin. *Lancet* 1991;337:326–7.

43. Mahone PR, Sherer DM, Abramowicz JS, Woods JR Jr. Twin–twin transfusion syndrome: rapid development of severe hydrops of the donor following selective feticide of the hydropic recipient. *Am J Obstet Gynecol* 1993;169:166–8.

44. Rodeck C, Deans A, Jauniaux E. Thermocoagulation for the early treatment of pregnancy with an acardiac twin. *N Engl J Med* 1998;339:1293–5.

45. Sepulveda W, Corral E, Gutierrez J. A simple device for vascular occlusion of acardiac twins. *Ultrasound Obstet Gynecol* 2003;21:386–8.

46. Tsao K, Feldstein VA, Albanese CT, Sandberg PL, Lee H, Harrison MR, *et al.* Selective reduction of acardiac twin by radiofrequency ablation. *Am J Obstet Gynecol* 2002;187:635–40.

47. Torok O, Lapinski R, Salafia CM, Bernasko J, Berkowitz RL. Multifetal pregnancy reduction is not associated with an increased risk of intrauterine growth restriction, except for very-high-order multiples. *Am J Obstet Gynecol* 1998;179:221–5.

48. Boulot P, Vignal J, Vergnes C, Dechaud H, Faure JM, Hedon B. Multifetal reduction of triplets to twins: a prospective comparison of pregnancy outcome. *Hum Reprod* 2000;15:1619–23.

49. Geva E, Fait G, Yovel I, Lerner-Geva L, Yaron Y, Daniel Y, *et al.* Second-trimester multifetal pregnancy reduction facilitates prenatal diagnosis before the procedure. *Fertil Steril* 2000;73:505–8.

50. Smith-Levitin M, Kowalik A, Birnholz J, Skupski DW, Hutson JM, Chervenak FA, *et al.* Selective reduction of multifetal pregnancies to twins improves outcome over nonreduced triplet gestations. *Am J Obstet Gynecol* 1996;175:878–82.

51. Kadhel P, Olivennes F, Fernandez H, Vial M, Frydman R. Are there still obstetric and perinatal benefits for selective embryo reduction of triplet pregnancies? *Hum Reprod* 1998;13:3555–9.

52. Skrablin S, Kuvacic I, Pavicic D, Kalafatic D, Goluza T. Maternal neonatal outcome in quadruplet and quintuplet versus triplet gestations. *Eur J Obstet Gynecol Reprod Biol* 2000;88:147–52.

53. Pons JC, Charlemaine C, Dubreuil E, Papiernik E, Frydman R. Management and outcome of triplet pregnancy. *Eur J Obstet Gynecol Reprod Biol* 1998;76:131–9.

54. Kaufman GE, Malone FD, Harvey-Wilkes KB, Chelmow D, Penzias AS, D'Alton ME. Neonatal morbidity and mortality associated with triplet pregnancy. *Obstet Gynecol* 1998;91:342–8.

55. Abu-Heija AT. Maternal and neonatal outcome of high order gestation. *Arch Gynecol Obstet* 2003;268:15–18.

56. Roest J, van Heusden AM, Verhoeff A, Mous HV, Zeilmaker GH. A triplet pregnancy after *in vitro* fertilization is a procedure-related complication that should be prevented by replacement of two embryos only. *Fertil Steril* 1997;67:290–5.

57. Barkehall-Thomas A, Woodward L, Wallace EM. Maternal and neonatal outcomes in 54 triplet pregnancies managed in an Australian tertiary centre. *Aust N Z J Obstet Gynaecol* 2004;44:222–7.

58. Leondires MP, Ernst SD, Miller BT, Scott RT Jr. Triplets: outcomes of expectant management versus multifetal reduction for 127 pregnancies. *Am J Obstet Gynecol* 2000;183:454–9.

Chapter 7
Preterm labour in multiple pregnancies

Sheri Lim, TG Teoh and Phillip Bennett

Introduction

Prematurity is the delivery of an infant before 37 weeks of gestation. It is associated with significant neonatal morbidity and is responsible for up to 85% of neonatal deaths in infants without any congenital malformations. The increased neonatal mortality is five times higher for twins and nine times higher for triplets.

With increasing neonatal expertise, the survival of very premature babies has improved but many are left with significant long-term disabilities such as cerebral palsy, mental retardation, deafness and blindness. Twenty percent of all triplet pregnancies and 50% of quadruplet pregnancies result in at least one child with a major long-term disability.[1,2] This places a great strain on the healthcare system and is a problem in both developing and developed countries. It remains one of the major obstetric concerns today.

The concept of the estimated due date is derived from singleton pregnancies. The majority of twins and triplets deliver at 37–38 and 32–34 weeks of gestation, respectively. There is a possibility that multiple pregnancies experience accelerated fetal maturation *in utero*. Perinatal mortality for twins is lowest at 38 weeks of gestation:[3] placental maturation appears to occur earlier in twins compared with singletons,[4] indicating a variation in fetal maturation points compared with singletons. It is from this viewpoint that we should consider preterm labour in multiple pregnancies.

Incidence and epidemiology

The background incidence of prematurity is 5–10%. Multiple births account for about 2% of births each year, with twins accounting for 94% of all multiple births. The overall incidence of prematurity in multiple pregnancies is 54% (50% of twins and 90% of triplets are born prematurely). Multiple pregnancies thus account for approximately 25% of preterm births, which represents a disproportionate share of preterm births and neonatal morbidity and mortality.

The overall incidence of preterm delivery has been slowly rising in developed countries over the last decade. A significant proportion of this is contributed to by the increase in the incidence of multiple gestation. The March of Dimes study[5] showed that multiple births account for a significant proportion of admissions to neonatal intensive care units. Seventeen percent of infants delivered before 27 weeks of gestation and 21% of infants delivered by 28–31 weeks were from multiple pregnancies. The main contributor to the increase in multiple gestations has been the increase in the use of assisted reproductive technologies (ART). Ovulation induction with either clomifene or pituitary gonadotrophins and *in vitro* fertilisation (IVF) are all significant risk factors for multiple gestation. In particular, the practice of implanting three or more embryos is a major risk factor for twin and higher order multiple gestations. Another factor contributing to the increase in multiple gestation rates is the trend towards delayed childbirth. Improving educational and job opportunities for women and a change in the family social structure, which means that divorce and remarriage are more common and more women restart families at a more advanced age, has increased the frequency of births among older mothers.

Aetiology

Preterm labour is a symptom rather than a disease. It can result from a number of different causes. There are well-known associations between multiple pregnancy, over-distension of the uterus by extensive amniotic fluid (polyhydramnios), abnormalities of the uterus or the cervix, and the presence of infection or colonisation of the genital tract with pathogenic bacteria, and the onset of labour before term. Exactly how or why these various associations cause preterm delivery is not fully understood and is the subject of ongoing research. There is, however, a sufficient understanding of what causes the onset of labour in the human to enable us to begin to understand the mechanisms of the onset of preterm labour.[6,7]

Throughout most of the pregnancy the uterus has to expand and grow to accommodate the growing fetus, placenta and amniotic fluid without contracting, while the cervix remains firm and closed to retain the pregnancy within the uterus. Near to term the cervix needs to become soft (identified clinically as cervical ripening) to allow it to be easily dilated and the uterus needs to become a contractile organ. This transition is associated with an increase in the expression of a number of proteins that will be needed to allow the uterus to contract. These include gap junction proteins, which provide electrical connections between the muscle cells of the uterus, and proteins that act as receptors for substances that stimulate the uterus to contract, such as prostaglandins and oxytocin. The biochemical changes that take place within the cervix, the fetal membranes and the myometrium in association with human labour are very similar to those which are seen at sites of inflammation.

It is currently believed that the mechanism which controls the length of human pregnancy is the release of a hormone known as corticotrophin-releasing hormone (CRH) from the placenta.[8,9] Outside pregnancy, CRH produced by the hypothalamus stimulates the release of a second hormone, adrenocorticotrophic hormone (ACTH), from the pituitary gland, which in turn controls the release of the stress hormone cortisol from the adrenal gland. There is negative feedback by cortisol upon ACTH and CRH, so that as cortisol levels rise CRH and ACTH levels fall. This represents the normal homeostatic mechanism controlling cortisol levels in nonpregnant women. During pregnancy CRH is also released into the maternal circulation by the placenta.

CRH, a 41 amino acid peptide initially found to be produced by the hypothalamus and later in placental, amnion, chorion and decidual cells, rises exponentially through pregnancy.[10] It acts on the fetal pituitary gland to release ACTH, which subsequently stimulates fetal adrenal steroidogenesis, i.e. production of cortisol and dehydro-epiandrosterone (DHEA-S). These steroids help hasten fetal organ maturation before labour. The steroids then travel back to the placenta through the umbilical circulation, amplifying further cortisol production through a positive feedback loop. DHEA-S is then converted to oestrogen, which promotes further CRH through its action on prostaglandins. CRH also acts directly on the placenta through paracrine effects to produce more ACTH, which adds to the fetal adrenal stimulation resulting in increased levels of cortisol. As there is greater placental mass in multiple pregnancies, and hence increased production of CRH, it is very likely that CRH plays an important role in the onset of preterm labour.

In the maternal circulation CRH is bound to a binding protein (CRH-BP), which renders it biologically inactive. CRH-BP is negatively regulated by CRH, so as CRH levels rise CRH-BP levels fall. Three to four weeks before the onset of human labour at term, CRH levels in the maternal circulation begin to exceed those of CRH-BP.[8,9] This means that there is, relatively suddenly, an excess of biologically active CRH in the maternal circulation. CRH is then believed to switch on the various genes that produce the proteins that are important for the onset of uterine contractions. These proteins include inflammatory mediators whose function is to cause ripening of the cervix and contractions of the uterus.

This simple model of the mechanism of the onset of labour, sometimes described as the 'placental clock',[9] helps to explain the onset of preterm labour in various situations. In a multiple pregnancy, where there is more placental mass, CRH concentrations rise more quickly, such that CRH exceeds CRH-BP earlier in the pregnancy; thus the average duration of a twin pregnancy is shorter than in a singleton. In general, twin pregnancies deliver approximately two weeks earlier than singleton pregnancies.

In the case of infection-associated preterm labour the presence of organisms within the uterus switch on inflammatory mediators prematurely.[11] This leads to ripening of the cervix, weakening of the fetal membranes, preterm prelabour rupture of the membranes and the onset of uterine contractions. Cervical incompetence, that is to say a weakness of the cervix leading to a degree of premature dilatation for mechanical reasons, is classically said to produce painless second-trimester miscarriage. It is likely, however, that a degree of cervical incompetence may contribute to the onset of preterm labour by enabling pathogenic bacteria, which are present within the vagina, to gain access to the lower pole of the uterus, where they set up an inflammatory reaction leading to cervical ripening and myometrial contractions and therefore to the onset of preterm labour.

It has been recognised recently that stress, either in the mother or in the fetus, may be associated with preterm delivery.[12] Placental CRH, unlike its hypothalamic counterpart, is positively upregulated by cortisol. The hypothesis is that fetal stress (as may be associated with growth restriction, infection or chronic disease) causes a chronic increase in the release of cortisol. This may then stimulate increased production of CRH by the placenta and the CRH 'placental clock' mechanism may be activated early. A similar mechanism has been proposed whereby chronic maternal stress may produce a premature rise in CRH and lead to the onset of preterm labour.

A larger number of twin pregnancies than singleton pregnancies are delivered before 37 weeks of gestation and therefore twin pregnancy is associated with preterm delivery. In this context, however, 'preterm delivery' is fairly late in the pregnancy and in modern practice is associated with a good outcome for the twins. It is also the case that there is a higher incidence of earlier preterm delivery in twin pregnancy. However, this cannot be simply because of the presence of two fetuses and placentas within the same uterus. An additional factor, which probably underlies the increased sensitivity of multiple pregnancies to factors that stimulate preterm labour, is the effect of stretch upon the expression of various labour-associated and contraction-associated genes.[13,14] Studies in both intact animal models and in human cells in culture have shown that mechanical stretch increases the expression of connexins, oxytocin receptor, inflammatory cytokines and inducible type 2 cyclooxygenase (COX-2) (the key enzyme in the synthesis of prostaglandins). This effect of stretch appears to apply not only in the myometrium but also in the amnion and it is possible that one of the explanations for the earlier upregulation of cytokines and prostaglandins in the lower pole of the uterus than in the upper pole is the increased effect of mechanical force on the lower segment and fetal membranes overlying the lower segment as the fetal head engages in the last few weeks of pregnancy.

Twin-to-twin transfusion syndrome represents a particular risk factor for preterm delivery because, when it becomes severe, polyhydramnios will develop in the sac of the recipient twin and this, together with the pre-existing stretch of the uterus from the multiple pregnancy itself, will combine to increase the expression of labour-associated and contraction-associated genes.

Risk factors may combine to increase the risk of preterm labour. Again, there are biochemical explanations for the epidemiological evidence that combining risk factors increases the risk. So, for example, if a woman has a mild degree of cervical incompetence, which results in only a degree of opening of the cervix during pregnancy, this may allow bacteria from the vagina to enter the uterus and stimulate the onset of preterm labour. If, at the same time, the woman has a large number of pathogenic bacteria in her vagina, then the chance of infection becoming established earlier is increased and preterm labour is likely to occur earlier. If the same woman is also carrying a twin pregnancy, then the earlier upregulation of contraction-associated proteins might mean that preterm labour would occur even earlier. Multiple gestation is therefore a risk factor that, when it combines with other factors that might stimulate preterm labour, results in earlier delivery than might occur in a singleton pregnancy under the same circumstances. In other words, the twin pregnancy primes the uterus to be more sensitive to other factors that cause preterm delivery.

Prediction

Risk scoring systems

Multiple gestation itself is a powerful risk factor for preterm birth. Other risk factors for preterm labour in singleton pregnancies such as previous preterm birth, recurrent second-trimester miscarriage, previous cone biopsy,[15,16] pelvic infection and demographic characteristics such as age and race will apply similarly in multiple gestation. This has led to attempts to develop risk scoring systems by assigning weighting to these various possible associated factors. A number of different risk scoring systems have been suggested, none of which have been shown to have sufficient specificity or sensitivity to make them clinically useful. Most systems place considerable weight on past obstetric history and so are of little value for nulliparous women who constitute approximately 45% of women in any antenatal cohort. Positive predictive values range from 15% to 30% and sensitivities from 35% to 60%. There have been no good-quality randomised controlled trials of the effectiveness or otherwise of risk scoring systems for preterm labour in multiple pregnancies. There is currently no evidence that the use of risk scoring systems improves the outcome for neonates following multiple gestation and they have not found their way into routine clinical practice in the UK.

Cervical length

The cervix is a dynamic organ that changes with pregnancy. One of the earliest clinically identifiable events associated with parturition is a change in the consistency and length of the cervix that precedes the onset of preterm labour in the majority of cases. Digital cervical assessment has a poor ability to assess the actual length of the cervix and therefore the risk of preterm labour. Similarly, although experiments were undertaken in the 1980s to use transabdominal ultrasound to measure cervical length, this also performed poorly, probably because without a full bladder the cervix will not be visualised in up to 50% of cases and a full bladder compresses the lower segment of the uterus and may give the impression of a longer cervix. Transvaginal ultrasound is a reliable method of measurement of cervical length and one that appears in general to be acceptable to pregnant women. Following the pioneering work of Owen et al.[17] in the USA, a large number of studies have been published in the last 15 years that have assessed the value of cervical length at various gestational ages to predict preterm delivery in both asymptomatic and symptomatic women (i.e. those with contractions). The relationship between cervical length and risk of preterm delivery is continuous, and the risk increases exponentially as cervical length decreases. It also appears that the earlier that cervical shortening is detected in pregnancy, the higher the risk of preterm delivery. So, for example, Honest et al.,[18] in a systematic review of the accuracy of cervical sonography in predicting preterm birth, found that the risk of spontaneous preterm delivery before 34 weeks of gestation following a measurement of cervical length of 25 mm or less was 21% if the measurement was made before 20 weeks, 15% if it was made between 20 and 24 weeks and 14% if the measurement was made after 24 weeks.

Transcervical ultrasound appears to be an effective method for determining the risk of preterm delivery in twin pregnancies. Honest et al.[18] found that in a twin pregnancy with a cervical length of 25 mm or less between 20 and 24 weeks there was a 47% risk of preterm delivery compared with a 16% risk in a singleton pregnancy. In six studies on the value of sonographic cervical assessment at 18–26 weeks in otherwise low-risk twin pregnancies, which enrolled a total of 1112 pregnancies, preterm delivery before 32 weeks occurred in 7.6% pregnancies overall but this increased to 30% if cervical length was less than 25 mm (or less than 20 mm in some studies).

Skentou et al.[19] studied the relationship between cervical length at 20–24 weeks of gestation and the risk of preterm delivery in asymptomatic women with both singleton and twin pregnancies. They found that at any given cervical length the risk of preterm delivery was higher for twin pregnancies than for singletons. The median cervical length in twin pregnancies was similar to that found in singleton pregnancies but there were higher proportions of twin pregnancies among the women whose cervical length was less than 25 mm or less than 15 mm. In singleton pregnancies a dramatic increase in the risk for early preterm delivery was seen in those women with a cervical length of 15 mm. However, in twin pregnancies this occurred at cervical lengths of less than 25 mm.

Measurement of cervical length may also be used in symptomatic women presenting with contractions to distinguish between those who are genuinely in preterm labour and are candidates for tocolysis and corticosteroid treatment and those who are not in preterm labour. Fuchs et al.[20] showed in a study of 532 singleton pregnancies that delivery within seven days occurs in 49% of women whose cervical length is less than 15 mm but in only 1% of women whose cervical length is greater than 15 mm. In singleton pregnancies no woman whose cervical length was longer than 20 mm delivered within seven days. However, in twin pregnancies this 'cut-off' value increased to 25 mm. Therefore, while a cervical length of either 15 or 20 mm might be considered to be the cut-off for treatment in symptomatic women with singleton pregnancies, this should probably be raised to 25 mm in twin pregnancies.

Fetal fibronectin and bacterial vaginosis

Fetal fibronectin (fFN) is a basement membrane adhesion protein synthesised by the fetal membranes. It is normally detected in the cervix and vagina up to 16–20 weeks of gestation, until the time of full fusion of the amnion chorion, after which it is not detected until close to delivery. Detection is considered positive when a swab taken from the posterior fornix of the vagina and cervix has an assay reading of greater than 50 ng/mL.[21] Oliveira et al.[22,23] reported that positive fFN between 24 and 34 weeks is useful for predicting twin deliveries before 37 weeks, but poorer in predicting deliveries before 34 weeks. Wennerholm et al.,[24] in a study of 121 women with twin pregnancies, showed the same association between a positive fFN and preterm delivery before 35 weeks of gestation. The positive predictive value of fFN for preterm labour in twins is high (67%) compared with singletons (29–50%). Conversely, the negative predictive value is lower in twins than singletons (70% versus 83–97%). Therefore, a negative result in a twin pregnancy is not as reassuring as in a singleton pregnancy (probably owing in part to the higher overall rate of preterm labour in multiple pregnancies).

Studies that have compared transcervical sonography for measurement of cervical length, detection of fFN or bacterial vaginosis in predicting preterm delivery in twin pregnancies have reported conflicting results and conclusions. The National Institutes of Health (NIH) preterm prediction study[25] prospectively screened 147 women with twin pregnancies at 24–28 weeks of gestation for more than 50 potential risk factors for spontaneous preterm birth. They measured cervical length by ultrasound, tested for the presence of bacterial vaginosis and measured fFN levels in vaginal secretions every two weeks from 24 to 30 weeks. They found that most of the known risk factors for spontaneous preterm birth were not significantly associated with spontaneous preterm birth in twin pregnancy. Measurement of cervical length at 24 weeks with a 'cut-off' of 25 mm was found to be the best predictor of spontaneous preterm birth. Fetal fibronectin was found to have a significant association with spontaneous preterm birth at less than 32 weeks when it was detected at 28 or 30 weeks. Wennerholm et al.[24] sampled vaginal or cervical fluid for measurement of fFN, bacterial endotoxin concentrations and the presence of bacterial vaginosis at two week intervals from 24 to 34 weeks and measured cervical length at the same time. They found that neither detection of bacterial endotoxin nor of bacterial vaginosis had any predictive power for preterm delivery and that the predictive value of cervical length measurement was also low. In their study the best predictor of preterm birth in twin pregnancies was the detection of fFN. Gibson et al.[26] performed measurements of cervical length and used a bedside assay for detection of fFN in vaginal secretions at 18, 24, 28 and 32 weeks. They found that the best predictors of preterm delivery were the measurement of cervical length of less than 25 mm at 18 weeks and 22 mm at 24 weeks but that there was no relationship between the detection of fFN and preterm delivery.

Although various studies have shown quite dramatic differences in the value of sonographic measurement of cervical length or detection of fFN in the prediction of preterm delivery in twin pregnancies, we would conclude that currently the best method for identification of a risk of preterm delivery in twin pregnancies that are otherwise asymptomatic is the measurement of cervical length. Measurement of cervical length earlier in pregnancy appears to be a better predictor than measurement later. The introduction of routine screening of cervical length to predict preterm delivery and how that screening will be undertaken, either by serial measurements during the second or third trimester, or by a single measurement at any given gestational age, is likely to be dictated by availability of resources. Refinement of the risk of preterm delivery in twin pregnancy may help to target the administration of corticosteroids but, until an effective 'prophylactic' treatment to prevent preterm delivery in those identified as being at high risk is found, there are no good economic arguments for introducing screening of cervical length in the general obstetric population (whether with singleton or multiple pregnancies).

It appears that currently f FN testing in the UK should be limited to patients who are symptomatic. Although there is good evidence that detection of bacterial vaginosis in the second trimester in singleton pregnancies predicts a risk of preterm delivery, there is controversy as to whether treating bacterial vaginosis improves the outcome. In multiple pregnancies it appears that bacterial vaginosis is poorly correlated with risk of preterm delivery and there is not, therefore, at this point, a strong case for routinely testing for bacterial vaginosis in women whose only risk factor for preterm delivery is a multiple pregnancy.

'Prophylaxis' for preterm labour

Nutrition

There is some evidence that nutritional intervention may reduce the risk of low birthweight and preterm delivery in twin pregnancies. In the Higgins Nutrition Intervention Program[27] the rate of preterm delivery was 30% lower in the group with nutritional intervention, which was associated with a six-fold reduction in neonatal mortality.

Bed rest

Earlier generations of obstetricians recommended bed rest for women with multiple pregnancies. However, in a systematic review, Crowther[28] identified six trials of bed rest in hospital for multiple pregnancy involving over 600 women and 1400 babies. In those women with an uncomplicated twin pregnancy the bed rest did not reduce the risk of preterm birth. Indeed, significantly more women gave birth before 34 weeks of gestation in the group allocated to bed rest. There were no significant differences in perinatal mortality or other neonatal outcomes. It is more difficult to assess the value of hospitalisation in triplets and higher order multiples since all of the studies include very low numbers and none have sufficient power to demonstrate any significant outcomes. As with many controversial areas in obstetric practice, a major difficulty in studying bed rest in triplets and higher order multiples has been poor recruitment rates among an already rare cohort of women. This has resulted in at least one study closing prematurely.

Cervical cerclage

Studies of prophylactic cervical cerclage in multiple pregnancies have not demon-strated any benefit. Several small studies that randomised women at high risk of spontaneous preterm delivery into cerclage or no cerclage failed to demonstrate a benefit of cervical cerclage and included multiple pregnancy as a risk factor. The Medical Research Council/Royal College of Obstetricians and Gynaecologists multicentre randomised controlled trial of cervical cerclage included 74 patients with twin pregnancies. Sixty patients had prophylactic cervical cerclage and 14 were treated conservatively. There was no difference between the groups. Sixty percent delivered prematurely in the cerclage group and 50% in the control group.[29]

It also appears that the potentially more sophisticated approach of performing serial transvaginal ultrasound measurements of cervical length and targeting cervical cerclage at those identified as at risk of preterm delivery because of cervical shortening, is not appropriate in twin pregnancy. Berghella et al.[30] undertook a meta-analysis of trials of cervical cerclage for short cervix using the individual patient level data. They concluded that in singleton pregnancies cervical cerclage does not prevent preterm birth in all women with a short cervical length but in a subgroup of women with singleton gestations, with a short cervix and with a history of prior preterm birth, cervical cerclage may reduce the preterm birth rate. In twin pregnancies, however, introduction of a cervical cerclage from identification of a short cervix actually increased the preterm birth rate at less than 35 weeks of gestation with a relative risk of 2.15. Cervical cerclage in women with multiple pregnancies should, therefore, be reserved for those whose past obstetric history points strongly at the probability of a mechanical cervical problem as the cause of previous pregnancy losses or preterm deliveries.

It is unclear why cervical cerclage in multiple pregnancies where there is a short cervix increases the risk of preterm delivery. This may be a reflection of the fact that a woman with a multiple pregnancy is no more likely to have a pre-existing cervical problem than is a woman with a low-risk singleton pregnancy and that the number of women in a cohort with multiple pregnancies who are likely to benefit from cervical cerclage is very small.

Nonsteroidal anti-inflammatory drugs

Nonsteroidal anti-inflammatory drugs (NSAIDs), particularly indometacin, are widely used both for prophylaxis for preterm delivery and for acute treatment. Their use is associated with significant fetal adverse effects including oligohydramnios, renal failure, premature closure of the ductus arteriosus, persistent pattern ductus arteriosus in the neonate and necrotising enterocolitis. NSAIDs are also associated with a range of maternal adverse effects including gastric ulceration, coagulation and renal impairment. There are no trials of NSAIDs for prophylaxis or treatment of contractions in multiple pregnancies. Although indometacin and other NSAIDs have been used for several decades for acute treatment in singleton pregnancies, there are no strong data to support their use. King et al.[31] undertook a systematic review of inhibitors for treating preterm labour and concluded that, because the overall numbers of women enrolled in these studies was small, all of the estimates of effect were imprecise and needed to be interpreted with caution.

Since it is the inducible type 2 cyclooxygenase that is principally associated with the synthesis of prostaglandins at the time of term and preterm labour, it has been hoped that COX-2-specific NSAIDs might be used to reduce the risk of preterm delivery but without the fetal adverse effects of non-selective NSAIDs. In the only currently published study of a COX-2-specific inhibitor (rofecoxib) for prophylaxis in women at risk of preterm labour, there was a higher risk of preterm delivery in the women randomised to treatment.[32] Although this study specifically excluded multiple pregnancy it is probably not unreasonable to extrapolate these data and to conclude that COX-2-specific NSAIDs are unlikely to be of prophylactic benefit in reducing the risk of preterm delivery in multiple pregnancy.

Progesterone

Progesterone is thought to act in pregnancy to inhibit myometrial contractility by inhibiting the expression of contraction-associated proteins. Progesterone also acts as an anti-inflammatory agent within the uterus, downregulating the synthesis of inflammatory cytokines and prostaglandins. In most animal species the onset of labour is heralded by a withdrawal of progesterone from the maternal circulation. Although such progesterone withdrawal is not seen in humans, it is currently thought that there may be 'functional progesterone withdrawal' mediated by various mechanisms including changes in the expression of progesterone receptor isoforms and their co-factors and interactions between the progesterone receptor and inflammatory mediators leading to a downregulation in progesterone receptor function.[6,7] Two recent studies have suggested that progesterone may reduce the risk of preterm delivery in women at high risk. Da Fonseca et al.[33] showed that daily administration of progesterone to women at high risk of preterm delivery reduced the risk of delivery before 34 weeks of gestation from 18.5% to 2.7%. Meis et al.[34] used weekly injections of 17 α-hydroxyprogesterone caproate in women at high risk of preterm delivery and showed that this reduced the risk of delivery before 32 weeks from 19.6% to 11%. Concern has been raised about the general applicability of the data from these studies, especially the study of Meis et al.,[34] because of the relatively high rates of preterm labour in the cohort studied. Whether or not progesterone supplementation will reduce the risk of preterm delivery in multiple pregnancies is not known. However, there are large multicentre clinical trials currently in progress which should resolve these questions.

Corticosteroid therapy

The value of administering corticosteroids to the mother 24 to seven days before preterm delivery in reducing the risk of neonatal respiratory distress syndrome, intraventricular haemorrhage and necrotising enterocolitis and therefore improving neonatal mortality is established.[35] There is an increase in respiratory distress syndrome in babies born preterm following multiple pregnancy, which is particularly marked in the second twin. The reason for this is currently unproven but it is possible that the increase in respiratory distress syndrome rates in the second twin is a reflection of the increased risk of perinatal hypoxia. Current practice is to use the same dose of dexamethasone or betamethasone in a multiple pregnancy as is used in the singleton. Birkett et al.[36] have demonstrated that the effects of antenatal corticosteroid therapy appear to be suboptimal in multiple pregnancy. This may be due to subtherapeutic maternal plasma corticosteroid levels or to an offsetting of the benefits of corticosteroid therapy by the effects of perinatal hypoxia in second twins, or it may simply be a type II error.[35]

Tocolysis

Atosiban, an oxytocin/arginine vasopressin (AVP) receptor antagonist, and nifedipine, a calcium channel blocker, have generally replaced the use of beta sympathomimetics for tocolysis in the UK because of their vastly improved maternal adverse effect profile. There continues to be controversy as to which of these agents is optimal.[37–39] However, the current evidence is that, whichever tocolytic is used in women in preterm labour with singleton pregnancies, there will be a high placebo response rate (because more than 50% women who experience preterm contractions are not actually in preterm labour) and that the majority of women who are genuinely in preterm labour will not experience any clinically useful delay from the use of tocolysis. The only tocolytic drug which has been shown to have any effect upon any marker of neonatal outcome is nifedipine, which has been shown to reduce the risk of respiratory distress syndrome.[39] There have been several case reports of hypotension associated with the use of nifedipine as a tocolytic, including in twin pregnancy, although often these are cases where very high doses have been used, or where there is doubt that the hypotension was directly caused by nifedipine.[40–42] The majority of studies of tocolytic drugs have excluded multiple pregnancies. There are no good-quality studies of tocolysis in preterm labour in multiple pregnancy and, given the difficulty of mounting such a study in singleton pregnancies, this situation is likely to remain unchanged. At the present time, therefore, tocolytic drugs should probably be used in multiple pregnancies in the same way that they are in singleton pregnancies in the hope of delaying delivery by at least 24 hours to allow *in utero* transfer and administration of corticosteroids. If nifedipine is used there must be intravenous access and close observation of maternal vital signs.

References

1. Pharoah PO, Price TS, Plomin R. Cerebral palsy in twins: a national study. *Arch Dis Child Fetal Neonatal Ed* 2002;87:F122–4.
2. Petterson B, Nelson KB, Watson L, Stanley F. Twins, triplets, and cerebral palsy in births in Western Australia in the 1980s. *BMJ* 1993;307:1239–43.
3. Hartley RS, Emanuel I, Hitti J. Perinatal mortality and neonatal morbidity rates among twin pairs at different gestational ages: optimal delivery timing at 37 to 38 weeks' gestation. *Am J Obstet Gynecol* 2001;184:451–8.
4. Ohel G, Granat M, Zeevi D, Golan A, Wexler S, David MP, et al. Advanced ultrasonic placental maturation in twin pregnancies. *Am J Obstet Gynecol* 1987;156:76–8.
5. Gardner MO, Goldenberg RL, Cliver SP, Tucker JM, Nelson KG, Copper RL. The origin and outcome of preterm twin pregnancies. *Obstet Gynecol* 1995;85:553–7.
6. Mohan AR, Loudon JA, Bennett PR. Molecular and biochemical mechanisms of preterm labour. *Semin Fetal Neonatal Med* 2004;9:437–44.
7. Terzidou V, Bennett PR. Preterm labour. *Curr Opin Obstet Gynecol* 2002;14:105–13.
8. Smith R, Mesiano S, McGrath S. Hormone trajectories leading to human birth. *Regul Pept* 2002;108:159–64.
9. McLean M, Smith R. Corticotrophin-releasing hormone and human parturition. *Reproduction* 2001;121:493–501.
10. Linton EA, Perkins AV, Woods RJ, Eben F, Wolfe CD, Behan DP, et al. Corticotropin releasing hormone-binding protein (CRH-BP): plasma levels decrease during the third trimester of normal human pregnancy. *J Clin Endocrinol Metab* 1993;76:260–2.
11. Gomez R, Romero R, Ghezzi F, Yoon BH, Mazor M, Berry SM. The fetal inflammatory response syndrome. *Am J Obstet Gynecol* 1998;179:194–202.
12. Gennaro S, Hennessy MD. Psychological and physiological stress: impact on preterm birth. *J Obstet Gynecol Neonatal Nurs* 2003;32:668–75.
13. Ou CW, Orsino A, Lye SJ. Expression of connexin-43 and connexin-26 in the rat myometrium during pregnancy and labor is differentially regulated by mechanical and hormonal signals. *Endocrinology* 1997;138:5398–407.
14. Terzidou V, Sooranna SR, Kim LU, Thornton S, Bennett PR, Johnson MR. Mechanical stretch up-regulates the human oxytocin receptor in primary human uterine myocytes. *J Clin Endocrinol Metab* 2005;90:237–46.
15. Creasy RK, Gummer BA, Liggins GC. System for predicting spontaneous preterm birth. *Obstet Gynecol* 1980;55:692–5.

16. Holbrook RH Jr, Laros RK Jr, Creasy RK. Evaluation of a risk-scoring system for prediction of preterm labor. *Am J Perinatol* 1989;6:62–8.

17. Owen J, Iams JD, Hauth JC. Vaginal sonography and cervical incompetence. *Am J Obstet Gynecol* 2003;188:586–96.

18. Honest H, Bachmann LM, Coomarasamy A, Gupta JK, Kleijnen J, Khan KS. Accuracy of cervical transvaginal sonography in predicting preterm birth: a systematic review. *Ultrasound Obstet Gynecol* 2003;22:305–22.

19. Skentou C, Souka AP, To MS, Liao AW, Nicolaides KH. Prediction of preterm delivery in twins by cervical assessment at 23 weeks. *Ultrasound Obstet Gynecol* 2001;17:7–10.

20. Fuchs I, Tsoi E, Henrich W, Dudenhausen JW, Nicolaides KH. Sonographic measurement of cervical length in twin pregnancies in threatened preterm labor. *Ultrasound Obstet Gynecol* 2004;23:42–5.

21. Goldenberg RL, Mercer BM, Meis PJ, Copper RL, Das A, McNellis D. The preterm prediction study: fetal fibronectin testing and spontaneous preterm birth. NICHD Maternal Fetal Medicine Units Network. *Obstet Gynecol* 1996;87(5 Pt 1):643–8.

22. Oliveira TA, Carvalho CM, de Souza E, Mariani-Neto C, Camano L. Detection of fetal fibronectin in twin pregnancies in relation to gestational age. *Sao Paulo Med J* 1999;117:121–4.

23. Oliveira T, de Souza E, Mariani-Neto C, Camano L. Fetal fibronectin as a predictor of preterm delivery in twin gestations. *Int J Gynaecol Obstet* 1998;62:135–9.

24. Wennerholm UB, Holm B, Mattsby-Baltzer I, Nielsen T, Platz-Christensen J, Sundell G, et al. Fetal fibronectin, endotoxin, bacterial vaginosis and cervical length as predictors of preterm birth and neonatal morbidity in twin pregnancies. *Br J Obstet Gynaecol* 1997;104:1398–40.

25. Goldenberg RL, Iams JD, Miodovnik M, van Dorsten JP, Thurnau G, Bottoms S, et al. The preterm prediction study: risk factors in twin gestations. National Institute of Child Health and Human Development Maternal–Fetal Medicine Units Network. *Am J Obstet Gynecol* 1996;175(4 Pt 1):1047–53.

26. Gibson JL, Macara LM, Owen P, Young D, Macauley J, Mackenzie F. Prediction of preterm delivery in twin pregnancy: a prospective, observational study of cervical length and fetal fibronectin testing. *Ultrasound Obstet Gynecol* 2004;23:561–6.

27. Dubois S, Dougherty C, Duquette MP, Hanley JA, Moutquin JM. Twin pregnancy: the impact of the Higgins Nutrition Intervention Program on maternal and neonatal outcomes. *Am J Clin Nutr* 1991;53:1397–403.

28. Crowther CA. Hospitalisation and bed rest for multiple pregnancy. *Cochrane Database Syst Rev* 2001;(1):CD000110.

29. Final report of the Medical Research Council/Royal College of Obstetricians and Gynaecologists multicentre randomised trial of cervical cerclage. MRC/RCOG Working Party on Cervical Cerclage. *Br J Obstet Gynaecol* 1993;100:516–23.

30. Berghella V, Odibo AO, To MS, Rust OA, Althuisius SM. Cerclage for short cervix on ultrasonography: meta-analysis of trials using individual patient-level data. *Obstet Gynecol* 2005;106:181–9.

31. King J, Flenady V, Cole S, Thornton S. Cyclo-oxygenase (COX) inhibitors for treating preterm labour. *Cochrane Database Syst Rev* 2005;(2):CD001992.

32. Groom KM, Shennan AH, Jones BA, Seed P, Bennett PR. TOCOX – a randomised, double-blind, placebo-controlled trial of rofecoxib (a COX-2-specific prostaglandin inhibitor) for the prevention of preterm delivery in women at high risk. *BJOG* 2005;112:725–30.

33. da Fonseca EB, Bittar RE, Carvalho MH, Zugaib M. Prophylactic administration of progesterone by vaginal suppository to reduce the incidence of spontaneous preterm birth in women at increased risk: a randomized placebo-controlled double-blind study. *Am J Obstet Gynecol* 2003;188:419–24.

34. Meis PJ, Klebanoff M, Thom E, Dombrowski MP, Sibai B, Moawad AH, et al.; National Institute of Child Health and Human Development Maternal–Fetal Medicine Units Network. Prevention of recurrent preterm delivery by 17 alpha-hydroxyprogesterone caproate. *N Engl J Med* 2003;348:2379–85. Erratum in: *N Engl J Med* 2003;349:1299.

35. Crowley P. Antenatal corticosteroids – current thinking. *BJOG* 2003;110 Suppl 20:77–8.

36. Birkett G, Bauer CR, Morrison JC, Curet LB. Effect of prenatal dexamethasone administration upon respiratory distress syndrome in twin pregnancies. *J Perinatol* 1986;6:304–8.

37. Papatsonis D, Flenady V, Cole S, Liley H. Oxytocin receptor antagonists for inhibiting preterm labour. *Cochrane Database Syst Rev* 2005;(3):CD004452.

38. King JF, Flenady VJ, Papatsonis DN, Dekker GA, Carbonne B. Calcium channel blockers for inhibiting preterm labour. *Cochrane Database Syst Rev* 2003;(1):CD002255.

39. Coomarasamy A, Knox EM, Gee H, Song F, Khan KS. Effectiveness of nifedipine versus atosiban

for tocolysis in preterm labour: a meta-analysis with an indirect comparison of randomised trials. *BJOG* 2003;110:1045–9.

40.   van Veen AJ, Pelinck MJ, van Pampus MG, Erwich JJHM. Severe hypotension and fetal death due to tocolysis with nifedipine. *BJOG* 2005;112:509–10.

41.   Papatsonis DNM, van Geijn HP, Bleker OP, Adèr HJ, Dekker GA. Hemodynamic and metabolic effects after nifedipine and ritodrine tocolysis. *Int J Gynecol Obstet* 2003;82:5–10.

42.   Papatsonis DNM, Carbonne B, Dekker GA, Flenady V, King JF. Severe hypotension and fetal death due to tocolysis with nifedipine. *BJOG* 2005;112:1582–3.

Chapter 8

Twin clinics: a model for antenatal care in multiple gestations

Andrew Carlin and James P Neilson

Introduction

Multiple pregnancy is a high-risk situation for both the mother and the fetuses. Adverse perinatal outcomes occur more frequently, with prematurity as the main cause and important contributions from intrauterine growth restriction (IUGR), malformation and twin-to-twin transfusion syndrome (TTTS). Cerebral palsy is also a significant problem, with a six-fold increased risk in twins and up to 24 times greater risk in triplets, with aetiologies not restricted to prematurity.[2]

Maternal mortality is more than double that of singleton gestations, mainly owing to the increase in pre-eclampsia and haemorrhage.[3] Up to 25% of multiple pregnancies are complicated by pregnancy-induced hypertension[4] and the incidence of gestational diabetes is 2–3 times that seen in singletons. The risk of pre-eclampsia with a twin pregnancy increases almost three-fold (relative risk 2.90, 95% CI 1.70–4.93), independently of chorionicity, and triplet pregnancy carries in turn a three-fold increased risk compared with twin pregnancy (RR 2.83, 95% CI 1.25–6.40).[5] Antepartum and postpartum haemorrhage, operative delivery and urinary tract infection are all more common and can lead to serious maternal morbidity or even mortality.

Maternal risks are all too often overshadowed by fetal considerations and this appears to be reflected in the medical literature, with only one study from the developed world that directly addresses the association between multiple pregnancy and maternal mortality.[6]

Rationale for the role of specialised care/specialised clinics

Evidence

Logic suggests that women with high-risk pregnancies should receive care in specialised clinics run by appropriately skilled healthcare professionals. However, there is only limited evidence for the benefits of such clinics. Special twin management protocols may improve outcome[7,8] but attendance at dedicated clinics has yet to be proven beneficial. The proposed advantages of specialised clinics are to:

- promote evidenced-based practices

- concentrate knowledge and skills, e.g. prenatal diagnosis and screening and dedicated and experienced sonography staff
- encourage a multidisciplinary approach to multiple pregnancies, with doctors (obstetric, anaesthetic and neonatal), midwives, counsellors and sonographers all within a dedicated clinic
- provide antenatal classes that address the specific needs of women with multiple pregnancies
- provide a continuity of care that is difficult to achieve in smaller units
- offer a good chance of delivery within the unit – tertiary fetal medicine centres usually have excellent neonatal support
- provide seamless transition into postnatal care
- have well-established links to independent support agencies
- provide opportunities for clinical research, including efficient recruitment into clinical trials.

To achieve all of the above in smaller units is difficult but not impossible, and one solution would be to have a named consultant with a special interest in fetal medicine coordinating patient care. Complications such as TTTS are uncommon in the general twin population; we see only 10–12 cases per year (including intra- and extra-regional referrals) at our unit, where the annual delivery rate is 8000 (with around 130 women with twin pregnancies). In less experienced hands, some of the subtle nuances of this condition may be overlooked, resulting in delays in diagnosis and appropriate action.

Early discordant IUGR can also be very complex to manage, when the needs (sometimes conflicting) of two or more fetuses must be considered together rather than in isolation as with singleton pregnancies.

We established a twin clinic in 1995 at Liverpool Women's Hospital. Women are referred directly by the sonographers who perform booking scans. Twenty-six percent of the women have a declared history of treatment for infertility.

Role of the midwife

The specialist midwife can provide a comprehensive package of care within the multiple pregnancy clinic, ensuring an individualised approach to each woman's needs, as well as continuity of care.

Special antenatal classes tackle all the usual aspects of antenatal education but also focus on the impact of multiple gestations, both during and after the pregnancy, providing a robust package that traditional parentcraft would struggle to achieve. Public health issues such as lifestyle, diet, sex, smoking and work are discussed and visits to the neonatal intensive care unit are arranged to lessen the emotional distress caused by unexpected admissions after delivery.

Awareness of the risks of multiple pregnancy lead to a certain level of anxiety in most patients and thus much emphasis is placed on providing a better understanding of the problems encountered antenatally, through to delivery, and the problems of caring for and supporting more than one child. The specialist midwife's role in this setting is to educate both individually and within groups, provide links with community midwifery and social support networks, and facilitate contacts with the various multiple pregnancy support groups such as the Twins and Multiple Births Association (TAMBA). In Liverpool we have an active local Twins Club whose members assist at antenatal classes to provide joint parent education sessions. These women provide a unique insight into multiple pregnancy, perfectly complementing the specialist midwives' own skills and experiences.

Role of the obstetrician

The obstetrician's role is to manage the complications of multiple pregnancy. Women may have pre-existing medical problems or develop conditions as a result of the pregnancy, such as pre-eclampsia and gestational diabetes. Other issues including prenatal diagnosis and counselling, malformations, growth restriction and TTTS must be coordinated by the lead clinician within the clinic.

Ideally, the clinician should be ultrasound-trained to tertiary level, thus offering a complete suite of imaging options such as nuchal translucency, recognition of TTTS, identification of structural and karyotypical abnormalities, and invasive testing and procedures such as amnioreduction or cord occlusion.

Serial growth scans of uncomplicated pregnancies will still be carried out by experienced sonographers with the clinician on hand to interpret and manage potential problems such as growth restriction. The obstetrician will also coordinate the management of medical disorders by effective liaison with the local obstetric medical clinic.

Obstetricians should be actively engaged in intrapartum care and experienced in surgical skills such as cervical cerclage and higher order operative deliveries. In our unit every effort is made to allow the obstetricians to personally manage such procedures, ensuring good continuity.

A proposed model for antenatal care in multiple pregnancy, for each trimester, is discussed below.

First trimester

Early routine ultrasound

The Royal College of Obstetricians and Gynaecologists (RCOG) recommends routine early ultrasound[9] although there is no evidence that it improves perinatal outcome. However, the policy does reduce post-term inductions by up to 70%.[10] An early scan, if performed in the first trimester, provides accurate dating, which is very useful in the management of growth restriction and prematurity. Coincidentally, it also reveals multiple pregnancies, which may benefit from more specialist care.

In multiple pregnancies the dating scan also determines fetal number, amnionicity and chorionicity[11] and is ideally performed in the first trimester when accuracy for chorionicity approaches 100%.[12] Many multiple pregnancies are induced prior to term and thus accurate dating is essential to prevent iatrogenic prematurity.

Early determination of chorionicity is important for several reasons, as discussed below.

Risk stratification and counselling

Monochorionic (MC) twins have increased risks of late miscarriage, perinatal mortality and genetic and structural abnormalities. Ten to 15 percent will develop TTTS, which results in up to 80% loss rates if left untreated. TTTS has also been reported in higher order pregnancies.[13–15]

Because of the risk of TTTS, MC pregnancies are managed more intensively than their dichorionic (DC) equivalents and are usually reviewed ultrasonographically from as early as 16 weeks to detect clinical disease, although discordant nuchal translucency at 11–14 weeks may be the earliest sign of this problem.[16]

One percent of MC pregnancies are also monoamniotic, which is associated with an extreme risk of perinatal mortality due to cord entanglement. Prenatal diagnosis, intensive surveillance and aggressive management of monoamniotic pregnancies has demonstrated an improved outcome.[17,18]

Knowledge of chorionicity promotes a full and open discussion about the specific risks associated with MC placentations and guides prenatal diagnosis and subsequent pregnancy management.

Multifetal pregnancy reduction

Higher order pregnancies are associated with increased risks for both the mother and the infants, and thus selective fetal reduction using intracardiac potassium chloride has been advocated in these circumstances.[19] A systematic review suggested pregnancy reduction to twins achieved outcomes comparable with those twin pregnancies conceived spontaneously or secondary to assisted reproduction.[20] However, no randomised controlled trials (RCTs) have assessed multifetal pregnancy reduction (MFPR) and this is likely to remain the case owing to anticipated recruitment problems.

For those wishing to embark on MFPR, the ultrasound-guided procedure is usually performed at 11–12 weeks by intrathoracic potassium chloride, after the main risk of miscarriage. Those fetuses with the largest nuchal translucencies or suspicious ultrasound features are selected for termination. The pregnancy is reduced to twins in most cases, as miscarriage rates are lowest when two fetuses are left alive.[21]

As experience with MFPR has improved, miscarriage rates post procedure have fallen to below those of unreduced pregnancies.[22]

Implications for selective termination

The presence of discordant abnormalities or higher order pregnancies may lead to discussions about selective termination. The preferred method in singletons and DC pregnancies is intracardiac potassium chloride, although for lethal anomalies, expectant management should be considered in view of the 5–10% risk of loss of the healthy twin if the selective termination is performed in the first or second trimester. The situation is more complicated in MC placentations as the numerous vascular connections between the fetuses make the use of potassium undesirable. In such cases, fetal reduction techniques must occlude all the cord vessels to avoid damage in or death of the co-twin. The method of cord occlusion is dependent upon gestation, with the best success rates being achieved by endoscopic or interstitial laser in the first trimester and ultrasound-guided bipolar diathermy thereafter.

However, despite all the apparent advantages of early diagnosis, knowledge of chorionicity has not yet been proven in prospective clinical trials to improve outcome.

Education

Once the diagnosis of multiple pregnancy is confirmed, early referral to a specialist clinic is arranged and adequate folate supplementation ensured. Where the pregnancy is at borderline gestation for nuchal translucency, i.e. approaching 14 weeks, every effort must be made to ensure that the woman is seen while this is still possible.

The first visit should focus on the unique nature of the pregnancy and the differences compared with singleton gestations. Initial discussions include:

- the importance of chorionicity and its implications
- prenatal screening and diagnosis
- an individualised scanning schedule
- specific risks of multiple pregnancy, with emphasis on preterm labour.

Discussions should be open and relaxed, with care taken to present the positive aspects of the pregnancy. Ideally, the patient will meet all members of the clinic team during the first few attendances, and later visits in conjunction with special antenatal classes should address all the issues relevant to the pregnancy, delivery and postnatal period.

The specific roles of the midwives and obstetricians have already been discussed.

Nutritional advice

The literature on the importance of adequate nutrition in pregnancy is primarily focused on singleton gestations and data are not easily extrapolated to multiple pregnancies. It is, however, important to remember that pre-existing nutritional deficiencies are more likely to be exacerbated by multiple gestations and these may contribute to any complications that may develop.[23,24]

Iron deficiency is associated with increased maternal mortality and reduced immunity, while neonatal effects include premature birth, lower birthweight and delayed psychomotor development.[25] Despite this, routine iron supplementation is not recommended in normal pregnancy as this practice is unproven and associated with unpleasant adverse effects.[26]

Moderate to severe anaemia occurs more frequently in developing countries and has been associated with adverse outcomes for both mother and fetus. However, a Cochrane review[27] suggested that routine iron supplementation has no detectable effect on any substantive measures of either maternal or fetal outcome. Routine oral iron supplementation for pregnant women in the industrialised world thus remains a controversial issue,[28] and the situation in multiple pregnancies is even less clear. Some units offer supplements only on the basis of documented deficiencies while others advocate routine oral iron from the second trimester onwards. Our unit prefers the latter approach in combination with folic acid throughout the pregnancy as the requirements for the latter during normal pregnancy increase 20- to 30-fold and it also improves utilisation of iron.[29] We also continue to monitor haemoglobin levels in the second and third trimesters in order to ensure adequate levels prior to delivery.

Nutritional status may also play a significant role in postnatal depressive illness. The depletion of nutrient reserves throughout pregnancy and the lack of recovery postnatally may increase a woman's risk of depression.[30]

Prenatal diagnosis

It is assumed that structural malformations are more common in multiple pregnancies and in general twins have a two- to three-fold greater risk than singletons, mainly because of the higher incidence of abnormalities (about 50%) in monozygotic twins compared with dizygotic twins.[31,32] Monozygotic pregnancies are associated with an increased risk of malformation owing to the unusual nature of the cleavage of the conceptus that generates monozygotic twins. There is however, little evidence for increased risks in dizygotic twins.

Screening

Serum screening for Down syndrome in multiple pregnancies has a poor detection rate. It also poses problems relating to the identification of which fetus is at higher risk. There is no strong evidence that multiple pregnancies are at increased risk of chromosomal aneuploidy. The complexities of screening in multiple gestations can be considerable and this is therefore best managed by experienced practitioners.

Monochorionic (i.e. monozygotic) twins have identical karyotypes, which makes the risk of aneuploidy the same as the maternal age related risk. In dizygotic twins, each fetus has its own independent risk of chromosomal abnormality and thus the risk is additive.

Nuchal translucency

Because of the limitations of serum screening, nuchal translucency (NT) should be offered as a more accurate alternative. Its efficacy in singletons is well established, with detection rates of 75% for Down syndrome for a false positive rate of 5%.[33]

The sensitivity of NT for detecting Down syndrome in DC twins is similar to that in singleton pregnancies.[34] However, false positive rates are higher in MC twins because approximately 8% of euploid MC fetuses have increased NT. In some cases this increase may reflect early cardiovascular compromise related to TTTS. A discordant NT greater than the 95th centile in MC twins increases the risk of TTTS four-fold.[35]

Recent data suggest that in MC twins effective screening for trisomy 21 is best provided by using the average NT measured in the two fetuses.[36]

Invasive testing

Invasive techniques such as amniocentesis and chorionic villus sampling (CVS) are now commonly performed in multiple pregnancies. Because of the possibility of discordant anomalies, even in MC pregnancies, and the management difficulties that may follow, the RCOG recommends that such testing should only be performed in specialist centres.[37]

Each fetus should ideally be tested individually, as even genetically identical MC twins can have post-zygotic mutations.[38]

Documentation is extremely important in the context of invasive testing. Careful fetal mapping before the test and accurate sample labelling should avoid disastrous errors. To improve on this aspect of risk management, it is now our practice to have two trained doctors present at all invasive testing procedures on multiple pregnancies.

In the estimation of procedural loss rates for amniocentesis and CVS, consideration of the higher background loss rates of multiple pregnancies is required. When this is taken into account the outcomes appear to be similar to that of singletons for amniocentesis,[39,40] although the data for CVS are less robust.

Second trimester

Serum α-fetoprotein

Although serum screening for the detection of Down syndrome and other aneuploidies is less sensitive in multiple pregnancies, maternal α-fetoprotein (AFP) measurements can provide a reasonable screen for neural tube, abdominal wall and renal defects and this test is therefore offered routinely to women attending our multiple pregnancy clinic. A correction factor needs to be applied to allow for the presence of more than one fetus and this is reflected in an MoM (multiples of the median) cut-off for normality in multiple pregnancies. Twins have twice the level of maternal AFP, triplets three times and quadruplets four times.[41] A meta-analysis of published studies gave twin median MoM levels of 2.18 on 1638 unaffected twin pregnancies.[42] As in singleton pregnancies, it can also be a potential marker of poor outcome.[43]

Anatomy scans

Multiple pregnancies are at increased risk of structural abnormalities, mainly owing to the contribution of monozygotic gestations with an overall prevalence of 1.2–2.0 times higher than in singletons.[44] Defects may be concordant or discordant but 80–90% are discordant regardless of zygosity.

Scanning schedules

Estimates vary but approximately 25–33% of infants born of multiple pregnancies are small for gestational age by standard definitions. This is more common in MC pregnancies and is associated with increased perinatal mortality and morbidity.[45,46] MC pregnancies also have the unique risk of TTTS and scanning schedules should be adjusted accordingly.

In twin pregnancies, a cervical length of less than 25 mm at 23 weeks of gestation is associated with an increased risk of early (before 32 weeks) spontaneous preterm delivery (OR 6.9, 95% CI 2.0–24.2). Because of the current lack of effective interventions,[47] we do not routinely perform cervical assessments in twin pregnancies. However, in view of the significantly increased risk of preterm delivery and the lack of data concerning reactive cervical cerclage in higher order pregnancies, it is our practice to screen and surgically treat cervical shortening in this small group of patients. Prophylactic cerclage, i.e. routine practice not based on cervical assessment, has not been shown to be helpful in triplet pregnancies.[48]

The role of uterine artery Doppler in twin pregnancies has been established.[49,50] It provides a useful screen for pre-eclampsia or growth restriction but at lower sensitivities than for singleton pregnancies.

As multiple pregnancies are already subjected to close fetal and maternal surveillance, and in the absence of proven interventions for either condition, it is difficult to argue for the routine inclusion of uterine artery Doppler assessments at 22–24 weeks in all patients.

Monochorionic twins

Ten percent to 15% of MC twins will develop TTTS and this may be detected ultrasonographically prior to 18–20 weeks, when most routine anatomy scans are performed. Early TTTS can therefore be missed along with opportunities for prompt treatment, although there is little evidence to guide the timing of first intervention. Nonetheless, most units begin their MC serial scans at around 16 weeks and this is our practice.

It may be useful during the course of this scan to establish the presence or absence of superficial arterio-arterial (AA) anastomoses along the chorionic plate using colour flow Doppler. Some authorities use a modified Quintero[51] staging system for classification of TTTS based on AA anastomoses, arguing that it improves prognostication and aids selection of treatment.[52] Larger studies are required before this practice is universally accepted.

Because of the reportedly higher risk of congenital cardiac disease in MC pregnancies,[53] cardiac echo should be offered at 22–23 weeks.

A suggested scanning schedule for MC twins is outlined below:

- 16 weeks: twin clinic (trained medical staff) assessment to detect early TTTS
- 19 weeks: twin clinic growth, liquor and anatomy scan
- 22 weeks: twin clinic completion of anatomy scan with fetal cardiac echo, growth and liquor.

The median gestational age for the development of TTTS is 21 weeks and thus if there is no evidence of TTTS by 22 weeks then further scans are performed by experienced sonographers at 25, 28, 31, 33 and 36 weeks for growth, liquor and umbilical artery Doppler.

Where there is even minor liquor discordance, scans should be performed more frequently. In most units, the frequency of serial scans varies from every two to every four weeks, while in others growth scans are alternated with assessments of liquor, bladder dynamics and umbilical artery Doppler.

There are currently no data to guide the optimal frequency of ultrasound assessment of fetal growth in multiple pregnancies. However, the addition of umbilical artery Doppler to serial growth scans is of proven benefit.[54,55]

Dichorionic twins

Unlike MC pregnancies, TTTS is not an issue in DC twins and thus scanning schedules are less intensive, with the main emphasis being on the early detection of fetal growth restriction. A suggested scanning schedule for DC twins is outlined below:

- 20 weeks: anatomy and baseline biometry
- 24 weeks: growth, liquor and umbilical artery Doppler
- 27, 30, 33 and 36 weeks: growth, liquor and umbilical artery Doppler.

Higher order multiples

In our unit triplets and quadruplets have intensive two-weekly ultrasound surveillance from 16 weeks of gestation onwards. All scans are performed by experienced medical staff within the multiple pregnancy clinic. These pregnancies also have routine cervical assessment from 20 weeks and cerclage is offered if significant cervical shortening is demonstrated on transvaginal ultrasound. Progressive changes in cervical length may be more important than the absolute measurement. Cerclage remains unproven in higher order pregnancies.

Preterm labour – prediction

Preterm labour is the most important fetal complication of multiple pregnancy, yet the optimal methods for prediction and prevention remain the subject of continuing debate. The aetiology of preterm labour is probably multifactorial with the most effective predictor being a previous preterm delivery, although this is not helpful in primigravidae.

Preterm labour is more common in multiple gestations, where the risk of delivery prior to 32 weeks of gestation is eight times that of singletons, with increasing risks for higher order multiples.

Cervical assessment

A mean cervical length of less than 25 mm (compared with 15 mm in singletons) is a good predictor of pregnancies destined to deliver before 32 weeks of gestation (OR 6.9, 95% CI 2.0–24.2).[56] Sensitivity falls away with increasing gestation but the vast majority of fetuses born after 32 weeks will survive with few complications. Transvaginal ultrasound is the gold standard and provides information about the state of the internal os, i.e. funnelling, and overall cervical length. It is easy to do and well tolerated by most women although the ideal frequency of assessment is unclear.

In the absence of proven and effective interventions in higher risk cases, it is difficult to justify routine cervical assessments in all twin pregnancies, particularly in the light of recent evidence which suggests that prophylactic cerclage may actually increase the risk of preterm delivery.[57]

In our unit we do not perform routine cervical assessment in twin pregnancies, but do offer screening of higher order multiples form 20 weeks, aggressively treating progressive shortening with cervical cerclage.

Fetal fibronectin

The presence of fetal fibronectin (f FN) in vaginal secretions in multiple pregnancies is less predictive of preterm delivery than in singletons, with only 50% of deliveries before 35 weeks of gestation detected at 28 weeks compared with 80–90% in mixed populations.[58,59] The value of the information derived has yet to be proved beneficial in guiding effective interventions to either reduce preterm delivery or improve fetal outcome. We do not currently recommend routine f FN assessment.

Stress and depression

Multiple pregnancy has been a neglected model for the study of the causes of and prevention of preterm birth. Our multiple pregnancy clinic has hosted a research project assessing the possible effects of depression and stress on preterm labour. It is recognised that clinical depression is not uncommon during pregnancy.[60] There are many animal studies that demonstrate a link between preterm birth and chronic stress. There are large epidemiological studies in humans that indicate a dose–response relation between psychological distress and preterm birth (in singleton pregnancies).[61] There are plausible biological models that may explain these links. For example, severely stressful life events, in the absence of clinical depression, may cause prolonged hypercortisolaemia. Depression is also associated with hypothalamic–pituitary–adrenal dysregulation. Cortisol stimulates rather than inhibits production of placental corticotrophin-releasing hormone (CRH). CRH levels are known to be elevated in both twin and singleton pregnancies before preterm labour.

This project is not yet complete but preliminary results indicate that the risk of preterm labour in twins is increased in the presence of subclinical depression and that the risks are also increased in women experiencing stressful life events and difficulties. Overall, the prevalence of subclinical and clinical anxiety in women with twin pregnancies is even higher than in women attending a colposcopy clinic for the first time. If these findings are confirmed on full analysis, they may have important implications for risk prediction and for developing preventative strategies.

Preterm delivery – prevention

Routine admission and bed rest

Routine admission paradoxically increases the risk of preterm delivery in twin pregnancies.[62] The situation in higher order pregnancies is less clear, with a single small RCT involving only 19 women suggesting a non-significant trend towards prolonged gestation and improved neonatal outcome.[63]

We have admitted women with quadruplet pregnancies in the second trimester because of the increased risk of preterm delivery and rapid access to high-quality neonatal intensive care facilities. The presence of such women as in-patients also allows us to minimise the risks of *in utero* transfer by advance planning and a close working relationship with our neonatal colleagues.

Home uterine activity monitoring

Some authorities advocate home uterine activity monitoring (HUAM) as a method of early detection of preterm labour to allow prompt treatment with antenatal corticosteroids and tocolysis.[64,65] A single small RCT[64] involving 45 women suggested a reduction in preterm delivery but this was contradicted by another study which not only increased the risk but also the frequency of antenatal visits and tocolytic use without apparent benefit.[65] In view of the conflicting data we do not support the routine use of HUAM.

Pharmacology

- **Prophylactic tocolysis:**
  There is very little evidence that prophylactic or emergency tocolysis are of any benefit in improving fetal outcome. A systematic review and a meta-analysis[66] has failed to demonstrate a significant reduction in preterm delivery or improved outcome and thus routine use is not recommended.

- **Antibiotics:**
  A recent systematic review has reported that the use of antibiotics to prevent preterm labour is not justified.[67] The outcome of this review might have been different had it included two RCTs published one month later, which showed a reduction in preterm delivery of 60% using clindamycin in low-risk unselected populations.[68,69] A prospective trial[70] assessing routine infection screening demonstrated reductions in preterm delivery but as multiple pregnancies were excluded from this study it is difficult to recommend this practice for all our patients.

- **Progesterone:**
  17-Hydroxyprogesterone is an effective treatment for the prevention of preterm delivery in those women with a history of spontaneous preterm delivery.[71,72] As there is no evidence to support its use as a tocolytic in multiple pregnancy, it cannot at present be recommended for this purpose. There are, however, clinical trials under way in Scotland and Denmark that should address this question.

Third trimester

Fetal monitoring – cardiotocography

Routine weekly cardiotocography (CTG) or biophysical assessment have not been prospectively assessed in multiple pregnancies. However, both of these methods are as reliable as in singleton pregnancies in identifying those fetuses at risk of hypoxic injury. A single retrospective study involving 665 twins compared a policy of third-trimester non-stress testing (NST) with no NST and found no statistically significant differences, although there was only one stillbirth in the monitored group compared with nine in those managed conservatively.[73]

It is our practice to monitor multiple pregnancies by weekly CTG at 36 weeks of gestation and beyond because of the increasing risk of stillbirth towards term. It is critically important that the traces are visually inspected to ensure that they come from different babies. Differing quantitative indices on computerised CTG readouts do not necessarily provide this reassurance.

Timing of delivery

Perinatal mortality rates in multiple pregnancies begin to rise at 39 weeks of gestation, with the intrauterine death rate surpassing that of singletons at 42 weeks.[74] A single randomised trial from Japan comparing expectant management with induction of labour at 37 weeks in twin pregnancies failed to demonstrate any differences between the two groups but was underpowered to detect differences in neonatal outcome.[75] In a study of 8150 twin pregnancies[76] the optimal timing of delivery was found to be 37–38 weeks, with the recommendation that twin pregnancies should not be allowed to go beyond 39 weeks. This view is opposed by a recent Cochrane review, which found no strong evidence to support this practice.[77] A large multicentre RCT, coordinated by the Maternal and Perinatal Clinical Trials Unit at the University of Adelaide, may clarify this important issue.

In our unit we continue to offer elective delivery after 37 weeks for uncomplicated DC or MC pregnancies. The very small risk of TTTS in labour does not, in our opinion, warrant elective caesarean section for all MC pregnancies.

The optimal mode of delivery of twins is a controversial issue.[78] Of those pregnancies where an attempt at vaginal delivery is made, 30–40% result in caesarean section and there is also a 7% risk of having to deliver the second twin by caesarean section.[79] A large retrospective study found an increased perinatal mortality in vaginally delivered second twins.[80] Further information is required and a large multicentre randomised trial (the Twin Birth Study) coordinated by the Maternal, Infant and Reproductive Health Research Unit in Toronto is currently addressing this issue.

There are merits in performing an ultrasound examination before caesarean section to check viability of both babies.

Delivery of higher order multiple is more complex than delivery of twins, and the vast majority of larger centres prefer the caesarean route. Cord prolapse, abruption, problems with achieving adequate monitoring, lower Apgar scores and higher perinatal death rates are all issues which make caesarean a more attractive option. Despite this, some studies have reported good outcomes for vaginally born triplets.[81,82] In our unit higher order pregnancies are delivered electively by caesarean section, as has been documented to occur in over 90% of triplets in Europe and the USA.[83]

Although intrapartum management of multiple pregnancies is beyond the scope of this article, our unit follows standard protocols in the absence of randomised data to inform practice.

Special circumstances

Monoamniotic pregnancies

Approximately 1–2% of MC pregnancies are monoamniotic and they are associated with high perinatal mortality owing to the complications of cord entanglement.[84] Historical studies quote stillbirth rates of 30–70%[85,86] but newer series are more optimistic with mortality rates of 10–15%.[18,87] Because of the rarity of the condition, optimal management has yet to be established and the current literature provides limited guidance regarding appropriate antepartum fetal surveillance and timing and mode of delivery.

Two recent publications advocate intensive in-patient monitoring and elective preterm delivery, suggesting that this lowers perinatal losses,[88,89] although caution should be exercised in interpreting this retrospectively collected data. Such intensive monitoring may reveal signs of cord compression but will not always prevent sudden death.[18]

Medical amnioreduction has been used to reduce the risk of cord complications,[90,91] but owing to the potential complications of sulindac, the most commonly used nonsteroidal anti-inflammatory drug (NSAID), it is recommended that this only be used in the context of clinical trials.

Most monoamniotic pregnancies are delivered by caesarean section but successful vaginal deliveries have been reported.[92,93] Timing of delivery remains controversial with some studies supporting elective preterm birth[17,88,89,91,94] but others holding out until term.[92]

Currently, there is no prospective evidence to guide the management of these high-risk pregnancies but a combination of routine intensive fetal monitoring using computerised fetal heart rate analysis, ultrasound and colour flow/power Doppler from 25 to 26 weeks of gestation with planned elective delivery at 32–33 weeks, following administration of steroids, seems a reasonable approach.

Twin reversed arterial perfusion

Twin reversed arterial perfusion (TRAP) sequence occurs in approximately 1% of MC twins. Because of the rarity of this condition, clinical management is based on case series (rather than RCTs) that recommend increased fetal surveillance with intervention being triggered by hydrops or polyhydramnios.[95,96] The perfused twin cannot survive, while mortality for the donor ranges from 50% to 70%.[97,98] TRAP is discussed in more detail in Chapter 13.

Death of a co-twin

Single fetal death occurs in 2–7% of spontaneous pregnancies and in up to 25% of pregnancies from assisted reproduction techniques (ART) most commonly in the first trimester.[99] The greater loss rates seen in latter group is attributed to the inherent fragility of pregnancies resulting from ART and the increased frequency of higher order multiples. The consequences of fetal loss after the first trimester are more severe in MC pregnancies, with stillbirth and neurological abnormality rates of 10% and 20%, respectively.[100] Neurological injuries probably result from either profound hypotension or thrombosis that occurs at the time of demise of the co-twin and is unlikely to be altered by immediate delivery, regardless of gestation. For both MC and DC pregnancies, death of a co-twin increases the risks of growth restriction, preterm delivery and perinatal mortality[101] (see Chapter 10).

Management depends on chorionicity, gestation and time since death. A conservative policy of increased surveillance with delivery at 37 weeks is recommended in DC pregnancies,[102] but optimal care in MC pregnancies has not been determined.

Patients should be appropriately counselled about the risks of long-term sequelae and follow-up with ultrasound of the fetal brain should be offered, with magnetic resonance imaging (MRI) in the event of abnormality.

Concerns surrounding maternal coagulopathy seem to have been grossly exaggerated and need play no role in the decision-making process.

Twin-to-twin transfusion syndrome

TTTS occurs in approximately 10–15% of MC pregnancies, most commonly presenting in the second trimester with discordant liquor volumes and biometry. If untreated, perinatal mortality can exceed 80%. The pathophysiology relates to unbalanced vascular connections within the placenta and a paucity of protective superficial AA anastomoses.

Until recently, optimal therapy for TTTS was controversial. The traditional treatment was amnioreduction, which reduces the risk of preterm delivery but does not address the underlying disease processes. Endoscopic laser ablation is now the treatment of choice for severe TTTS, with similar success rates to amnioreduction but significantly better neurological outcomes.[103] We have moved to laser ablation for severe TTTS, but are not yet convinced that the advantages outweigh the disadvantages in mild TTTS.

TTTS is discussed in more detail in Chapter 12.

Summary

Multiple pregnancies are of high risk for both mother and fetuses and we believe that these sometimes complex pregnancies are best managed on an individual basis by a multidisciplinary team within a specialist clinic. Each member of the team has an important role to play in order to maximise maternal and fetal outcomes.

Our proposed model of care incorporates much of what is routine practice at the Liverpool Women's Hospital Multiple Pregnancy Clinic, in addition to more controversial issues. It is certainly not definitive but merely aims to blend evidence-based practice – where available – with an element of pragmatism, and we hope that it stimulates positive discussion and debate.

Acknowledgements

We thank Lorna Wood, specialist midwife at the Multiple Pregnancy Clinic, for her thoughts about the role of the midwife, and Dr David Owen, who leads the psychosocial stress/depression preterm labour research project.

References

1. Petterson B, Blair E, Watson L, Stanley F. Adverse outcome after multiple pregnancy. *Baillieres Clin Obstet Gynaecol* 1998;12:1–17.
2. Pharoah PO, Cooke T. Cerebral palsy and multiple births. *Arch Dis Child Fetal Neonatal Ed* 1996;75:F174–7.
3. Lewis G, editor. *Why Mothers Die 2000–2002. Report on Confidential Enquiries into Maternal Deaths in the United Kingdom.* 8th ed. London: RCOG Press; 2004.
4. Long PA, Oats JN. Preeclampsia in twin pregnancy – severity and pathogenesis. *Aust N Z J Obstet Gynaecol* 1987;27:1–5.
5. Duckitt K, Harrington D. Risk factors for pre-eclampsia at antenatal booking: systematic review of controlled studies. *BMJ* 2005;330:565.
6. Senat MV, Ancel PY, Bouvier-Colle MH, Breart G. How does multiple pregnancy affect maternal mortality and morbidity? *Clin Obstet Gynecol* 1998;41:78–83.
7. Vergani P, Ghidini A, Bozzo G, Sirtori M. Prenatal management of twin gestation. Experience with a new protocol. *J Reprod Med* 1991;36:667–71.
8. Luke B, Brown MB, Misiunas R, Anderson E, Nugent C, van de Ven C, *et al.* Specialized prenatal care and maternal and infant outcomes in twin pregnancy. *Am J Obstet Gynecol* 2003;189:934–8.
9. Royal College of Obstetricians and Gynaecologists. *Ultrasound Screening for Fetal Abnormalities.* Report of the RCOG Working Party. London: RCOG Press; 2000.
10. Neilson JP. Ultrasound for fetal assessment in early pregnancy. *Cochrane Database Syst Rev* 2000;(2):CD000182.
11. Mahony BS, Filly RA, Callen PW. Amnionicity and chorionicity in twin pregnancies: prediction using ultrasound. *Radiology* 1985;155:205–9.
12. Sepulveda W. Chorionicity determination in twin pregnancies: double trouble. *Ultrasound Obstet Gynecol* 1997;10:79–81.
13. Berg C, Baschat AA, Geipel A, Germer U, Smrcek J, Krapp M, *et al.* First trimester twin-to-twin transfusion syndrome in a trichorionic quadruplet pregnancy – a diagnostic challenge. *Fetal Diagn Ther* 2002;17:357–61.
14. Giles W, O'Callaghan S, Cole S, Bisits A. Triplet pregnancy complicated by feto-feto-fetal transfusion with very rapid deterioration and fetal demise in all three triplets. *Aust N Z J Obstet Gynaecol* 2002;42:408–9.
15. Van Schoubroeck D, Lewi L, Ryan G, Carreras E, Jani J, Higueras T, *et al.* Fetoscopic surgery in triplet pregnancies: a multicenter case series. *Am J Obstet Gynecol* 2004;191:1529–32.
16. Nicolaides K, Sebire N, Snijders RJ. *The 11-14 Weeks Scan: the Diagnosis of Fetal Abnormalities.* New York: The Parthenon Publishing Group; 1999.
17. Rodis JF, McIlveen PF, Egan JF, Borgida AF, Turner GW, Campbell WA. Monoamniotic twins: improved perinatal survival with accurate prenatal diagnosis and antenatal fetal surveillance. *Am J Obstet Gynecol* 1997;177:1046–9.
18. Beasley E, Megerian G, Gerson A, Roberts NS. Monoamniotic twins: case series and proposal for antenatal management. *Obstet Gynecol* 1999;93:130–4.
19. Evans MI, Dommergues M, Timor-Tritsch I, Zador IE, Wapner RJ, Lynch L, *et al.* Transabdominal versus transcervical and transvaginal multifetal pregnancy reduction: international collaborative experience of more than one thousand cases. *Am J Obstet Gynecol* 1994;170:902–9.
20. Dodd JM, Crowther CA. Reduction of the number of fetuses for women with triplet and higher order multiple pregnancies. *Cochrane Database Syst Rev* 2003;(2):CD003932.
21. Dodd J, Crowther C. Multifetal pregnancy reduction of triplet and higher-order multiple pregnancies to twins. *Fertil Steril* 2004;81:1420–2.
22. Stone J, Eddleman K, Lynch L, Berkowitz RL. A single center experience with 1000 consecutive cases of multifetal pregnancy reduction. *Am J Obstet Gynecol* 2002;187:1163–7.
23. Brown JE, Carlson M. Nutrition and multifetal pregnancy. *J Am Diet Assoc* 2000;100:343–8.
24. Elster N. Less is more: the risks of multiple births. The Institute for Science, Law, and Technology Working Group on Reproductive Technology. *Fertil Steril* 2000;74:617–23.
25. Roem K. Nutritional management of multiple pregnancies. *Twin Res* 2003;6:514–9.
26. National Institute for Clinical Excellence. *Antenatal Care Clinical Guideline.* 6th ed. London: NICE; 2003.
27. Mahomed K. Iron and folate supplementation in pregnancy. *Cochrane Database Syst Rev* 2000;(2):CD001135.
28. Roodenburg AJ. Iron supplementation during pregnancy. *Eur J Obstet Gynecol Reprod Biol* 1995;61:65–71.
29. Juarez-Vazquez J, Bonizzoni E, Scotti A. Iron plus folate is more effective than iron alone in the

treatment of iron deficiency anaemia in pregnancy: a randomised, double blind clinical trial. *BJOG* 2002;109:1009–14.

30. Bodnar LM, Wisner KL. Nutrition and depression: implications for improving mental health among childbearing-aged women. *Biol Psychiatry* 2005;58:679–85.

31. Edwards MS, Ellings JM, Newman RB, Menard MK. Predictive value of antepartum ultrasound examination for anomalies in twin gestations. *Ultrasound Obstet Gynecol* 1995;6:43–9.

32. Schinzel AA, Smith DW, Miller JR. Monozygotic twinning and structural defects. *J Pediatr* 1979;95:921–30.

33. Snijders RJ, Noble P, Sebire N, Souka A, Nicolaides KH. UK multicentre project on assessment of risk of trisomy 21 by maternal age and fetal nuchal-translucency thickness at 10–14 weeks of gestation. Fetal Medicine Foundation First Trimester Screening Group. *Lancet* 1998;352:343–6.

34. Sebire NJ, Snijders RJ, Hughes K, Sepulveda W, Nicolaides KH. Screening for trisomy 21 in twin pregnancies by maternal age and fetal nuchal translucency thickness at 10–14 weeks of gestation. *Br J Obstet Gynaecol* 1996;103:999–1003.

35. Sebire NJ, D'Ercole C, Hughes K, Carvalho M, Nicolaides KH. Increased nuchal translucency thickness at 10–14 weeks of gestation as a predictor of severe twin-to-twin transfusion syndrome. *Ultrasound Obstet Gynecol* 1997;10:86–9.

36. Vandecruys H, Faiola S, Auer M, Sebire N, Nicolaides KH. Screening for trisomy 21 in monochorionic twins by measurement of fetal nuchal translucency thickness. *Ultrasound Obstet Gynecol* 2005;25:551–3.

37. Alfirevic Z, Walkinshaw S. *Amniocentesis and Chorionic Villus Sampling.* RCOG Green Top Guideline No 8. London: RCOG; 2005.

38. Gonsoulin W, Copeland KL, Carpenter RJ Jr, Hughes MR, Elder FF. Fetal blood sampling demonstrating chimerism in monozygotic twins discordant for sex and tissue karyotype (46, XY and 45, X). *Prenat Diagn* 1990;10:25–8.

39. Ghidini A, Lynch L, Hicks C, Alvarez M, Lockwood CJ. The risk of second-trimester amniocentesis in twin gestations: a case–control study. *Am J Obstet Gynecol* 1993;169:1013–6.

40. Ko TM, Tseng LH, Hwa HL. Second-trimester genetic amniocentesis in twin pregnancy. *Int J Gynaecol Obstet* 1998;61:285–7.

41. Wald N, Cuckle H, Stirrat G. Maternal serum alpha-fetoprotein levels in triplet and quadruplet pregnancy. *Br J Obstet Gynaecol* 1978;85:124–6.

42. Aitken DA. *Biochemical Screening in Twins.* London: RCOG Press; 1995.

43. Strigini F, Melis GB, Gasperini M, Fioretti P. Raised maternal plasma alpha-fetoprotein and pregnancy outcome. *J Nucl Med Allied Sci* 1989;33(3 Suppl):77–80.

44. Baldwin VJ. *Anomalous Development of Twins.* New York: Springer-Verlag; 1994.

45. Lynch A, McDuffie R, Stephens J, Murphy J, Faber K, Orleans M. The contribution of assisted conception, chorionicity and other risk factors to very low birthweight in a twin cohort. *BJOG* 2003;110:405–10.

46. Minakami H, Honma Y, Matsubara S, Uchida A, Shiraishi H, Sato I. Effects of placental chorionicity on outcome in twin pregnancies. A cohort study. *J Reprod Med* 1999;44:595–600.

47. Newman RB, Krombach RS, Myers MC, McGee DL. Effect of cerclage on obstetrical outcome in twin gestations with a shortened cervical length. *Am J Obstet Gynecol* 2002;186:634–40.

48. Mordel N, Zajicek G, Benshushan A, Schenker JG, Laufer N, Sadovsky E. Elective suture of uterine cervix in triplets. *Am J Perinatol* 1993;10:14–16.

49. Yu CK, Papageorghiou AT, Boli A, Cacho AM, Nicolaides KH. Screening for pre-eclampsia and fetal growth restriction in twin pregnancies at 23 weeks of gestation by transvaginal uterine artery Doppler. *Ultrasound Obstet Gynecol* 2002;20:535–40.

50. Geipel A, Berg C, Germer U, Katalinic A, Krapp M, Smrcek J, et al. Doppler assessment of the uterine circulation in the second trimester in twin pregnancies: prediction of pre-eclampsia, fetal growth restriction and birth weight discordance. *Ultrasound Obstet Gynecol* 2002;20:541–5.

51. Quintero RA, Morales WJ, Allen MH, Bornick PW, Johnson PK, Kruger M. Staging of twin–twin transfusion syndrome. *J Perinatol* 1999;19(8 Pt 1):550–5.

52. Tan TY, Taylor MJ, Wee LY, Vanderheyden T, Wimalasundera R, Fisk NM. Doppler for artery-artery anastomosis and stage-independent survival in twin–twin transfusion. *Obstet Gynecol* 2004;103:1174–80.

53. Karatza AA, Wolfenden JL, Taylor MJ, Wee L, Fisk NM, Gardiner HM. Influence of twin–twin transfusion syndrome on fetal cardiovascular structure and function: prospective case–control study of 136 monochorionic twin pregnancies. *Heart* 2002;88:271–7.

54. Johnstone FD, Prescott R, Hoskins P, Greer IA, McGlew T, Compton M. The effect of introduction of umbilical Doppler recordings to obstetric practice. *Br J Obstet Gynaecol* 1993;100:733–41.

55. Giles W, Bisits A, O'Callaghan S, Gill A. The Doppler assessment in multiple pregnancy randomised controlled trial of ultrasound biometry versus umbilical artery Doppler ultrasound and biometry in twin pregnancy. *Bjog* 2003;110:593–7.

56. Goldenberg RL, Iams JD, Miodovnik M, Van Dorsten JP, Thurnau G, Bottoms S, *et al*. The preterm prediction study: risk factors in twin gestations. National Institute of Child Health and Human Development Maternal-Fetal Medicine Units Network. *Am J Obstet Gynecol* 1996;175(4 Pt 1):1047–53.

57. Berghella V, Odibo AO, To MS, Rust OA, Althuisius SM. Cerclage for short cervix on ultrasonography: Meta-analysis of trials using individual patient-level data. *Obstet Gynecol* 2005;106:181–9.

58. Wennerholm UB, Holm B, Mattsby-Baltzer I, Nielsen T, Platz-Christensen J, Sundell G, *et al* Fetal fibronectin, endotoxin, bacterial vaginosis and cervical length as predictors of preterm birth and neonatal morbidity in twin pregnancies. *Br J Obstet Gynaecol* 1997;104:1398–404.

59. Maymon R, Herman A, Jauniaux E, Frenkel J, Ariely S, Sherman D. Transvaginal sonographic assessment of cervical length changes during triplet gestation. *Hum Reprod* 2001;16:956–60.

60. Deater-Deckard K, Pickering K, Dunn JF, Golding J. Family structure and depressive symptoms in men preceding and following the birth of a child. The Avon Longitudinal Study of Pregnancy and Childhood Study Team. *Am J Psychiatry* 1998;155:818–23.

61. Hedegaard M, Henriksen TB, Sabroe S, Secher NJ. The relationship between psychological distress during pregnancy and birth weight for gestational age. *Acta Obstet Gynecol Scand* 1996;75:32–9.

62. Crowther CA. Hospitalisation and bed rest for multiple pregnancy. *Cochrane Database Syst Rev* 2001;(1):CD000110.

63. Crowther CA, Verkuyl DA, Ashworth MF, Bannerman C, Ashurst HM. The effects of hospitalization for bed rest on duration of gestation, fetal growth and neonatal morbidity in triplet pregnancy. *Acta Genet Med Gemellol (Roma)* 1991;40:63–8.

64. Knuppel RA, Lake MF, Watson DL, Welch RA, Hill WC, Fleming AD, *et al*. Preventing preterm birth in twin gestation: home uterine activity monitoring and perinatal nursing support. *Obstet Gynecol* 1990;76(1 Suppl):24S–27S.

65. Dyson D, Danbe K, Bamber J. A multicentre randomised trial of three levels of surveillance in patients at risk for preterm labour – twin gestation subgroup analysis. *Am J Obstet Gynecol* 1997;176:S118.

66. Keirse M, Grant A, King J. Preterm labour. In: Chalmers I, Enkin M, Keirse M, editors. *Effective Care in Pregnancy and Childbirth*. Oxford: Oxford University Press; 1989. p. 694–749.

67. McDonald H, Brocklehurst P, Parsons J, Vigneswaran R. Antibiotics for treating bacterial vaginosis in pregnancy. *Cochrane Database Syst Rev* 2003;(2):CD000262. Update in: *Cochrane Database Syst Rev* 2005;(1):CD000262.

68. Lamont RF, Duncan SL, Mandal D, Bassett P. Intravaginal clindamycin to reduce preterm birth in women with abnormal genital tract flora. *Obstet Gynecol* 2003;101:516–22.

69. Ugwumadu A, Manyonda I, Reid F, Hay P. Effect of early oral clindamycin on late miscarriage and preterm delivery in asymptomatic women with abnormal vaginal flora and bacterial vaginosis: a randomised controlled trial. *Lancet* 2003;361:983–8.

70. Kiss H, Petricevic L, Husslein P. Prospective randomised controlled trial of an infection screening programme to reduce the rate of preterm delivery. *BMJ* 2004;329:371.

71. Meis PJ, Klebanoff M, Thom E, Dombrowski MP, Sibai B, Moawad AH, *et al*. Prevention of recurrent preterm delivery by 17 alpha-hydroxyprogesterone caproate. *N Engl J Med* 2003;348:2379–85. Erratum in: *N Engl J Med* 2003;349:1299.

72. Meis PJ, Klebanoff M, Dombrowski MP, Sibai BM, Leindecker S, Moawad AH, *et al*. Does progesterone treatment influence risk factors for recurrent preterm delivery? *Obstet Gynecol* 2005;106:557–61.

73. Sherman SJ, Kovacs BW, Medearis AL, Bear MB, Paul RH. Nonstress test assessment of twins. *J Reprod Med* 1992;37:804–8.

74. Sairam S, Costeloe K, Thilaganathan B. Prospective risk of stillbirth in multiple-gestation pregnancies: a population-based analysis. *Obstet Gynecol* 2002;100:638–41.

75. Suzuki S, Otsubo Y, Sawa R, Yoneyama Y, Araki T. Clinical trial of induction of labor versus expectant management in twin pregnancy. *Gynecol Obstet Invest* 2000;49:24–7.

76. Hartley RS, Emanuel I, Hitti J. Perinatal mortality and neonatal morbidity rates among twin pairs at different gestational ages: optimal delivery timing at 37 to 38 weeks' gestation. *Am J Obstet Gynecol* 2001;184:451–8.

77. Dodd JM, Crowther CA. Elective delivery of women with a twin pregnancy from 37 weeks' gestation. *Cochrane Database Syst Rev* 2003;(1):CD003582.

78. Hogle KL, Hutton EK, McBrien KA, Barrett JF, Hannah ME. Cesarean delivery for twins: a systematic review and meta-analysis. *Am J Obstet Gynecol* 2003;188:220–7.

79. Persad VL, Baskett TF, O'Connell CM, Scott HM. Combined vaginal-cesarean delivery of twin pregnancies. *Obstet Gynecol* 2001;98:1032–7.

80. Smith GC, Pell JP, Dobbie R. Birth order, gestational age, and risk of delivery related perinatal death in twins: retrospective cohort study. *BMJ* 2002;325:1004.

81. Pheiffer EL, Golan A. Triplet pregnancy. A 10-year review of cases at Baragwanath Hospital. *S Afr Med J* 1979;55:843–6.

82. Ron-El R, Mor Z, Weinraub Z, Schreyer P, Bukovsky I, Dolphin Z, et al. Triplet, quadruplet and quintuplet pregnancies. Management and outcome. *Acta Obstet Gynecol Scand* 1992;71:347–50.

83. Dommergues M, Mahieu-Caputo D, Dumez Y. Is the route of delivery a meaningful issue in triplets and higher order multiples? *Clin Obstet Gynecol* 1998;41:24–9.

84. Nyberg DA, Filly RA, Golbus MS, Stephens JD. Entangled umbilical cords: a sign of monoamniotic twins. *J Ultrasound Med* 1984;3:29–32.

85. Timmons JD, Dealvarez RR. Monoamniotic twin pregnancy. *Am J Obstet Gynecol* 1963;86:875–81.

86. Benirschke K. The placenta in twin gestation. *Clin Obstet Gynecol* 1990;33:18–31.

87. Allen VM, Windrim R, Barrett J, Ohlsson A. Management of monoamniotic twin pregnancies: a case series and systematic review of the literature. *BJOG* 2001;108:931–6.

88. Ezra Y, Shveiky D, Ophir E, Nadjari M, Eisenberg VH, Samueloff A, et al. Intensive management and early delivery reduce antenatal mortality in monoamniotic twin pregnancies. *Acta Obstet Gynecol Scand* 2005;84:432–5.

89. Heyborne KD, Porreco RP, Garite TJ, Phair K, Abril D. Improved perinatal survival of monoamniotic twins with intensive inpatient monitoring. *Am J Obstet Gynecol* 2005;192:96–101.

90. Sebire NJ, Souka A, Skentou H, Geerts L, Nicolaides KH. First trimester diagnosis of monoamniotic twin pregnancies. *Ultrasound Obstet Gynecol* 2000;16:223–5.

91. Shveiky D, Ezra Y, Schenker JG, Rojansky N. Monoamniotic twins: an update on antenatal diagnosis and treatment. *J Matern Fetal Neonatal Med* 2004;16:180–6.

92. Tessen JA, Zlatnik FJ. Monoamniotic twins: a retrospective controlled study. *Obstet Gynecol* 1991;77:832–4.

93. Dubecq F, Dufour P, Vinatier D, Thibault D, Lefebvre C, Tordjeman N, et al. Monoamniotic twin pregnancies. Review of the literature, and a case report with vaginal delivery. *Eur J Obstet Gynecol Reprod Biol* 1996;66:183–6.

94. Su LL. Monoamniotic twins: diagnosis and management. *Acta Obstet Gynecol Scand* 2002;81:995–1000.

95. Moore TR, Gale S, Benirschke K. Perinatal outcome of forty-nine pregnancies complicated by acardiac twinning. *Am J Obstet Gynecol* 1990;163:907–12.

96. Brassard M, Fouron JC, Leduc L, Grignon A, Proulx F. Prognostic markers in twin pregnancies with an acardiac fetus. *Obstet Gynecol* 1999;94:409–14.

97. Malinowski W, Wierzba W. Twin reversed arterial perfusion syndrome. *Acta Genet Med Gemellol (Roma)* 1998;47:75–87.

98. Sullivan AE, Varner MW, Ball RH, Jackson M, Silver RM. The management of acardiac twins: a conservative approach. *Am J Obstet Gynecol* 2003;189:1310–13.

99. Dickey RP, Taylor SN, Lu PY, Sartor BM, Storment JM, Rye PH, et al. Spontaneous reduction of multiple pregnancy: incidence and effect on outcome. *Am J Obstet Gynecol* 2002;186:77–83.

100. Pharoah PO, Adi Y. Consequences of in-utero death in a twin pregnancy. *Lancet* 2000;355:1597–602.

101. Prompeler HJ, Madjar H, Klosa W, du Bois A, Zahradnik HP, Schillinger H, et al. Twin pregnancies with single fetal death. *Acta Obstet Gynecol Scand* 1994;73:205–8.

102. Santema JG, Swaak AM, Wallenburg HC. Expectant management of twin pregnancy with single fetal death. *Br J Obstet Gynaecol* 1995;102:26–30.

103. Senat MV, Deprest J, Boulvain M, Paupe A, Winer N, Ville Y. Endoscopic laser surgery versus serial amnioreduction for severe twin-to-twin transfusion syndrome. *N Engl J Med* 2004;351:136–44.

Chapter 9
Impact of twins on neonatal care

David Field

Introduction

Twin pregnancies present a number of special challenges to obstetricians in terms of how to manage the pregnancy and delivery. Actions and interventions often have to be considered in terms of the balance of effect on the two babies as well as on the health of the mother. There is also often the issue of previous infertility. Parents who may have been waiting years for a baby suddenly have the prospect of two. Handling the expectations of the couple, which may well conflict with the obstetrician's view of what is likely to produce the most satisfactory outcome from the pregnancy, adds another layer of complexity to obstetric management. In contrast, the neonatal management is about the care of two babies who can be treated quite independently without concern about reciprocal effects from any particular intervention. What does affect neonatal care in relation to twins is the need to manage the birth of two, sometimes highly dependent, babies at once.

Events during twin pregnancy do predispose to an increase risk of certain neonatal problems. Some of these are unique to twins (e.g. twin-to-twin transfusion syndrome (TTTS)) while others are also seen in singletons (e.g. prematurity). In relation to other issues such as cerebral palsy and congenital anomalies, there is uncertainty about the extent to which twinning adds to the risk of these problems occurring. This chapter will focus on the full range of organisational and medical challenges posed by twins to the neonatal service:

- managing the 'resuscitation' and stabilisation of twins
- the neonatal effects of TTTS
- birthweight discordance
- prematurity in twins
- neurological damage in twins
- congenital anomalies including conjoined twins
- normal care of twins (natural and artificial).

Resuscitation and stabilisation of twins

As will be discussed later, twins are at increased risk of being born significantly preterm (≤ 32 weeks of gestation). In this situation, the neonatal unit responsible for the babies will need to be able to cope with the arrival of two, potentially highly dependent, babies at once. While this may seem obvious, the decision about whether the babies can or cannot be cared for locally often depends on a whole range of conflicting factors, such as:

- the current availability of intensive care cots in the neonatal unit
- the risk of the babies' needing intensive care (based largely on the gestation and known additional complications during the pregnancy)
- the staffing profile over the following few days (coping with two highly dependent babies will occupy a significant proportion of the whole neonatal nursing team in most neonatal units in the UK, where no more than ten intensive care cots are likely to be available in total at any one time)
- the availability of an alternative unit capable of accepting both babies within a reasonable journey time. The balance of risk involved in keeping babies whose care after birth cannot be guaranteed to be optimal versus a difficult transfer with delivery imminent should be assessed by the most senior neonatologist and obstetrician available. There are examples in the literature where things have gone badly wrong, for example twins have been split after delivery only to die in different hospitals separated by miles or that delivery has occurred en route during an *in utero* transfer.[1]

For units supervising a twin preterm birth it is important to remember to prepare well and to have two of everything available, including resuscitation teams and all types of equipment likely to be needed. Having additional back-up staff, in particular someone senior that can oversee what is going on, is also important, especially where the babies are very preterm or one baby is very growth restricted.

Planning of care, in terms of who is going to do what, should also extend into the early hours of care so that lines are placed efficiently and surfactant given promptly, etc.

Where a twin delivery involves more mature babies, the situation is a little less pressured as the problems of prematurity will not complicate matters. However, since delivery of twins is often difficult and may involve delay in delivery of the second twin, the same principles should apply, with adequate staff and equipment for the resuscitation of both babies if necessary.

On some occasions, it will be necessary to transfer the babies for neonatal care after delivery. Whenever possible, both babies should be moved to the same hospital even if the move is precipitated by the needs of just one of the twins, for example where one baby has a congenital anomaly requiring surgery and the other does not. Separating the babies places enormous pressure on the family, who may have other young children who have to stay somewhere else. Traditionally, hospitals providing transport teams have at least two sets of equipment to deal with such an occasion, i.e. the simultaneous transfer of twins. At the present time, the current regulation of working hours poses a more major difficulty than the availability of equipment. Unless both babies are unstable despite support from the local team or alternatively the babies have been delivered away from neonatal support of any kind, it is often preferable to move one baby and then the other. Where the transport personnel are being provided from the complement of staff on duty in the base unit, such an approach should not compromise the care of existing babies in that unit.

Neonatal effects of twin-to-twin-transfusion syndrome

The implications of the vascular connections between twins *in utero* have been and continue to be the focus of a great deal of study by obstetric teams around the world.

A number of intervention strategies have been evaluated in order to establish the best way to deal with the situation, in particular to try to prevent TTTS from occurring (see Chapters 3, 11 and 12). From the neonatal perspective, once delivery has occurred the acute implications of TTTS are very straightforward. One twin is anaemic and, unless the situation has arisen acutely, is also typically growth restricted. The other twin is polycythaemic and at risk of hyperviscosity.

For the anaemic twin, birth stabilises the situation and transfusion can proceed electively almost always without haste. If the anaemia is particularly severe, partial exchange transfusion is felt to be the most appropriate first step in raising the haemoglobin. Attention to nutrition then becomes the priority but here the exact approach will follow unit policy as there is no clear consensus about the merits of intravenous versus enteral feeds in the first few days after delivery in babies who have suffered this type of insult *in utero*. There is consensus that where milk is to be given, breast milk is the first choice.

For the polycythaemic twin the situation is somewhat more complex. In a variety of circumstances babies can be born polycythaemic (e.g. growth restriction, maternal diabetes, Down syndrome) and all of these babies are at risk of hyperviscosity syndrome.[2] Where this is present, the increased resistance to flow results in reduced circulatory efficiency and ultimately reduced oxygen delivery and impaired function of a variety of organs. This can manifest acutely with a variety of symptoms such as respiratory distress, hypoglycaemia and impaired renal function. However, it is the data on longer term outcome in babies affected in this way that cause most concern.[3,4] The situation is a little confused since, in general, neonatal units use the haematocrit to estimate the risk of hyperviscosity being present with venous values of ≥ 70 felt to indicate the need for treatment. However, recent reviewers of this topic have drawn attention to the fact that:

- the relationship between haematocrit and viscosity is variable
- the normal treatment (partial exchange transfusion) is itself associated with a number of complications
- the risk from the presence of hyperviscosity operates not just after birth but may also have been present for a significant period *in utero*.[5]

This last point is particularly important since it highlights the fact that the circulatory disturbances that may be present *in utero* can result in important long-term neurological problems irrespective of how efficiently they are treated after birth. Therefore, while concerns about hyperviscosity remain valid, it may be that our current approach after delivery is unnecessarily aggressive.

Birthweight discordance

Irrespective of whether the twins suffer TTTS, it is common for there to be a discrepancy in the birthweights. For the obstetrician, this is clearly a challenge since there is, within the obstetric literature, evidence that if the estimated weights of the babies show a greater than 15% discrepancy then there is an increased risk of adverse outcome.[6,7] This is a difficult situation to interpret since the presence of such discordance is rarely an isolated event. For example, one or both twins may also meet the criteria for intrauterine growth restriction while in other pairs weight discordance will be present in two appropriately grown twins. For the obstetrician faced with this situation, there is an obligation to monitor the pregnancy particularly closely, and there is certainly an increased risk of such pregnancies ending prematurely. For the neonatologist, it is important to understand that in twins where there is birthweight discordance but no evidence of TTTS the risks of major morbidities such as respiratory distress syndrome (RDS) and intraventricular haemorrhage appear to be independently increased. It is true to say that not all studies have found such an effect but in this situation, where prematurity and growth restriction as well as a range of other risk factors for poor outcome may be present, interpreting studies examining this issue poses considerable difficulties.[8]

Prematurity in twins

There is no doubt that multiple births are associated with preterm delivery.[9] It seems to be generally accepted that the mechanism for this association is a combination of the physical space constraints of the uterus and of obstetric intervention to end the pregnancy where there are concerns about the health of the mother and/or one or more of the babies. This is of course different from singleton preterm births where 'infection' is felt to play a major role in the aetiology of spontaneous preterm labour.[10] This is important in that any health interventions that increase the rate of multiple pregnancy will inevitably increase the rate of preterm birth related to twins and higher order multiples. In contrast, it would appear that 'social factors and deprivation' are linked to spontaneous preterm labour and hence rates of premature delivery from this mechanism are unlikely to be linked to any specific type of medical care.

Around the world, the introduction of assisted reproductive technologies (ART) has led to increased rates of multiple birth (twins and higher order) although the size of this effect and its timing has varied. The exact size of this effect is difficult to estimate precisely since obtaining reliable data about all types of ART is extremely difficult. These technologies vary from the highly sophisticated *in vitro* fertilisation to the relatively low-tech prescription of clomifene by family doctors. Nonetheless, there is generally agreement that ART has affected multiple birth rates. For example, in the USA twin births rose by nearly 60% between 1980 and 2001,[11] and in the UK the rise was 25% between 1980 and 1993.[12] It is probably worth commenting that the differences in the preterm multiples population and the preterm singleton population is further compounded by the relative unavailability of ART to low-income groups in society.

While there is general acceptance that the preterm population in neonatal units is of lower weight than the equivalent population of babies whose pregnancy is continuing, the problem of growth restriction is common in preterm twins. Indeed, it may be the cause of expedited delivery. Clearly growth restriction brings its own problems but in relation to twins the presence of a significant discrepancy between the two babies has been suggested as a major factor predicting adverse outcome, as discussed above. The exact mechanisms for the difference in size will vary between individual pairs of twins and is certainly affected by zygosity. However, in some cases it seems certain that vascular 'maldistribution' is a factor and as a result may have important implications for various organs, particularly the brain.

All of the these factors make it clear that prematurity in relation to twins is likely to be the result of a number of different aetiologies and similarly there are likely to be a variety of risk factors for major adverse outcome that may or may not affect individual twins. It is, therefore, reasonable to expect preterm twins to behave differently to preterm singleton babies. In relation to survival after preterm birth, the situation is confusing, with the majority of certainly older studies indicating a worse survival rate for preterm twins compared with preterm singletons.[13,14] It is difficult to interpret these reports as a number did not adjust for major differences in gestation between the singleton and twin groups and this approach adversely affected the twin results. Some studies that have corrected for gestation have found no difference in mortality between preterm twins and preterm singletons[15] but again this is not a general finding.[16] These studies did, however, draw attention to additional major confounding variables present in the two groups. In particular, mothers carrying twins presented for antenatal care earlier and had more visits than mothers of singletons and in addition were more likely to receive antenatal steroids before a premature birth. Delivery by caesarean section was also more likely in twin pregnancies ending prematurely. Despite these management differences, RDS was more common among preterm twins. However, other important short-term morbidities (chronic lung disease and intraventricular haemorrhage) were not increased.

Current data from my own group based on a complete UK population indicate that preterm twins are associated with a small reduction in the risk of death. Further analysis has shown a differential effect with improved survival between 26 and 32 weeks of gestation but no effect, either way, below 26 weeks (Figure 9.1). The true situation for any one setting is likely to be determined by the exact nature of the population under study, for example the overall level of deprivation, the exact inclusion criteria, the extent of ART use, etc.

The situation with regard to later health status is rather more complex, as additional issues need to be considered.

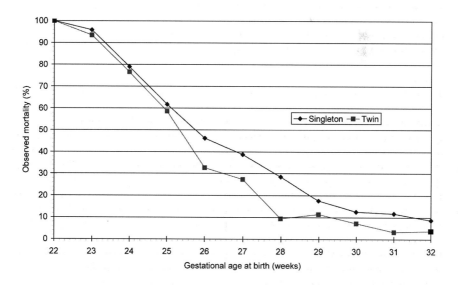

Figure 9.1.   Survival rates of preterm twins and singletons based on all births in the UK health region previously termed 'Trent' during the five years 1999–2003

Neurological outcome

It has long been established that twins are at increased risk of cerebral palsy – overall the increased risk in all twins versus all singletons is perhaps five-fold.[17] The nature and timing of the insult that leads to a brain injury manifesting as cerebral palsy remains a matter of debate.

As discussed above, twins are at increased risk of preterm delivery. Current evidence would suggest that premature twins are at a similar risk of developing cerebral palsy as equivalent singleton preterm babies.[17] This impression is not apparent in all studies as it is only when various confounding factors, such as the tendency for twins to be of lower birthweight, are taken into account that this pattern is seen. It is important also to recall that some factors that tend to encourage a more favourable outcome, such as the greater use of antenatal steroids and more frequent antenatal visits, are noted more commonly in the care of twins than singletons who deliver preterm.

Among babies born at term, twins represent a much higher proportion of the population of babies who develop cerebral palsy. In these babies it seems unlikely that delivery difficulties or other events around the time of birth could account for the cerebral insult, and a vascular aetiology seems more plausible. A good deal of attention has focused on the evidence indicating a particularly high risk of adverse neurological outcome among monozygous monochorionic twins, where vascular connection between the two fetuses is common.[18,19] A clear understanding of the exact risk attached to this situation is hard to establish since around the world precise information about the zygosity, or even chorionicity, of twin births is not recorded accurately and consistently. In general, the effect of zygosity is dealt with by looking at the group who are same-sex (a proportion of whom will be monozygous) and then comparing with the group that are opposite-sex (and who have to be dizygous).[17]

Given these problems, other evidence has been sought in relation to the risks of vascular connections being present between the placentas of the two babies. The outcome of monochorionic twins in which one baby has died has been the subject of considerable study since the risk of cerebral palsy in the surviving twin is particularly high.[20] It was initially thought that thromboplastic material generated by the dead twin might enter the circulation of the live twin and lead to infarction. Alternatively, thrombi formed after death might simply embolise from one twin to the other. Certainly, there are cases in the literature where the timescale of observed change would be appropriate for such a mechanism.[21] So too would the distribution of lesions noted, with changes having been recorded in the kidneys, liver and spleen as well as the brain.[18]

However, while this mechanism appears plausible it does not account for the increased risk of cerebral palsy in monochorionic twins where they are both born alive or where one twin dies after birth. To explain this phenomenon it is necessary to consider that problems with the blood supply to either twin can occur at any time prior to delivery if the vascular connections are sufficiently developed to permit dynamic changes to occur – although it is difficult to guess what would be the trigger to such changes in blood flow leading to damage but not death.[22]

This mechanism also does not explain the increased risk of cerebral palsy in unlike twin pairs where they must be dizygous. The recent interest in the predictive ability of birthweight discordance in relation to poor outcome suggests that placental function can be affected not simply by vascular connections between the two fetuses[23] but perhaps also by the effectiveness of placentation per se.

While the focus of most research in relation to neurological impairment in twins has been on cerebral palsy, the overall risk of other neurological problems such as learning disability and epilepsy is also increased. There are too few data outside the area of cerebral palsy to assess adequately the plausibility of a vascular aetiology. However, there are data in relation to congenital anomalies, thought to have a vascular aetiology, to suggest that vascular problems may well be occurring in twins. For example, renal agenesis, intestinal atresias and aplasia cutis are all more common in monozygous twins.[24–26]

For those who have to care for pregnant mothers having twins or deal with the infants after delivery, it is important to consider this information in context. There is no doubt that twins are at increased risk of adverse neurodevelopmental outcome but this still only equates to perhaps 1 per 100 compared with perhaps 1 per 500 in the general population of singletons. This general figure includes particularly high-risk subgroups, such as where the babies are born preterm or the pregnancy is mono-zygous, and thus it may be possible to modify the risk during the course of the pregnancy. For example, where the obstetrician feels that preterm delivery is inevitable and the estimated fetal weight is below 1500 g, the risk of cerebral palsy approaches 1 in 10.[17]

Congenital anomalies

Where one or both twins suffer a congenital anomaly it clearly has a major influence on their neonatal course (see Chapter 4). Issues relating to specific congenital anomalies will not be covered here but three points are worth making:

1. Twins, particularly monozygous twins, are at increased risk of a range of congenital anomalies. In general these types of anomaly are compatible with a vascular aetiology.
2. Twins resulting from ART are at increased risk of congenital anomalies compared with natural twins. However, evidence to quantify this risk is not entirely conclusive.[27]
3. Conjoined twins represent a very rare problem which can readily be identified *in utero*. Where such a diagnosis is made *in utero* the involvement of a centre that has experience in treating conjoined twins may well be appropriate in helping parents to decide whether to continue the pregnancy.[28] Where parents opt to continue the pregnancy in the hope of definitive surgery, they should be warned that:
   - they are likely to have to confront complex medical and ethical problems
   - it may not be possible to save both babies
   - in many cases, multiple operations will be required in childhood
   - referral to a specialist unit for assessment is essential.

Normal care

Of course, the majority of twins have no specific problems in the newborn period and in most cases in the UK, where antenatal care has a very high take-up rate, mothers know that they are carrying twins. In these circumstances, there is an opportunity to prepare for two babies and perhaps also arrange for additional support in the early days after delivery when families are trying to adjust to the major change in their day-to-day life. However, caring for normal-term twins is a challenge and many families will need additional support in adapting.[29] In relation to breastfeeding, particular help is needed so that the mother can decide what works best for her. This can involve feeding one baby and then the other or alternatively using one of the techniques that enables both babies to be fed at once.[30] This type of advice requires input from a specialist adviser (although not necessarily a health professional) and is most useful if such help is available away from the hospital setting.

Other contributors to this publication have focused on the development of twins but it is important to say here that midwifery and neonatal staff have a responsibility to set a good example in relation to the psychological development of the two babies. Many twins, especially monozygous twins, have trouble in establishing their independent identity in later life. Emphasising aspects of care such as not always dressing the babies alike and using both first names instead of referring to 'the twins' are examples of simple things that, even very early in life, will help the babies grow into separate individuals who share certain characteristics rather than twins who always have to do everything together.

Finally, an anecdotal comment in relation to the parents of twins conceived following artificial reproductive help. These parents by definition will have waited a long time for a baby and have often undergone much hardship. For years, their focus may have been on becoming pregnant. They may well have thought little about what it will be like in reality to have two babies or indeed that one or both of those babies may need some kind of help. Such parents may need extra support and counselling before they adjust to family life with twins.

References

1. Parmanum J, Field D, Rennie J, Steer P. National census of the availability of neonatal intensive care. *BMJ* 2000;321:727–9.
2. Gross GP, Hathaway WE, McGaughey HR. Hyperviscosity in the neonate. *J Pediatr* 1973;82:1004–12.
3. Delaney-Black V, Camp BW, Lubchenco LO, Swanson C, Roberts L, Gaherty P, et al. Neonatal hyperviscosity association with lower achievement and IQ scores at school age. *Pediatrics* 1989;83:662–7.
4. Drew JH, Guaran RL, Cichello M, Hobbs JB. Neonatal whole blood hyperviscosity: the important factor influencing later neurologic function is the viscosity and not the polycythemia. *Clin Hemorheol Microcirc* 1997;17:67–72.
5. Schimmel MS, Bromiker R, Soll RF. Neonatal polycythemia: is partial exchange transfusion justified? *Clin Perinatol* 2004;31:545–53.
6. Sebire NJ, D'Ercole C, Soares W, Nayar R, Nicolaides KH. Intertwin disparity in fetal size in monochorionic and dichorionic pregnancies. *Obstet Gynecol* 1998;91:82–5.
7. Vergani P, Locatelli A, Ratti M, Scian A, Pozzi E, Pezzullo JC, et al. Preterm twins: what threshold of birth weight discordance heralds major adverse neonatal outcome? *Am J Obstet Gynecol* 2004;191:1441–5.
8. Yinon Y, Mazkereth R, Rosentzweig N, Jarus-Hakak A, Schiff E, Simchen MJ. Growth restriction as a determinant of outcome in preterm discordant twins. *Obstet Gynecol* 2005;105:80–4.
9. Shinwell ES. Neonatal and long-term outcomes of very low birth weight infants from single and multiple pregnancies. *Semin Neonatol* 2002;7:203–9.
10. Mohan AR, Loudon JA, Bennett PR. Molecular and biochemical mechanisms of preterm labour. *Semin Neonatol* 2004;9:437–44.
11. MacDorman MF, Minino AM, Strobino DM, Guyer B. Annual summary of vital statistics – 2001. *Pediatrics* 2002;110:1037–52.
12. Doyle P. The outcome of multiple pregnancy. *Hum Reprod* 1996;11 Suppl 4:110–17; discussion 118–20.
13. Luke B, Keith LG. The contribution of singletons, twins and triplets to low birth weight, infant mortality and handicap in the United States. *J Reprod Med* 1992;37:661–6.
14. Martin JA, Park MM. Trends in twin and triplet births. *Natl Vital Stat Rep* 1980–97. 1999;47:1–16.
15. Donovan EF, Ehrenkranz RA, Shankaran S, Stevenson DK, Wright LL, Younes N, et al. Outcomes of very low birth weight twins cared for in the National Institute of Child Health and Human

Development Neonatal Research Network's intensive care units. *Am J Obstet Gynecol* 1998;179:742–9.

16. Botting BJ, Davies IM, Macfarlane AJ. Recent trends in the incidence of multiple births and associated mortality. *Arch Dis Child* 1987;62:941–50.

17. Pharoah POD. Neurological outcome in twins. *Semin Neonatol* 2002;7:223–30.

18. Bejar R, Vigliocco G, Gramajo H, Solana C, Benirschke K, Berry C, *et al.* Antenatal origin of neurologic damage in newborn infants. II. *Multiple gestations Am J Obstet Gynecol* 1990;162:1230–6.

19. Denbow ML, Battin MR, Cowan F, Azzopardi D, Edwards AD, Fisk NM. Neonatal cranial ultrasonographic findings in preterm twins complicated by severe fetofetal transfusion syndrome. *Am J Obstet Gynecol* 1998;178:479–83.

20. Pharoah POD, Cooke T. Cerebral palsy and multiple births. *Arch Dis Chld* 1996;75:F174–7.

21. Moore CM, McAdams AJ, Sutherland J. Intrauterine disseminated intravascular coagulation: a syndrome of multiple pregnancy with a dead twin fetus. *J Pediatr* 1969;74:523–8.

22. Pharoah PO, Price TS, Plomin R. Cerebral palsy in twins: a national study. *Arch Dis Child Fetal Neonatal Ed* 2002;87:F122–4.

23. Blickstein I. Twin-twin transfusion syndrome *Obstet Gynecol* 1990;76:714–22.

24. Schinzel AA, Smith DW, Miller JR. Monozygotic twinning and structural defects. *J Pediatr* 1979;95:921–30.

25. Hoyme HE, Higginbottom MC, Jones KL. Vascular etiology of disruptive structural defects in monozygotic twins. *Pediatrics* 1981;67:288–91.

26. Mannino FL, Jones KL, Benirschke K. Congenital skin defects and fetus papyraceus. *J Pediatr* 1977;91:559–64.

27. Hansen M, Bower C, Milne E, de Klerk N, Kurinczuk JJ. Assisted reproductive technologies and the risk of birth defects – a systematic review. *Hum Reprod* 2005;20:328–38.

28. Spitz L, Kiely EM. Conjoined twins. *JAMA* 2003;289:1307–10.

29. Bryan E. Educating families, before, during and after a multiple birth. *Semin Neonatol* 2002;7:241–6.

30. Flidel-Rimon O, Shinwell ES. Breast-feeding multiples. *Semin Neonataol* 2002;7:231–9.

Chapter 10

Single-twin demise: consequences for the survivor

Stephen Ong, Javier Zamora, Khalid S Khan
and Mark D Kilby

Introduction

Perinatal mortality is increased considerably in multiple compared with singleton pregnancies. Monochorionic placentation, with its high prevalence of inter-twin vasculature, has particular perinatal risks. The incidence of single-twin demise after 20 weeks of pregnancy is estimated to be between 2.6% and 6.2% of all twin pregnancies.[1,2] Its occurrence may result in a poor outcome for both monochorionic and dichorionic surviving twins, with the consequences for the surviving fetus being profound in monochorionic pregnancy.[3] Monochorionic monozygotic twins are particularly at risk as they are associated with an increase risk of associated inter-twin growth discrepancy[4] and discordant congenital anomalies.[5]

Morbid sequelae may include preterm delivery (whether by the onset of spontaneous labour or iatrogenic intervention), death after the demise of the first twin or survival with perinatal morbidity. In monochorionic pregnancies, single-twin demise may be associated with multi-organ injury, including ischaemic injury to the central nervous system of the surviving twin.[6] A large epidemiological survey (of both monochorionic and dichorionic twins) has suggested that the risk of a surviving co-twin suffering cerebral impairment is 20%.[3] Data from Australia suggest that single-twin demise confers an eight-fold increase in risk of cerebral palsy compared with the background twin population.[7]

Management of pregnancies complicated by intrauterine death in a twin may be challenging as there is controversy regarding the optimal time of delivery, the frequency of antenatal surveillance, the appropriate investigations to determine cerebral impairment and the effects on maternal wellbeing (both physical and psychological) of retaining one dead fetus.

In this review, we will discuss the determinants of these risks to the survivor, the pathophysiology of potential morbidity and current obstetric practice regarding management. Within this chapter, we have also provided preliminary data from our continuing systematic review (and meta-analysis) of the literature, which we believe may be useful in imparting information on prognosis for the surviving twin.

Determinants of risk to the surviving co-twin

The surviving co-twin is at risk of the underlying pathological condition (e.g. pre-eclampsia) that led to the demise of its sibling. Aside from this, the risk to the surviving fetus is dependent on two factors:

■ timing and gestation of intrauterine demise
■ chorionicity of the placenta.

Timing of intrauterine demise

Twins occur in 12% of all spontaneous conceptions. Only 14% of twin pregnancies survive to term and this process is thus associated with considerable attrition.[8] A proportion of twin pregnancies detected in the first trimester will result in spontaneous loss of the entire pregnancy with a further percentage complicated by the early demise of one fetus and delivery as a singleton pregnancy. This is known as the 'vanishing twin' phenomenon and is now perhaps recognised more frequently because of the more frequent use of ultrasound examinations within the first trimester.

In general terms, first-trimester fetal loss in a twin pregnancy does not result in an adverse outcome for the surviving co-twin,[9] although controversy surrounds this area of epidemiological research.[3,10] In contrast, single intrauterine demise in the second and third trimester is associated with the potential for considerable significant morbidity in the surviving twin.

Data from the US National Center of Health Statistics examining 152 233 sets of twins noted that survival of the remaining fetus was inversely related to the time of single-twin demise (Table 10.1).[1] In dichorionic twins, single-twin demise at 20–24 weeks of gestation was associated with a survival of 12% (95% CI 8–16%). This rose to 98% (95% CI 92–100%) after 37 weeks.[1]

Chorionicity

It appears that placentation rather than zygosity per se is the important factor with respect to mortality and morbidity. Monochorionic twins in which the placentas have a high proportion of inter-twin vascular connections have a worse outcome compared with dichorionic twins. Recent epidemiological data derived from the Office for National Statistics and from the Northern Perinatal Survey in the UK have highlighted the magnitude of the problem.[3,11] These data have to be interpreted with caution as the data are reported as the prevalence of cerebral palsy between same-sex and opposite-sex twin pairs. Data derived from the Office of National Statistics suggest that in the presence of single-twin demise, with survival of the co-twin to infancy, the prevalence of cerebral palsy in same-sex twin pairs is 106 per 1000 (95% CI 70–151). In opposite-sex twin pairs, this figure is 29 per 1000 (95% CI 6–83).[3] A similar but separate epidemiological study with data derived from the Northern Perinatal Survey was consistent with these findings. In this study, in the presence of a single-twin demise, with survival of the co-twin to infancy, the prevalence of cerebral palsy in same-sex twin pairs was reported as 114 per 1000 (95% CI 51–213) compared with 45 per 1000 (95% CI 1–228) in opposite-sex twin pairs (Table 10.2).[11] This is in keeping with clinical experience, where a higher rate of neurological complications and death would be expected following monochorionic single-twin demise. With histological data confirming chorionicity, Bajoria et al.[12]

Table 10.1. Outcome of the remaining fetus and the time of single-twin demise; adapted from Johnson and Zhang[1]

Time of first fetal death (weeks)	n	Outcome of remaining fetus		
		Surviving infant (%) (95% CI)	Fetal death (%) (95% CI)	Infant death (%) (95% CI)
Same-sex twins				
20–24	1278	8 (6–9)	69 (66–71)	23 (21–26)
25–28	48	36 (31–40)	49 (44–54)	15 (12–19)
29–32	423	64 (59–68)	31 (27–36)	5 (3–7)
33–36	479	76 (71–79)	21 (18–25)	3 (2–5)
≥ 37	227	85 (79–89)	15 (11–20)	0 (0–2)
Opposite-sex twins				
20–24	351	12 (8–16)	59 (54–65)	29 (24–34)
25–28	70	64 (52–75)	16 (8–26)	20 (11–31)
29–32	96	86 (77–92)	10 (5–18)	4 (1–10)
33–36	135	94 (89–97)	4 (2–9)	2 (0–5)
≥ 37	92	98 (92–100)	0 (0–4)	2 (0–8)

reported 13 of 31 cases of monochorionic co-twin deaths *in utero* and only 1 of 41 dichorionic co-twin deaths following single-twin demise.

Pathophysiology

Aetiology of single-twin demise

There is a multitude of reasons for single-twin demise. These may include the discordant presence of congenital malformations (whether of genetic or anatomical abnormalities), placental insufficiency and abruption, cord abnormalities such as

Table 10.2. Cerebral palsy prevalence rates in the surviving co-twin one year after delivery; adapted from Glinianaia *et al.*[11]

Gestational age at delivery (weeks)	Number with cerebral palsy	Cerebral palsy rate (per 1000 survivors) (95%CI)
Same-sex twins		
< 32	1	111 (3–482)
≥ 32	7	115 (47–222)
Total	8	114 (51–213)
Opposite-sex twins		
< 32	1	500 (13–987)
≥ 32	0	–
Total	1	45 (1–228)

velamentous cord insertion, infection, and maternal disease such as diabetes and hypertensive disorders of pregnancy.[13–16] In monochorionic twins, single-twin demise may also be the end result in the highly morbid twin-to-twin transfusion syndrome (TTTS). In monoamniotic twins, cord entanglement is another cause. As with singletons, the aetiology of single-twin demise is often elusive.[17]

Effects of single in utero fetal demise on the surviving co-twin

In monochorionic twins, the surviving co-twin is at risk of multi-organ damage and multicystic encephalomalacia. In these instances, ischaemic changes have been documented in the spleen, kidney, gastrointestinal tract, skin and brain of the surviving co-twin.[18–21] Multicystic encephalomalacia is a term used to describe the presence of cystic lesions in cerebral white matter in the area of distribution of the anterior and middle cerebral artery.[22] The incidence probably varies between 1 in 9[23] and 1 in 5.[24]

There are two theories that have been advanced to explain multicystic encephalomalacia and co-twin demise in monochorionic pregnancies. The first is that there is passage of thrombotic material from the dead to healthy twin.[25] In support of this concept, there are angiographic data from neonates with neurological damage and perinatal autopsy data that suggest arteriolar occlusion as the cause of end-organ damage.[19] Others have noted multi-organ injury consistent with infarction ranging from a few days to eight weeks old in co-twin survivors.[21] There is little doubt that intravascular thrombi may be seen in the viscera of the surviving co-twin. The question, however, is whether the thrombi arose from circulating thromboplastins from the dead twin or whether there is an alternative mechanism to explain its presence. In 1989, Patten et al.[26] reported de novo ultrasound intracranial abnormalities in survivors as early as seven days after prenatal demise of the co-twin and the question was raised as to whether intravascular coagulopathy could have arisen this quickly.

The second theory is the 'haemodynamic imbalance theory'. This states that the placental anastomoses (frequently present in monochorionic placentas) allow transfer of blood from the surviving twin to the dead co-twin, giving rise to periods of hypo-perfusion, hypotension and acute fetal anaemia resulting in neurological damage.[27] This theory was first proposed by Fusi et al.[28] in a case report describing the occurrence of fetal cerebral and renal lesions without any derangement in coagulation. Furthermore, severe anaemia was found in the surviving fetus at delivery. This proposition was further supported by data from Okamura et al.[29] that again indicated the absence of coagulopathy and the presence of anaemia in the surviving co-twins.[29] In this study, an intrauterine fetal blood sample was obtained from five mono-chorionic survivors following single-twin demise. In all five cases, the fetus was anaemic and none showed evidence of coagulopathy. All five fetuses suffered cerebral injury. One fetus was sampled twice, once before and once after the death of its co-twin. The authors demonstrated a decline in haemoglobin from 15 to 10 g/dL within three hours of single-twin demise.

A recent study[30] from Italy reported similar findings, lending further weight to the theory that the high mortality in monochorionic pregnancies complicated by single-twin demise was related to haemodynamic changes. Nicolini et al.[30] demonstrated that all four monochorionic twin survivors sampled within 24 hours of death of their co-twins had low haematocrits. All four fetuses suffered a poor outcome. One of these four fetuses was sampled before and after the demise of its co-twin. In this instance, a drop in haematocrit from 40% to 17% was reported (Figure 10.1).

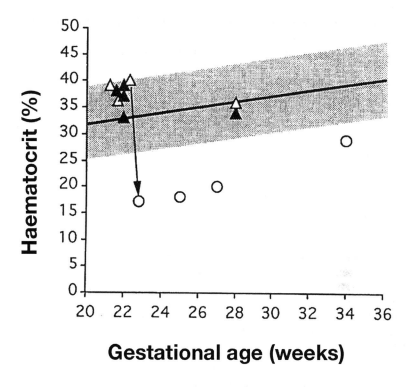

Gestational age (weeks)

Figure 10.1. Fetal haematocrit in the umbilical vein of monochorionic twins who underwent sampling after death of one twin; filled triangles = twins who died; open triangles = survivors who underwent sampling before death; open circles = haematocrit values in survivors who underwent sampling within 24 hours after the death of the co-twin; the case connected by the arrow represents a twin who was sampled before and after the death of the co-twin; shaded area = reference range; adapted from *Am J Obstet Gynecol*, vol. 179, Nicolini *et al.*, Fetal blood sampling immediately before and within 24 hours of death in monochorionic twin pregnancies complicated by single intrauterine death, pages 800–3, © 1998, with permission from Elsevier

It is tempting to speculate that this acute phenomenon is more marked in monochorionic twins with TTTS and will depend on the number and size of vascular placental anastomoses. However, histological data to support this is lacking.

Bajoria *et al.*[12] have conducted some analyses of placental injection studies in order to relate the vascular anatomy of monochorionic placentas to fetal demise. It appears that for monochorionic twins without TTTS, perinatal mortality was higher in patients with superficial arterio-arterial (AA)/veno-venous (VV) channels than in those with only bidirectional arterio-venous anastomosis (AVA) (12/15 versus 0/8; $P < 0.001$). In pregnancies complicated by TTTS, perinatal outcome of the surviving twin was dependent on whether the recipient or donor died first. The incidence of intrauterine death of the co-twin was higher if the recipient died first (9/16 versus 0/10; $P < 0.001$). Similarly, the incidence of neurological sequelae in the co-twin was higher if the recipient died first (6/7 versus 2/10; $P < 0.001$).

Two recent case reports are in line with the data produced by Bajoria *et al.*[12] In both these cases the donor died first and the recipient had a successful outcome. Gembruch *et al.*[31] describe a case of severe TTTS where the donor died at 25 weeks of gestation. The authors used Doppler ultrasound insonation of the fetal vasculature and reported that blood from the umbilical arteries of the surviving fetus was pumped into both umbilical arteries of the dead twin through superficial artery-to-artery placental shunts. In the dead twin, the route of blood flow from the umbilical arteries was as follows: descending aorta, aortic arch, aortic valve, left ventricle, mitral valve, left atrium, foramen ovale, right atrium, inferior vena cava, ductus venosus, and back to the placenta through the umbilical vein. The authors also performed cordocentesis 45 minutes and 105 minutes after demise of the donor, which revealed haemoglobin of 13.7 and 13.1 g/dL, respectively. Twelve hours later, the reversed arterial perfusion sequence disappeared. The surviving fetus was delivered at 30 weeks of gestation with a haemoglobin of 15.1 g/dL and had normal neurological examination at three years of age. Ohkuchi *et al.*[32] also reported on a twin pregnancy complicated by severe TTTS at 26 weeks of gestation. Both donor and recipient were severely compromised, with the recipient in cardiac failure and at risk of imminent demise as diagnosed by venous and arterial Doppler studies. In this case report, the donor had also died first. The authors reported the remarkable sequential improvement in Doppler indices following demise of the donor. The recipient was delivered alive with haemoglobin of 17.8 g/dL at 28 weeks and was neurologically normal. They proposed that haemorrhage from the recipient to the dead donor twin contributed to the good outcome in the recipient.

Prognosis following single-twin demise: results from a systematic review

In this section we provide preliminary data regarding prognosis from a systematic review of the literature on this subject.

Methods

Research questions

Following single-twin demise after 14 weeks of gestation, what is the incidence of:

- co-twin intrauterine demise
- neurological abnormality of co-twin survivors
- preterm delivery before 34 weeks (either iatrogenic or spontaneous)?

Sources and study selection

Literature was identified by searching the bibliographic databases Medline (1990–2005) and EMBASE (1990–2005). A hand search of relevant literature was also conducted from specialist journals. The search term combination captured citations with the relevant population (e.g. single twin demise; surviving twin). There was no language restriction.

Selection criteria

The selection criteria were as follows:

- Population: twin pregnancies with demise of one twin.
- Outcome: perinatal death and/or neurodevelopmental delay.
- Study design: case series with fewer than five cases were rejected.

The electronic searches yielded 632 potentially relevant citations on the subject. Full manuscripts of all 53 potentially relevant citations were then obtained (Figure 10.2). Twenty-seven studies were included in the systematic review (Table 10.3).[1–3,5,9,11,12,17,33–51]

Quality assessment and data extraction

The studies were assessed for quality (Figure 10.3) by the following criteria:

- Description of population: documentation of timing of single-twin demise was considered ideal.
- Prognostic factors considered: such as congenital anomalies, chorionicity.
- Outcome ascertainment: documentation of death and neurological abnormality was considered ideal.

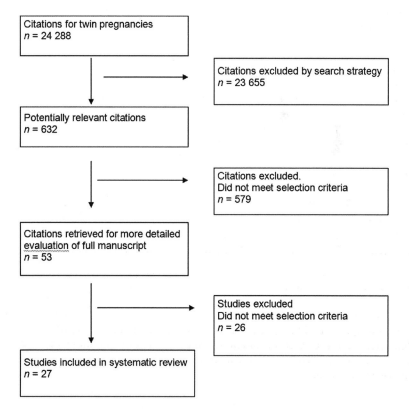

Figure 10.2.   Flow diagram of study selection for the systematic review

Table 10.3. Studies selected for the systematic review and availability of data for extraction and analysis

Study	n	Data extractable		
		Intrauterine death	Preterm delivery	Neurological abnormality
Case series				
van Heteren *et al.* (1998)[36]	11	Y	Y	Y
Aslan *et al.* (2004)[34]	25	N	N	Y
Saito *et al.*(1999)[2]	30	N	Y	Y
Fusi and Gordon (1990)[37]	16	Y	Y	Y
Petersen and Nyholm (1999)[35]	12	Y	Y	Y
Santema *et al.* (1995)[17]	29	Y	N	Y
Kilby *et al.* (1994)[5]	20	Y	N	Y
Axt *et al.* (1999)[33]	7	Y	Y	Y
Zorlu *et al.* (1997)[38]		Y	N	N
Prompeler *et al.* (1994)[9]	43	N	N	N
Woo *et al.* (2000)[39]	7	Y	Y	Y
Liu *et al.* (2000)[51]	3	N	N	N
Malinowski *et al.* (1996)[40]	15	N	N	N
Lin *et al.* (1999)[41]	17	N	N	Y
Wang *et al.* (2000)[42]	9	N	Y	Y
Gaucherand *et al.* (1994)[43]	9	Y	Y	Y
Jou *et al.* (1996)[46]	12	Y	Y	Y
Eglowstein and D'Alton (1993)[47]	20	Y	N	Y
Sonneveld and Correy (1992)[48]	25	Y	Y	N
Ishimatsu *et al.* (1994)[49]	15	Y	Y	Y
Abdal-Khalig and Sobande (2004)[50]	35	Y	N	Y
Birth register				
Rydhstrom and Ingemarsson (1993)[44]	206	Y	N	N
Rydhstrom (1994)[45]	326	Y	N	N
Pharoah and Adi (2000)[3]	597	Y	N	N
Glinianaia *et al.* (2002)[11]	164	Y	N	N
Johnson and Zhang (2002)[1]	3599	Y	N	N
Other				
Bajoria *et al.* (1979)[12]	92	Y	N	N

Data extraction sought information regarding the risk of intrauterine death, neurodevelopmental delay and preterm labour. Data were analysed by stratifying for gestational age of single–twin demise, chorionicity and the presence of TTTS. The extracted data were inspected for clinical and methodological heterogeneity. All studies were case series (cohort studies) or published data derived from registers (Table 10.3). In total there were 5353 cases of single–twin demise, from which some data were extractable in 4493 cases. The extracted data were tabulated to allow

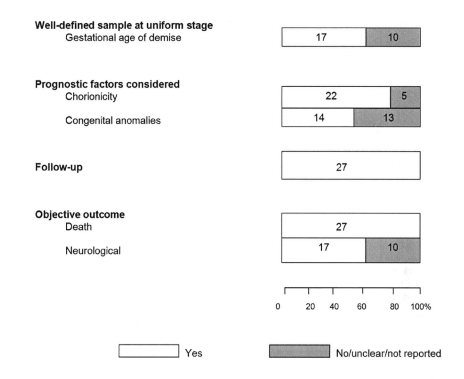

Figure 10.3. Quality assessment of studies in systematic review

qualitative inspection for various sources of heterogeneity. For different events (intrauterine death, neurological abnormality, preterm delivery) we calculated the proportion of events and the exact 95% confidence interval and then depicted this graphically in a Forrest plot. With the exception of intrauterine death, we were not able to compare event rates according to chorionicity owing to small sample sizes and the considerable heterogeneity among the studies.

Results

Risk of co-twin demise in utero

To assess the risk of co-twin demise, data were derived from 11 studies (4493 twin pregnancies). Following the death of one twin after 14 weeks of gestation, the overall risk (monochorionic and dichorionic) of intrauterine death of the co-twin was 39% (95% CI 38–40%) (Figures 10.4 and 10.5). Only three studies allowed for the comparison between monochorionic and dichorionic pregnancies (Figure 10.6). Tests for heterogeneity were not significant. The odds of monochorionic twin demise following single-twin demise after 20 weeks of gestation was nine times higher compared with dichorionic twins (OR 9.46; 95% CI 2.41–37.16).

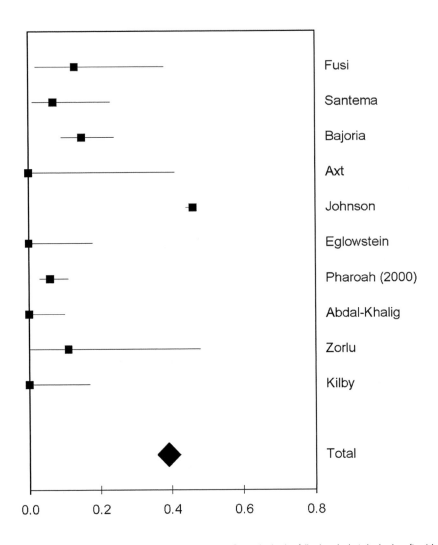

Figure 10.4.   Forrest plot of studies of the incidence of co-twin demise following single-twin demise after 14 weeks of gestation

Risk of neurological sequelae

To assess the risk of neurological abnormality, data were derived from 16 studies (267 twin pregnancies). Following the death of one twin after 14 weeks of gestation, the overall risk (monochorionic and dichorionic) of neurological abnormality four weeks after delivery was 9% (95% CI 6–13%) (Figure 10.5). Neurological abnormality appeared to be higher in monochorionic pregnancies compared with dichorionic pregnancies (19/108 (17.6%) versus 1/78 (1.2%)).

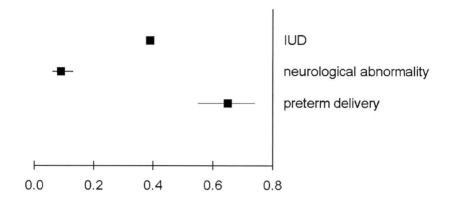

Figure 10.5.   Risk of co-twin intrauterine demise, neurological abnormality and preterm delivery before 34 weeks of gestation following single-twin demise after 14 weeks of gestation

Preterm delivery

To assess the risk of preterm delivery, data were derived from 11 studies (100 twin pregnancies). Following the death of one twin after 14 weeks of gestation, the overall risk (monochorionic and dichorionic) of preterm delivery before 34 weeks of gestation was 65% (95% CI 55–74%) (Figure 10.5). This figure for preterm delivery includes both iatrogenic and spontaneous preterm delivery. Preterm delivery before 34 weeks of gestation appeared to be marginally higher in monochorionic pregnancies compared with dichorionic pregnancies (52/77 (68%) versus 13/23 (57%)).

Review: Test
Comparison: Monochorionic vs Dichorionic
Outcome: IUD

Study or sub-category	Monochorionic n/N	Dichorionic n/N	OR (fixed) 95% CI	Weight %	OR (fixed) 95% CI
Abdal- Khalig	0/19	0/16			Not estimable
Kilby	0/7	0/13			Not estimable
Eglowstein	0/8	0/11			Not estimable
Axt	0/4	0/3			Not estimable
Fusi	1/7	1/7		47.62	1.00 [0.05, 19.96]
Santema	2/11	0/16		18.20	8.68 [0.38, 200.55]
Bajoria	13/37	1/41		34.19	21.67 [2.66, 176.22]
Total (95% CI)	93	107		100.00	9.46 [2.41, 37.16]

Total events: 16 (Monochorionic), 2 (Dichorionic)
Test for heterogeneity: Chi² = 2.77, df = 2 (P = 0.25), I² = 27.7%
Test for overall effect: Z = 3.22 (P = 0.001)

0.001 0.01 0.1   1   10   100 1000
Monochorionic better   Dichorionic better

Figure 10.6   Meta-analysis of studies providing information of intrauterine death following single-twin demise after 20 weeks of gestation, with a comparison of the odds of intrauterine death between monochorionic and dichorionic pregnancies.

Management strategy

In the majority of studies, data were not available concerning the type of management strategy employed. Where the pregnancy was monochorionic, a conservative approach following single-twin demise resulted in a 20% (12/60) attrition rate four weeks after delivery. Where the pregnancy was dichorionic this figure was 13% (5/38). There were insufficient data concerning aggressive/immediate delivery following single-twin demise.

Management

General principles in management

Clinical management depends on gestational age and the detection of *in utero* compromise of the surviving twin. The principle is to optimise outcome for the surviving twin while avoiding prematurity and its potential sequelae. Because of the paucity of evidence, recommendations are based largely on expert opinion.[1,52,53] In all cases, consultations with paediatric services are indicated and a detailed paediatric examination, particularly in monochorionic pregnancies, is important. Following delivery, histological examination of the placenta and postmortem of the dead fetus may reveal useful information.

Viable pregnancies

If an intrauterine fetal death occurs in a viable pregnancy, management is similar for both dichorionic and monochorionic pregnancies. Most workers would counsel a conservative approach for both mono- and dichorionic twins. In the case of mono-chorionic pregnancies, the exact timing of multi-organ injury or multicystic encephalomalacia is unknown but thought to be at the time of death.[54,55] This is consistent with the fact that immediate delivery of the surviving co-twin does not convey a better outcome.[37,54]

Following the demise of one twin in monochorionic pregnancies, prediction of cerebral injury in the surviving twin becomes an important issue, particularly if the mother is uncertain about continuing the pregnancy. Although ultrasound could suggest a diagnosis of multicystic encephalomalacia, this mode of imaging is generally thought to require the support of other modalities,[55] such as magnetic resonance imaging (MRI).[22,56] It is uncertain whether a negative MRI scan could lead to false reassurance,[57] and the patient should be counselled accordingly. It is known that cavitating lesions appear two or more weeks after the initial insult and brain atrophy appears weeks later.[58,59] In some units an MRI scan is thus scheduled at least three weeks after single-twin demise.[57]

The continued surveillance for fetal wellbeing is variously described by different authors. Cardiotocograms and biophysical profiles have been suggested by some as these investigations give insight into the physiological status of the fetus and are thought to be a reflection of the autonomic system.[57] However, evidence to support this approach is not available. Most would advocate weekly cardiotocograms and biophysical profiles[57] and others would suggest weekly umbilical artery Doppler insonation, although the frequency and timing of such surveillance is not well researched.

Some authors would recommend prophylactic steroids (betamethasone to induce type 2 pneumocyte maturation and surfactant production)[57] and most would suggest delivery by 38 weeks of gestation and others even earlier at 34 weeks.[57]

Vaginal delivery of the surviving co-twin is considered to be a reasonable option[37] but, because of the high prevalence of vascular anastomosis in monochorionic twin placentas, many elect for caesarean delivery to avoid the potential risks of an acute TTTS.

Pre-viable pregnancies

In dichorionic pregnancies complicated by single-twin demise, the same principles apply and expectant management is advocated to between 34 and 38 weeks of gestation.

In monochorionic pregnancies, the risks pertaining to multicystic encephalomalacia and multi-organ damage are present. The lack of specificity of the predictive investigations available means that some patients may opt to terminate the pregnancy.

Fetal blood sampling and intrauterine transfusion

The gradual understanding that co-twin demise may be a consequence of acute haemodynamic changes has led some workers to suggest a role for fetal blood sampling and intrauterine transfusion. These attempts have resulted in mixed outcomes. Tanawattanacharoen et al.[60] assessed ten cases over a four year period where fetal blood sampling was performed within 24 hours of death of the monochorionic co-twin. In three cases, the fetus was not anaemic, was not transfused and had a normal outcome. Intrauterine transfusion was performed in all seven anaemic fetuses where the haematocrit was below 30%. Two fetuses that were severely acidaemic at sampling died *in utero* 24 hours after transfusion. In two cases, the pregnancies continued uneventfully until 35 and 40 weeks with good outcomes. In another two cases, the surviving transfused twins had abnormal brain scans and were terminated. In one other case, the co-twin delivered a week after transfusion at 29 weeks and died. The authors suggested that intrauterine transfusion before severe acidaemia in anaemic surviving monochorionic co-twins may prevent death but may not necessarily prevent brain injury.

Senat et al.[61] managed 12 cases of single intrauterine death in monochorionic twins complicated by TTTS. Following the demise of one twin, a fetal blood sample was performed on the surviving twin within 24 hours. Of these 12 fetuses, six were anaemic (two donors, four recipients) and were transfused. All six fetuses survived the procedure and four were alive and well one year after delivery. One fetus had an abnormal brain scan and the pregnancy was terminated. One baby delivered at 34 weeks and was subsequently diagnosed with periventricular leukomalacia. In all six non-anaemic fetuses, the outcome was normal.

Although the number of cases is small, the combined data from studies by Tanawattanacharoen and Senat suggest that a good outcome may be achieved in six of 13 anaemic fetuses. It may be that this method of management deserves greater consideration.

The vanishing twin

It is generally believed that multicystic encephalomalacia and/or monochorionic co-twin demise is the result of single-twin demise in the second or third trimester,[55] with first-trimester losses being a lesser complication. Other workers have argued that a proportion of cases of a 'vanishing twin' in first-trimester monochorionic twin pregnancies secondary to acute TTTS could be the explanation of unexplained cerebral palsy. The concept was first put forward in the form of a letter to *The Lancet* in 1977.[62] The subject was raised again in 1990 and in 1992.[6,63] Pharoah and Cooke[10] brought the subject to prominence in 1997. While it is true that recent epidemiological evidence describes an inverse relation between time of single-twin demise and neurological morbidity for the co-twin,[1] and a number of large surveys have been consistent in their findings that like-sex twins have a greater morbidity and mortality than unlike-sex twins,[3,11] the issue as to whether twin demise in the first trimester has a significant impact on neurological development of its co-twin remains unresolved.[64] Interestingly, a recent report details the demise of a single fetus at 12 weeks of a monochorionic twin pregnancy, resulting in the development of multicystic encephalomalacia at 20 weeks of gestation of the surviving co-twin.[56]

Conclusion

The demise of one twin has profound consequences for the surviving co-twin, especially in the presence of monochorionic placentation. Following single-twin demise, the incidence of preterm delivery before 34 weeks is 65%. Overall, the incidence of co-twin demise *in utero* is 39%. Of survivors, the incidence of neurological abnormality is 9%, but is significantly higher in studies focusing on monochorionic sets (up to 30% risk). The principle guiding management is optimisation of outcome for the surviving twin while avoiding the consequences of iatrogenic prematurity. At present, there are no reliable tools for surveillance, nor are there predictors of cerebral impairment. However, the use of MRI has gained acceptance in many units and may demonstrate encephalomalacia even in the presence of an apparently normal ultrasound scan 2–4 weeks after single fetal death. Our understanding of why and when co-twin demise and injury occur is incomplete, but they are probably due to a state of altered acute fetal haemodynamics between the monochorionic twin pair. At present, the place of fetal blood sampling and intrauterine transfusion to reduce long-term morbidity in co-survivors has not been established.

The data from our systematic review has highlighted the need:

- for more data from regional databases on outcome of multiple pregnancies
- to prospectively and retrospectively confirm chorionicity of multiple pregnancy and relate this to epidemiological outcome
- for data to assist in surveillance of the surviving twin when one twin has died
- for evaluation of potential therapies to prevent end-organ damage in co-twin survivors.

Note

The full details of this systematic review of the literature on the topic of single twin demise has been accepted for publication and is in press with *BJOG*.

References

1.   Johnson CD, Zhang J. Survival of other fetuses after a fetal death in twin or triplet pregnancies. *Obstet Gynecol* 2002;99:698–703.
2.   Saito K, Ohtsu Y, Amano K, Nishijima M. Perinatal outcome and management of single fetal death in twin pregnancy: a case series and review. *J Perinat Med* 1999;27:473–7.

3.   Pharoah PO, Adi Y. Consequences of in-utero death in a twin pregnancy. *Lancet* 2000;355:1597–602.

4.   Ghai V, Vidyasagar D. Morbidity and mortality factors in twins. An epidemiologic approach. *Clin Perinatol* 1988;15:123–40.

5.   Kilby MD, Govind A, O'Brien PM. Outcome of twin pregnancies complicated by a single intrauterine death: a comparison with viable twin pregnancies *Obstet Gynecol*;1994:107–9.

6.   Anderson RL, Golbus MS, Curry CJ, Callen PW, Hastrup WH. Central nervous system damage and other anomalies in surviving fetus following second trimester antenatal death of co-twin. Report of four cases and literature review. *Prenat Diagn* 1990;10: 513–18.

7.   Petterson B, Nelson KB, Watson L, Stanley F. Twins, triplets, and cerebral palsy in births in Western Australia in the 1980s. *BMJ* 1993;307:1239–43.

8.   Boklage CE. Survival probability of human conceptions from fertilization to term. *Int J Fertil* 1990;35:79–80, 81–94.

9.   Prompeler HJ, Madjar H, Klosa W, du Bois A, Zahradnik HP, Schillinger H, *et al.* Twin pregnancies with single fetal death. *Acta Obstet Gynecol Scand* 1994;73:205–8.

10.   Pharoah PO, Cooke RW. A hypothesis for the aetiology of spastic cerebral palsy – the vanishing twin. *Dev Med Child Neurol* 1997;39:292–6.

11.   Glinianaia SV, Pharoah PO, Wright C, Rankin JM. Fetal or infant death in twin pregnancy: neurodevelopmental consequence for the survivor. *Arch Dis Child Fetal Neonatal Ed* 2002;86:F9–15.

12.   Bajoria R, Wee LY, Anwar S, Ward S. Outcome of twin pregnancies complicated by single intrauterine death in relation to vascular anatomy of the monochorionic placenta. *Hum Reprod* 1999;14:2124–30.

13.   Simpson LL. Maternal medical disease: Risk of antepartum fetal death. *Semin Perinatol* 2002;26:42–50.

14.   Ogunyemi D, Jackson U, Buyske S, Risk A. Clinical and pathologic correlates of stillbirths in a single institution. *Acta Obstet Gynecol Scand* 1998;77:722–8.

15.   Craven C, Ward K. Stillbirth: Tissue findings with environmental and genetic links. *Semin Perinatol* 2002;26:36–41.

16.   Collins JH. Umbilical cord accidents: human studies. *Semin Perinatol* 2002;26:79–82.

17.   Santema JG, Swaak AM, Wallenburg HC. Expectant management of twin pregnancy with single fetal death. *Br J Obstet Gynaecol* 1995;102:26–30.

18.   Bulla M, von Lilien T, Goecke H, Roth B, Ortmann M, Heising J. Renal and cerebral necrosis in survivor after *in utero* death of co-twin. *Arch Gynecol* 1987;240:119–24.

19.   Yoshioka H, Kadomoto Y, Mino M, Morikawa Y, Kasubuchi Y, Kusunoki T. Multicystic encephalomalacia in liveborn twin with a stillborn macerated co-twin. *J Pediatr* 1979;95:798–800.

20.   Moore CM, McAdams AJ, Sutherland J. Intrauterine disseminated intravascular coagulation: a syndrome of multiple pregnancy with a dead twin fetus. *J Pediatr* 1969;74:523–8.

21.   Szymonowicz W, Preston H, Yu VY. Surviving monozygotic twin. *Arch Dis Child* 1986;61:454–8.

22.   D'Alton ME, Dudley DK. The ultrasonographic prediction of chorionicity in twin gestation. *Am J Obstet Gynecol* 1989;160:557–61.

23.   Carlson NJ, Towers CV. Multiple gestation complicated by the death of one fetus. *Obstet Gynecol* 1989;73:685–9.

24.   Wessel J, Schmidt-Gollwitzer K. Intrauterine death of a single fetus in twin pregnancies. *J Perinat Med* 1988;16:467–76.

25.   Benirschke K. Intrauterine death of a twin: mechanisms, implications for surviving twin, and placental pathology. *Semin Diagn Pathol* 1993;10:222–31.

26.   Patten RM, Mack LA, Nyberg DA, Filly RA. Twin embolization syndrome: prenatal sonographic detection and significance. *Radiology* 1989;173:685–9.

27.   Bajoria R, Kingdom J. The case for routine determination of chorionicity and zygosity in multiple pregnancy. *Prenat Diagn* 1997;17:1207–25.

28.   Fusi L, McParland P, Fisk N, Nicolini U, Wigglesworth J. Acute twin–twin transfusion: a possible mechanism for brain-damaged survivors after intrauterine death of a monochorionic twin. *Obstet Gynecol* 1991;78:517–20.

29.   Okamura K, Murotsuki J, Tanigawara S, Uehara S, Yajima A. Funipuncture for evaluation of hematologic and coagulation indices in the surviving twin following co-twin's death. *Obstet Gynecol* 1994;83:975–8.

30.   Nicolini U, Pisoni MP, Cela E, Roberts A. Fetal blood sampling immediately before and within 24 hours of death in monochorionic twin pregnancies complicated by single intrauterine death. *Am J Obstet Gynecol* 1998;179:800–3.

31.   Gembruch U, Viski S, Bagamery K, Berg C, Germer U. Twin reversed arterial perfusion sequence

in twin-to-twin transfusion syndrome after the death of the donor co-twin in the second trimester. *Ultrasound Obstet Gynecol* 2001;17:153–6.

32. Ohkuchi A, Minakami H, Shiraishi H, Suzuki I, Ohki T, Sato I. Intrauterine death of one twin, with rescue of the other, in twin–twin transfusion syndrome. *Ultrasound Obstet Gynecol* 2002;19:293–6.

33. Axt R, Mink D, Hendrik J, Ertan K, von Blohn M, Schmidt W. Maternal and neonatal outcome of twin pregnancies complicated by single fetal death. *J Perinat Med* 1999;27:221–7.

34. Aslan H, Gul A, Cebeci A, Polat I, Ceylan Y. The outcome of twin pregnancies complicated by single fetal death after 20 weeks of gestation. *Twin Res* 2004;7:1–4.

35. Petersen IR, Nyholm HC. Multiple pregnancies with single intrauterine demise. Description of twenty-eight pregnancies. *Acta Obstet Gynecol Scand* 1999;78:202–6.

36. van Heteren CF, Nijhuis JG, Semmekrot BA, Mulders LG. van den Berg PP. Risk for surviving twin after fetal death of co-twin in twin–twin transfusion syndrome. *Obstet Gynecol* 1998;92:215–19.

37. Fusi L, Gordon H. Twin pregnancy complicated by single intrauterine death. Problems and outcome with conservative management. *Br J Obstet Gynaecol* 1990;97:511–16.

38. Zorlu CG, Yalcin HR, Caglar T, Gokmen O. Conservative management of twin pregnancies with one dead fetus: is it safe? *Acta Obstet Gynecol Scand* 1997;76:128–30.

39. Woo HH, Sin SY, Tang LC. Single foetal death in twin pregnancies: review of the maternal and neonatal outcomes and management. *Hong Kong Med J* 2000;6:293–300.

40. Malinowski W, Dec W, Biskup I. The assessment of the umbilical blood flow of the surviving twin after the intrauterine death of the other twin. *Acta Genet Med Gemellol (Roma)* 1996;45:383–6.

41. Lin IJ, Chen CH, Wang TM, Fu LS, Chi CS. Infants of twin pregnancies with one twin demise in the uterus: a retrospective study. *Acta Paediatr Taiwan* 1999;40:92–6.

42. Wang KC, Yuan CC, Chao HT, Chang SP, Yang ML, Hung JH, *et al.* Brain-damaged survivors after intrauterine death of a monochorionic twin. *Zhonghua Yi Xue Za Zhi (Taipei)* 2000;63:673–8.

43. Gaucherand P, Rudigoz RC, Piacenza JM. Monofetal death in multiple pregnancies: risks for the co-twin, risk factors and obstetrical management. *Eur J Obstet Gynecol Reprod Biol* 1994;55:111–15.

44. Rydhstrom H, Ingemarsson I. Prognosis and long-term follow-up of a twin after antenatal death of the co-twin. *J Reprod Med* 1993;38:142–6.

45. Rydhstrom H. Discordant birthweight and late fetal death in like-sexed and unlike-sexed twin pairs: a population-based study. *Br J Obstet Gynaecol* 1994;101:765–9.

46. Jou H, Teng R, Shyu M, Shih J, Su C, Chen H, *et al.* Perinatal outcome in monochorionic twin pregnancy complicated with one fetal death after 20 weeks. *J Matern Fetal Invest* 1996;6:145–7.

47. Eglowstein M, D'Alton ME. Single intrauterine demise in twin gestation. *J Matern Fetal Med* 1993;2:272–5.

48. Sonneveld SW, Correy JF. Antenatal loss of one of twins. *Aust N Z J Obstet Gynaecol* 1992;32:10–13.

49. Ishimatsu J, Hori D, Miyajima S, Hamada T, Yakushiji M, Nishimi T. Twin pregnancies complicated by the death of one fetus in the second or third trimester. *J Matern Fetal Invest* 1994;4:141–5.

50. Abdal-Khalig MM, Sobande AA. Maternal and neonatal outcome of twin pregnancies complicated by a single intrauterine dead fetus. *Saudi Med J* 2004;25:1770–1.

51. Liu J, Yang J, Bian X, Zhang Y. Conservative management of twin pregnancy with single fetal death. *Chin Med Sci J* 2000;15:103–6.

52. Enbom JA. Twin pregnancy with intrauterine death of one twin. *Am J Obstet Gynecol* 1985;152:424–9.

53. Landy HJ, Weingold AB. Management of a multiple gestation complicated by an antepartum fetal demise. *Obstet Gynecol Surv* 1989;44:171–6.

54. D'Alton ME, Newton ER, Cetrulo CL. Intrauterine fetal demise in multiple gestation. *Acta Genet Med Gemellol (Roma)* 1984;33:43–9.

55. D'Alton ME, Simpson LL. Syndromes in twins. *Semin Perinatol* 1995;19:375–86.

56. Weiss JL, Cleary-Goldman J, Tanji K, Budorick N, D'Alton ME. Multicystic encephalomalacia after first-trimester intrauterine fetal death in monochorionic twins. *Am J Obstet Gynecol* 2004;190:563–5.

57. Cleary-Goldman J, D'Alton M. Management of single fetal demise in a multiple gestation. *Obstet Gynecol Surv* 2004;59:285–98.

58. Levine D. Case 46: encephalomalacia in surviving twin after death of monochorionic co-twin. *Radiology* 2002;223:392–5.

59. Bejar R, Vigliocco G, Gramajo H, Solana C, Benirschke K, Berry C, *et al.* Antenatal origin of

neurologic damage in newborn infants. II. Multiple gestations. *Am J Obstet Gynecol* 1990;162:1230–6.

60. Tanawattanacharoen S, Taylor MJ, Letsky EA, Cox PM, Cowan FM, Fisk NM. Intrauterine rescue transfusion in monochorionic multiple pregnancies with recent single intrauterine death. *Prenat Diagn* 2001;21:274–8.

61. Senat MV, Bernard JP, Loizeau S, Ville Y. Management of single fetal death in twin-to-twin transfusion syndrome: a role for fetal blood sampling. *Ultrasound Obstet Gynecol* 2002;20:360–3.

62. Melnick M. Brain damage in survivor after in-utero death of monozygous co-twin. *Lancet* 1977;2:1287.

63. Scheller JM, Nelson KB. Twinning and neurologic morbidity. *Am J Dis Child* 1992;146:1110–13.

64. Blickstein I. Reflections on the hypothesis for the etiology of spastic cerebral palsy caused by the 'vanishing twin' syndrome. *Dev Med Child Neurol* 1998;40:358.

Chapter 11

Scientific basis of twin-to-twin transfusion syndrome

William JB Dennes, Mark FH Sullivan and
Nicholas M Fisk

Introduction

Twin-to-twin transfusion syndrome (TTTS) represents arguably the greatest challenge we face in fetal therapy. This is because: (i) untreated, the disease is characterised by inordinately high perinatal mortality and morbidity; (ii) TTTS affects not one but two fetuses; (iii) unlike other conditions warranting surgical intervention, these fetuses are intrinsically entirely structurally normal and thus eminently suitable for salvage; and (iv) the disease arises anatomically in the placenta and thus should be amenable to curative intervention.

Although there has been considerable progress in unravelling the pathophysiological basis of TTTS in the decade since the last Study Group on this topic,[1] much remains poorly understood. In 1995, our chapter focused on the clinical phenotype, with early insights into anastomotic and cardiovascular associations. Since then there have been considerable advances in delineating the anastomotic basis of unbalanced intertwin transfusion, as well as in understanding the seemingly counterproductive compensatory cardiovascular responses in the recipient.[2] However, there is no unique anastomotic signature in TTTS and a number of important questions remain unanswered. For instance, why do 15% of monochorionic (MC) twins develop TTTS and the rest do not? What is the relationship between fetal fluid imbalance, donor uteroplacental insufficiency and recipient cardiovascular dysfunction? What determines progression/regression? And why has a cure proved so elusive, if this is simply a surgical problem of maldistributed or aberrantly connected anastomoses?

Much of the progress over the last ten years has been in substantial improvements in treatment. However, even now, just how far we are from optimal therapy is illustrated by the recent randomised trial[3] which showed that two-thirds of TTTS pregnancies still result in at least one dead or brain-injured baby with the better of the two first-line treatments, a sobering figure supported by subsequent series.[4]

In addition to the usual difficulties of ethics and inaccessibility that restrain fetal medicine research, there are a number of other barriers to progressing our understanding of TTTS. These include the lack of a suitable animal model and limited access to tissues (both in the first trimester, when anastomoses are developing, and in later pregnancy, now that severe cases are increasingly treated definitively by methods that interrupt the disease process). On the other hand, there are a number of opportunities provided by the modern research tools of genomics and proteomics, by observing the natural experiment of interruption to anastomotic flow by laser ablation, and the ability to observe physiological processes *in vivo* in humans using minimally invasive approaches. This chapter reviews what is known and not known regarding the pathophysiological mechanisms underlying TTTS.

Clinical syndrome

TTTS affects around 15% of MC twin pregnancies in the mid trimester or, more rarely, the early third trimester, and untreated it is associated with an 80% perinatal mortality.[5] TTTS is a complex cardiovascular condition unique to MC twin pregnancies and which principally results from unbalanced inter-twin transfusion. Although placental vascular anastomoses are ubiquitous in MC placentation, TTTS placentas are typically associated with an imbalance in unidirectional arterio-venous anastomoses and absent bidirectional anastomoses.

Phenotype

The clinical syndrome results in mid-trimester discordance in amniotic fluid volumes, with signs of hypovolaemia and uteroplacental insufficiency in the donor and hypervolaemia and cardiac dysfunction in the recipient. The usual ultrasound definition requires both oligohydramnios (deepest vertical pool less than 2 cm) in the donor and polyhydramnios (deepest vertical pool greater than 8 cm) in the recipient. Additional supportive features indicative of greater severity include a small or non-visible bladder and abnormal umbilical artery Dopplers (absent or reversed end diastolic flow (EDF) in the donor, and an enlarged bladder, cardiac hypertrophy, abnormal venous Doppler (umbilical vein or ductus venosus) and hydrops in the recipient. Marked discordance in amniotic fluid volume between the donor and recipient may result in the inter-twin septum becoming closely adherent to the donor twin, a phenomenon known as the 'stuck twin' syndrome.

Staging

Quintero *et al.*[6] proposed an intuitive staging system for classifying disease severity:

- Stage I represents the mildest form, with amniotic fluid discordance only and where the donor bladder is still visible on ultrasound.
- In stage II, the donor bladder is no longer visible.
- Stage III is indicated by abnormal Doppler waveform patterns: absent or reversed EDF in the donor umbilical artery, and/or reversed ductus venosus flow or pulsatile umbilical venous flow in the recipient.
- Stage IV is characterised by fetal hydrops in the recipient.
- Stage V, denoting single intrauterine death, has largely been abandoned as the disease process is by then over.

Staging was proposed as a system to allow comparison of outcome data between different centres but it may also have a role in individualising therapeutic options and in counselling parents about likely outcome. However, attempts to validate this classification system suggest that it may be more relevant to monitoring disease progression rather than prognostication based on stage at presentation.[7] In a stage-dependent survival analysis[7] of 52 consecutive cases (median 21 weeks of gestation at presentation), there was no significant influence of stage on survival, once stage V disease and elective terminations were excluded. Forty-five percent of cases progressed and survival was intuitively worse where stage increased (27%) compared with when stage decreased (94%).[7]

The adoption of staging in clinical practice led to two important observations. The first is that 20–30% of early-stage disease regresses with simple therapy, such as amnioreduction or septostomy.[7,8] The second is the empirical difference in perinatal survival between early-stage (I–II, 58% and 60%, respectively) and late-stage disease (III–IV, 42% and 43%, respectively).[7] Accordingly, there has been broad consensus over recent years that advanced-stage disease warrants definitive treatment by laser or cord occlusion.

The use of a cancer-like staging system implies that the disease progresses from early through to later stages, but this has not strictly been established. Indeed, staging has raised a number of pathophysiological questions. For instance, can cardiovascular changes develop before amniotic fluid imbalance? Does uteroplacental insufficiency predispose to advanced disease? And is there a difference in prognosis depending on whether the donor or recipient has abnormal Dopplers in stage III disease? While the answer to all these questions may well be yes, formal investigation is required.

Long-term sequelae

In addition to the immediate *in utero* effects, TTTS carries a significant risk of long-term neurodevelopmental and cardiovascular complications.

With respect to neurological sequelae, initial concerns were based on imaging series, with an empirical 8% average incidence of lesions (range 4–23%) in TTTS neonates.[9–13] Neurological morbidity is the result of both antenatal insults and the sequelae of preterm birth, such as periventricular leucomalacia and intraventricular haemorrhage. The likely pathogenesis of antenatally acquired lesions is ischaemia, attributable to haemodynamic imbalance via placental vascular anastomoses. Polycythaemia and vascular stasis in the recipient and anaemia and hypotension in the donor are potential mechanisms for neurological insults. Intriguingly, given their disparate pathophysiology, donors and recipients seem to have a broadly equal incidence of neurological lesions.[14,15] Death of one twin is associated with a particularly increased risk of neurological sequelae in the co-twin,[16–19] as in non-TTTS MC twins. Although neurological sequelae are increased in those with abnormalities on antenatal or early postnatal imaging studies, an ultrasound abnormality does not equate to neurological sequelae. Highly sensitive ultrasound studies have identified minor antenatally acquired white matter lesions in around one in three TTTS neonates,[20] compared with a 6% incidence in control infants at term.[21] Abnormal postnatal ultrasounds are also relatively common in non-TTTS MC twins, with one study reporting an incidence of 23%.[15]

A number of long-term follow-up cohort studies have now been published. In contrast to the trend from poorly controlled observational series, which suggested increased largely imaging-based sequelae in those treated with serial amnioreduction compared with laser, there is no clear trend in the formal follow-up cohorts. Sutcliffe *et al.*[22] and Banek *et al.*[23] reported incidences of cerebral palsy of 11% and 13% in two cohorts of laser-treated survivors, totalling 45 and 89 children, respectively. In contrast, Dickinson *et al.*[24] found an incidence of only 6% in 49 children treated *in utero* predominantly by serial amnioreduction; those authors concluded that there seems to be no increase in cerebral palsy prevalence in TTTS.

MC twins have an increased prevalence of structural congenital heart defects (2.3%), which increases to 12% in recipients with TTTS.[25] In addition, all recipients have some degree of biventricular hypertrophy (secondary to hypervolaemia).[26] Serial fetal echocardiography found evidence of cardiac dysfunction in over 80% of recipient twins[27] compared with none in donor twins. Cardiac function deteriorated in 70% of recipient twins with increasing gestational age. The resultant hypertrophic cardiomyopathy may result in sub-valvular stenosis, leading to right ventricular out-flow tract obstruction, necessitating postnatal valvotomy.[25,26] Right ventricular outflow tract obstruction in the recipient twin occurred in at least 9% of 73 pregnancies complicated by TTTS in one series.[28] It is thought to arise as a result of altered fetal haemodynamics, resulting in muscular hypertrophy in the right ventricular outflow tract and leading to a direct obstructive effect, decreased forward flow and subsequent progression to pulmonary stenosis or pulmonary atresia. Fesslova *et al.*[29] found evidence of variable degrees of biventricular hypertrophy and dilatation, with tricuspid regurgitation in all recipient twin fetuses. Cardiac dysfunction resolved in nine of 17 cases after amnioreduction and in a further two following death of the co-twin. In recipient twins that survived, ventricular function normalised within 40 days to six months postnatally. In contrast, Lougheed *et al.*[28] found that four of seven recipients with right ventricular outflow tract obstruction succumbed. We have observed that this complication is rarely seen now that ongoing transfusion is seldom allowed to continue in advanced-stage disease, at least in the mid trimester.

Postnatal follow-up in the offspring of TTTS pregnancies has shown lower arterial distensibility in donor twins (in TTTS survivors) compared with recipients, suggest-ing raised cardiac afterload might result in intrauterine remodelling, influencing later cardiovascular health.[30,31]

Placental angioarchitecture

TTTS is typically due to unbalanced deep arterio-venous anastomoses with absent compensatory superficial anastomoses. Three types of interplacental anastomosis exist: arterio-arterial (AAA), veno-venous (VVA) and arterio-venous (AVA). AAAs and VVAs are superficial, running along the chorionic plate, often with bidirectional flow and with net transfusion dependent on hydrostatic pressure at the two ends. In contrast, AVAs consist of a chorionic artery from one twin dipping into the placenta to supply an underlying cotyledon, with the draining chorionic vein running to the contralateral twin. Thus, in contrast to AAAs and VVAs, an AVA has an intervening capillary bed and is thus not strictly an anastomosis. *Ex vivo* placental dye injection studies confirm that almost all MC placentas contain vascular anastomoses.[32–34] Inter-twin transfusion is thus the norm in MC pregnancies, which is confirmed by fetal blood sampling studies where the passage of a marker agent injected into one twin's circulation is demonstrated soon afterwards in the co-twin's.[35–38] Early studies suggested that TTTS was associated with absent superficial anastomoses.[39,40] Denbow *et al.*[34] found in a large *ex vivo* injection series that 96% of all MC placentas had AVAs and 70% also had an AAA. In the 30% with absent AAA, 78% of cases developed TTTS, confirming their protective role. MC twins usually have broadly similar numbers of arterio-venous compared with counterdirectional veno–arterial anastomoses,[41] and a trend towards imbalance, in TTTS. However, the precise relationship between AVA number and development of TTTS remains unclear, presumably because anastomotic diameter as well as number will influence the resultant flow. The importance of AAAs in protecting against TTTS is supported by the rarity of TTTS in monoamniotic twins, which have all been shown to have AAAs.[41]

In support of postnatal injection studies, *in vivo* fetoscopic observations have shown that the presence of at least one unidirectional AVA is a prerequisite for the development of TTTS.[42,43] AVAs were found in all MC placentas with a preponderance of blood flow towards the recipient.[42] However, the overall number seen with fetoscopy was higher than that seen in *ex vivo* studies, suggesting that either small AVAs are more visible at endoscopy or they were false positives.

Computer modelling of dynamic MC twin fetoplacental units supports the hypothesis that unbalanced AVAs, with a lack of superficial anastomoses, are responsible for the development of TTTS.[44,45] Umur *et al.*[45] demonstrated that an AAA of an equal size to the feeding artery of an AVA has significantly lower resistance, therefore mediating higher flow rates. This helps explain why AAAs play a greater compensatory role than oppositely directed AVAs.

Approximately 85% of AAAs can be visualised antenatally using colour Doppler. They can be detected as early as 12 weeks of gestation as arterial vessels on the chorionic plate, often identified between the cord insertions, displaying a characteristic speckled appearance on colour Doppler (Figure 11.1).[46,47] Their bidirectional waveform pattern on spectral Doppler reflects the summation of two chorionic arterial waveforms, with the periodicity being a function of the net difference in fetal heart rates. When an AAA is identified, 15% of pregnancies develop TTTS, compared with 61% where no AAA is seen (odds ratio 8.6).[46] Both *ex vivo* and endoscopic studies show that an AAA is present in around one-quarter to one-third of cases with TTTS.[42,48] The protective role of AAAs is further supported by a case report where TTTS developed acutely after thrombotic occlusion of an AAA.[49] Where TTTS does develop, detection of an AAA on ultrasound confers a survival advantage.[50] The presence of an AAA has been used to modify clinical staging,[51] because perinatal survival is significantly better stage-for-stage in the presence compared with the absence of an AAA. However, in stage IV TTTS outcomes appear paradoxically to be poorer in the presence of an AAA.[51] This concurs with an earlier study[52] that suggested that when intrauterine death occurs an AAA may mediate rapid agonal transfusion from the surviving twin to the dying co-twin, predisposing to death or neurological injury.[53,54] This raises the clinical dilemma of whether to ablate AAAs during endoscopic laser. In favour of ablation is the reduced risk of death or injury to the co-twin if one fetus does die *in utero*. Conversely, ablation of an AAA might worsen TTTS by halting haemodynamic compensation, precipitating worsening disease in the event of incomplete AVA ablation. This situation rarely arises clinically as AAAs are found predominantly in early-stage disease with good prognosis.

We know very little of how anastomoses form, and in particular what leads to the unbalanced patterns associated with TTTS. Sebire *et al.*[55] have suggested that TTTS results from a progressive (asymmetric) reduction of bidirectional arterio-venous connections during embryonic development of placental and fetal vessels in MC twins; this may explain why the classical features of TTTS do not develop in the first trimester. During the first trimester the placenta is still in the process of expanding and placental size is much larger relative to the fetus, facilitating compensation for vascular imbalances. Then in the second trimester the recipient's villous capillaries distend under an increased luminal pressure, as available intervillous space decreases, compared with the first trimester,[56] and colloid osmotic pressure and viscosity in fetal

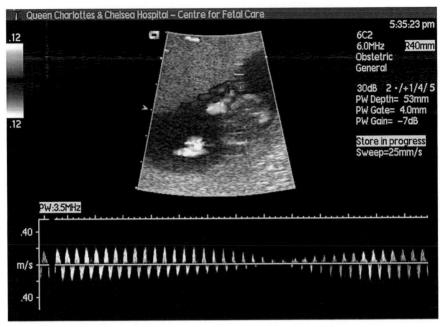

Figure 11.1. Colour Doppler imaging of an artery to artery anastomosis, showing typical bidirectional flow and periodicity

blood increases.[57] Finally, fetal kidneys are not fully functional at 12 weeks when the skin is still highly permeable to amniotic fluid, and thus amniotic volume discordance as a result of discordant urine output only occurs later.

The rate of flow through an AVA must be sufficiently high, presumably several mL/hour, to avoid thrombosis from stasis. However, this magnitude of flow, if uncompensated (and placentas from TTTS and non-TTTS cases have been reported with only a single AVA),[32] would lead to a physiologically implausible daily inter-twin transfusion that is several times the recipient's circulating volume. Quantisation of anastomotic flow would help resolve this dilemma and improve understanding of why gestation at presentation is so variable and why some disease regresses and others progress with advancing gestation. There have been several unrefined attempts to measure anastomotic blood flow, which have given some insight into the order of magnitude of transfusional flow.

Denbow et al.,[58] using colour Doppler, derived an approximate mean flow along an AAA of 4.5×10^{-3} mL/min at 28 weeks of gestation. Although unidirectional flow increased with gestation, net flow did not did not change significantly. We investigated flow in AVAs based on the assumption that AAA flow compensated for net imbalance in AVA flow equally divided among surplus AVAs documented at later injection study, and derived mean flow velocities of 4.6×10^{-3} mL/min at 28 weeks, consistent with 6.5 mL/day.[58] Nakata et al.[59] tried to measure AVA blood flow using an unvalidated invasive intraamniotic Doppler technique. However, their resultant total flow of 25 mL/min (36 litres per day) seems biologically implausible. Such transfusional blood loss would cause exsanguination of a 20 week fetus within three minutes. This overestimation may have been contributed to by failing to identifying all the AVAs during endoscopy.[60] As has been recently described, small deep AVAs cannot be visualised from the chorionic plate.[61] Nevertheless, this would be unlikely to account for the differences of several orders of magnitude.

Fetal vascular compensation

The characteristic discordance in amniotic fluid volume is attributed to hyper-volaemia in the recipient leading to polyuria and polyhydramnios, with hypovolaemia in the donor leading to oliguria and oligohydramnios.[62] The increase in the recipient's central blood volume and thus atrial pressure is thought to mediate an increase in cardiac atrial natriuretic peptide (ANP) synthesis. ANP, which increases glomerular filtration rates and reduces reabsorption of sodium from the proximal renal tubule resulting in polyuria, has been found to be elevated in the recipient's blood and amniotic fluid.[63] There is some evidence to suggest that this may lead to suppression of antidiuretic hormone (ADH), further increasing urine output and recipient polyuria.[64] Conversely, in the donor hypovolaemia mediates oliguria. In addition, chronic under-perfusion in the donor may result in renal degenerative changes with reduced tubular mass. Loss of proximal medullary tubules by apoptosis may be a precursor of more diffuse renal tubular atrophy and renal dysgenesis which accounts for the renal failure observed in a small proportion of donors with ongoing disease at birth.[12,65] Fetal blood and amniotic fluid studies have shown that brain natriuretic peptide (BNP) is also higher in the recipient than in the donor.[66] BNP, while structurally similar to ANP, is transcriptionally distinct with diverse actions including regulation of amniotic fluid volumes, although the mechanism by which BNP regulates fetal fluid balance remains unclear.

Discordant fluid balance fails to explain all of the cardiovascular effects of TTTS, such as systemic hypertension in the recipient and reversibly increased downstream placental resistance in the donor, as discussed below. Instead, fetal endocrine responses have been implicated, which may accelerate the disease process and also have impli-cations for cardiovascular disease in later life.[31] Recent evidence[67] suggests that cell-free mRNA in amniotic fluid is derived from the fetus (rather than the placenta), which may allow investigation of altered fetal gene expression in TTTS. These authors found in TTTS recipients' amniotic fluid increased expression of a*quaporin 1*, a water transporter gene transcript. Aquaporin 1 has been postulated to play a role in water movement from the amniotic cavity across the placenta into the fetal circulation. The increase in aquaporin 1 in recipients suggests it may play a role in the polyhydramnios associated with TTTS but not hydrops.[67]

Hypervolaemia in the recipient results in cardiac overload. Increased preload is further compounded by elevated afterload.[26,68] Systemic hypertension was found in all recipients, whether or not associated with atrio-ventricular regurgitation.[68,69] Endo-thelin 1 (ET-1) may be one of the mediators involved in hypertension in recipients. ET-1 expression is increased in recipient fetuses with TTTS, especially those with hydrops.[70] Other vasoactive mediators such as nitric oxide or prostacyclin may also be involved

Vascular tone in the feto-placental bed, a major contributor to fetal vascular resistance, is mainly regulated, in the absence of neural innervation, by endocrine/paracrine mediators. There is evidence that placental vascular resistance is increased in the donor, with absent EDF seen in severe TTTS donors.[71] Acute return of positive

EDF in the umbilical arteries of surviving donors following cord occlusion of the recipient suggests that these Doppler changes are a function of more-acute TTTS-related placental vascular dysfunction rather than chronic intrauterine growth restriction (IUGR)-associated placental pathology.[72] Clinically, this supports the recipient as the preferred target for cord occlusion (and it is usually technically easier) where indicated in advanced TTTS. The observation that EDF in the donor returns following laser ablation or cord occlusion suggests that it is not only placental resistance but also inter-twin connections that affect umbilical artery Doppler waveforms.[73] In this light we have recently observed that MC twins with discordant IUGR have increased latency (time to delivery or intrauterine death) compared with singletons and dichorionic twins.[74] Based on comparative data, abnormal vascular function in donors in infancy seems largely preventable by timely laser treatment *in utero*.[31] This is perhaps surprising as these donors still had severe cardiovascular discordance prior to laser treatment (although duration may play an important role).

Recent evidence suggests that discordant renin–angiotensin system (RAS) activation may contribute to the phenotypic features of TTTS and explain some of the pathophysiology not attributable to either anatomical or physiological anomalies. Both immunohistochemistry and *in situ* hybridisation studies show upregulation of renin in donor and downregulation in recipient kidneys (Figure 11.2).[75,76] While RAS upregulation in the donor might be a beneficial pressor adaptation to hypovolaemia, raised angiotensin II could potentially decrease renal and placental blood flow, worsening donor oliguria, oligohydramnios and IUGR. The recipient's kidneys have reduced renin expression, as expected, in response to hypervolaemia.[76,77]

Mahieu-Caputo *et al.*[77] investigated postmortem kidneys from recipients to find congested haemorrhagic infarcts and hypertensive microangiopathy consistent with RAS overactivity (rather than underactivity). They speculated that RAS mediators produced in the donor twin, by renal renin upregulation, might transfer to the donor via placental anastomoses. This is supported by a recent case report[78] that showed similar levels of renin and aldosterone in donor and in recipient plasma. However, simple trans-anastomotic transfer alone is unlikely to explain the significant RAS effects in the recipient, because of both the small volumes of donor blood involved in inter-twin flux and the short half-life of RAS mediators (angiotensin II). While therapeutic manipulation with RAS blockers may one day be an option, pharmacological manipulation of RAS overactivity in the recipient remains a challenge owing to the adverse fetal side effects of both angiotensin converting enzyme (ACE) inhibitors and angiotensin receptor blockers[79] and to the difficulties in selective administration to twins with opposite pathologies.

Insights from treatment

There is clear evidence from laser studies that interrupting the inter-twin vascular anastomoses can, and often does, lead to resolution of the disease phenotype. Non-selective laser ablation of all placental vessels crossing the placental equator has been abandoned by most, if not all, centres owing to the high procedure-related losses, particularly of the donor, as a result of inadvertent devitalisation of normal cotyledons. Selective laser ablation of AVAs only is associated with fewer procedure-related losses, better survival and better short-term neurological outcome, at least for advanced disease.[80] The only completed randomised controlled trial to date comparing endoscopic laser with serial amnioreduction found that laser was associated with improved perinatal survival (76% versus 56% survival of at least one

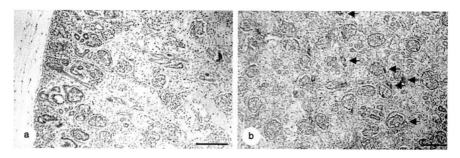

Figure 11.2. Renin immunolabelling in monochorionic twins complicated with TTTS: (a) in the recipient twin, all juxtaglomerular apparatus are renin negative; (b) in the donor twin, most juxtaglomerular apparatus are renin positive (arrows); scale bars = 100 μm; reproduced with permission from Mahieu-Caputo *et al.*[78]

twin) and a reduced incidence of short-term, predominantly imaging-based, neurological abnormalities (6% versus 14%).

Donor anuria and absent EDF can disappear after laser ablation, while recipients show reappearance of positive velocities during atrial contraction and even disappearance of hydrops.[81] Although the curative nature of laser ablation clearly supports the role of vascular anastomoses as pivotal in TTTS causation, only a third of treated pregnancies resulted in two healthy survivors.[82] This high level of failure suggests either technical limitations in laser ablation or that other underlying non-associated mechanisms may be involved. In terms of technical limitations, it is widely recognised that persistent or even reverse TTTS may recur many weeks after an apparently successful procedure.[61,83] Ville *et al.*[84] measured middle cerebral artery peak systolic velocities (MCA-PSV) as an indicator of fetal anaemia in double survivors of severe TTTS treated with selective laser. They found that eight of 55 (15%) recipient twins had an increased MCA-PSV between two and 28 days following laser ablation, and confirmed fetal anaemia by fetal blood sampling. They suggested that anaemia results from exsanguination of a hypervolaemic recipient into a hypovolaemic donor, and advocated MCA-PSV Doppler measurements following laser therapy. This may be the result of incomplete ablation or recanalisation of placental vessels. In this light, De Paepe *et al.*[60] showed, using post-procedure injection studies, that on average more than two AVAs are missed per procedure. Atypical, deep AVA connections lying beneath the chorionic plate may also be missed by fetoscopy.[85] Vascular casting (Figure 11.3) has shown that 53% of MC placentas had atypical AVAs (vascular connections between two apparently normal cotyledons) hidden beneath the chorionic plate with a mean diameter of 0.19 mm, and a mean length (distance between non-co-termination of the chorionic artery and vein) of 18.2 mm.[85] These atypical AVAs, while frequent, are small in size compared with chorionic plate vessels and convent-ional AVAs, and therefore their functional significance in terms of ability to mediate pathological inter-twin transfusion is unclear. Histomorphometric characterisation of shared and non-shared cotyledons in MC twins has shown that shared cotyledons in TTTS placentas are morphologically intermediate between donor and recipient cotyledons, and similar to cotyledons from MC twins discordant for IUGR, suggest-ing that these changes are not an isolated feature of TTTS.[86] Alternative explanations

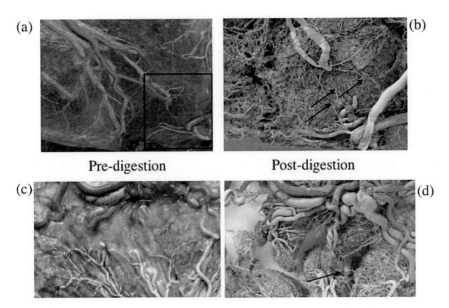

Figure 11.3. Atypical arterio-venous anastomoses (AVAs): (b) is a magnified post-digestion view of the area outlined by the black square in (a) and shows vessels transiting between the two normal cotyledons revealed by digestion (black arrows) that were not seen beforehand (a); in a further example, two apparently normal cotyledons on the surface (c) were revealed by digestion (d) to be communicating beneath the chorionic surface; the arrow in (d) indicates the vascular connection; reprinted from *Placenta*, vol. 26, Wee LY *et al.*, Characterisation of deep arterio-venous anastomoses within monochorionic placentae by vascular casting, pages 19–24, © 2005. with permission from Elsevier

for the imperfect outcome following laser ablation include inherent treatment-independent limitations such as donor placental insufficiency, or pre-existing stretch effects on membranous integrity or cervical ripening.

Conclusion

The last decade has seen considerable progress in our understanding of twin-to-twin transfusion syndrome. This has mainly been in the characterisation of the disease phenotype and in clinical management. In contrast, and notwithstanding some advance, much of the pathophysiological basis of TTTS remains poorly understood. TTTS is attributed to trans-anastomotic transfusion between twins. Anastomoses are ubiquitous in MC placentas yet TTTS develops in only 15%. Although both *ex vivo* and *in vivo* studies have failed to identify a unique anastomotic signature, TTTS placentas are typically associated with an imbalance in unidirectional arterio-venous anastomoses, with absent bidirectional anastomoses. Doppler detection of an arterio-arterial anastomosis reduces the chance of TTTS, whereas in those that develop disease, it improves stage-independent survival. Selective laser is often curative, but an increasingly recognised risk of persistent or reverse TTTS may be attributable to atypical arterio-venous anastomoses not identifiable from the chorionic plate. Simple dysvolaemia fails to explain several phenotypic features, including haematological concordance, recipient hypertension and reversibly absent EDF in the donor. The renin–angiotensin system is upregulated in the donor and downregulated in the recipient's kidneys, while paradoxically raised renin levels, along with endothelin, may contribute to raised afterload in the recipient.

In conclusion, current research suggests that the process is likely to be more complicated than a simple vascular developmental anomaly, and may represent a result of a combination of aberrant placental angioarchitecture, uteroplacental insufficiency, altered placental vascular reactivity and maladaptive expression of fetal vasoactive and humoral factors. Although research is limited in humans by therapy and the lack of a suitable experimental model, further studies of placental and vascular pathophysiology may not only refine current treatment modalities but also suggest further avenues for downstream management, such as genetic predisposition testing or pharmacological intervention.

Acknowledgements

We acknowledge programme funding for our work from the Richard & Jack Wiseman Trust and other support from SPARKS, Action Medical Research, Children Nationwide Medical Research Fund, Wellbeing and the Institute of Obstetrics & Gynaecology Trust.

References

1. Fisk NM. The scientific basis of feto-fetal transfusion syndrome and its treatment. In: Ward RHT, Whittle MJ, editors. *Multiple Pregnancy*. London: RCOG Press; 1995. p. 235–50.
2. Galea P, Jain V, Fisk NM. Insights into the pathophysiology of twin–twin transfusion syndrome. *Prenat Diagn* 2005;25:777–85.
3. Senat MV, Deprest J, Boulvain M, Paupe A, Winer N, Ville Y. Endoscopic laser surgery versus serial amnioreduction for severe twin-to-twin transfusion syndrome. *N Engl J Med* 2004;351:136–44.
4. Robyr R, Yamamoto M, Ville Y. Selective feticide in complicated monochorionic twin pregnancies using ultrasound-guided bipolar cord coagulation. *BJOG* 2005;112:1344–8.
5. Fisk NM, Taylor MJO. The fetus with twin–twin transfusion syndrome. In: Harrison MR, Evans MI, Adzick NS, Holzgreve W, editors. *The Unborn Patient: the Art and Science of Fetal Therapy*. 3rd ed. Philadelphia: WB Saunders; 2001.
6. Quintero RA, Morales WJ, Allen MH, Bornick PW, Johnson PK, Kruger M. Staging of twin–twin transfusion syndrome. *J Perinatol* 1999;19:550–5.
7. Taylor MJ, Govender L, Jolly M, Wee L, Fisk NM. Validation of the Quintero staging system for twin–twin transfusion syndrome. *Obstet Gynecol* 2002;100:1257–65.
8. Duncombe GJ, Dickinson JE, Evans SF. Perinatal characteristics and outcomes of pregnancies complicated by twin–twin transfusion syndrome. *Obstet Gynecol* 2003;101:1190–6.
9. Ville Y, Van Peborgh P, Gagnon A, Frydman R, Fernandez H. [Surgical treatment of twin-to-twin transfusion syndrome: coagulation of anastomoses with a Nd:YAG laser, under endosonographic control. Forty four cases]. *J Gynecol Obstet Biol Reprod (Paris)* 1997;26:175–81.
10. Trespidi L, Boschetto C, Caravelli E, Villa L, Kustermann A, Nicolini U. Serial amniocenteses in the management of twin–twin transfusion syndrome: when is it valuable? *Fetal Diagn Ther* 1997;12:15–20.
11. De Lia JE, Kuhlmann RS, Lopez KP. Treating previable twin–twin transfusion syndrome with fetoscopic laser surgery: outcomes following the learning curve. *J Perinat Med* 1999;27:61–7.
12. Cincotta RB, Gray PH, Phythian G, Rogers YM, Chan FY. Long term outcome of twin–twin transfusion syndrome. *Arch Dis Child Fetal Neonatal Ed* 2000;83:F171–6.
13. Haverkamp F, Lex C, Hanisch C, Fahnenstich H, Zerres K. Neurodevelopmental risks in twin-to-twin transfusion syndrome: preliminary findings. *Eur J Paediatr Neurol* 2001;5:21–7.
14. Mari G, Roberts A, Detti L, Kovanci E, Stefos T, Bahado-Singh RO, *et al.* Perinatal morbidity and mortality rates in severe twin–twin transfusion syndrome: results of the International Amnioreduction Registry. *Am J Obstet Gynecol* 2001;185:708–15.

15. Bejar R, Vigliocco G, Gramajo H, Solana C, Benirschke K, Berry C, et al. Antenatal origin of neurologic damage in newborn infants. II. Multiple gestations. *Am J Obstet Gynecol* 1990;162:1230–6.

16. Dickinson JE, Evans SF. Obstetric and perinatal outcomes from the Australian and New Zealand Twin–Twin Transfusion Syndrome Registry. *Am J Obstet Gynecol* 2000;182:706–12.

17. Mari G, Detti L, Oz U, Abuhamad AZ. Long-term outcome in twin–twin transfusion syndrome treated with serial aggressive amnioreduction. *Am J Obstet Gynecol* 2000;183:211–7.

18. Nicolini U, Poblete A. Single intrauterine death in monochorionic twin pregnancies. *Ultrasound Obstet Gynecol* 1999;14:297–301.

19. Wee LY, Taylor MJ, Vanderheyden T, Talbert D, Fisk NM. Transmitted arterio-arterial anastomosis waveforms causing cyclically intermittent absent/reversed end-diastolic umbilical artery flow in monochorionic twins. *Placenta* 2003;24:772–8.

20. Denbow ML, Battin MR, Cowan F, Azzopardi D, Edwards AD, Fisk NM. Neonatal cranial ultrasonographic findings in preterm twins complicated by severe fetofetal transfusion syndrome. *Am J Obstet Gynecol* 1998;178:479–83.

21. Mercuri E, Cowan F, Gupte G, Manning R, Laffan M, Rutherford M, et al. Prothrombotic disorders and abnormal neurodevelopmental outcome in infants with neonatal cerebral infarction. *Pediatrics* 2001;107:1400–4.

22. Sutcliffe AG, Sebire NJ, Pigott AJ, Taylor B, Edwards PR, Nicolaides KH. Outcome for children born after in utero laser ablation therapy for severe twin-to-twin transfusion syndrome. *BJOG* 2001;108:1246–50.

23. Banek CS, Hecher K, Hackeloer BJ, Bartmann P. Long-term neurodevelopmental outcome after intrauterine laser treatment for severe twin–twin transfusion syndrome. *Am J Obstet Gynecol* 2003;188:876–80.

24. Dickinson JE, Duncombe GJ, Evans SF, French NP, Hagan R. The long term neurologic outcome of children from pregnancies complicated by twin-to-twin transfusion syndrome. *BJOG* 2005;112:63–8.

25. Karatza AA, Wolfenden JL, Taylor MJ, Wee L, Fisk NM, Gardiner HM. Influence of twin–twin transfusion syndrome on fetal cardiovascular structure and function: prospective case-control study of 136 monochorionic twin pregnancies. *Heart* 2002;88:271–7.

26. Zosmer N, Bajoria R, Weiner E, Rigby M, Vaughan J, Fisk NM. Clinical and echographic features of in utero cardiac dysfunction in the recipient twin in twin–twin transfusion syndrome. *Br Heart J* 1994;72:74–9.

27. Simpson LL, Marx GR, Elkadry EA, D'Alton ME. Cardiac dysfunction in twin–twin transfusion syndrome: a prospective, longitudinal study. *Obstet Gynecol* 1998;92(4 Pt 1):557–62.

28. Lougheed J, Sinclair BG, Fung Kee Fung K, Bigras JL, Ryan G, Smallhorn JF, et al. Acquired right ventricular outflow tract obstruction in the recipient twin in twin–twin transfusion syndrome. *J Am Coll Cardiol* 2001;38:1533–8.

29. Fesslova V, Villa L, Nava S, Mosca F, Nicolini U. Fetal and neonatal echocardiographic findings in twin–twin transfusion syndrome. *Am J Obstet Gynecol* 1998;179:1056–62.

30. Cheung YF, Taylor MJ, Fisk NM, Redington AN, Gardiner HM. Fetal origins of reduced arterial distensibility in the donor twin in twin–twin transfusion syndrome. *Lancet* 2000;355:1157–8.

31. Gardiner HM, Taylor MJ, Karatza A, Vanderheyden T, Huber A, Greenwald SE, et al. Twin–twin transfusion syndrome: the influence of intrauterine laser photocoagulation on arterial distensibility in childhood. *Circulation* 2003;107:1906–11.

32. Bajoria R, Wigglesworth J, Fisk NM. Angioarchitecture of monochorionic placentas in relation to the twin–twin transfusion syndrome. *Am J Obstet Gynecol* 1995;172:856–63.

33. Machin GA. Placental vascular anatomy and twin transfusion syndrome. *Am J Obstet Gynecol* 1996;174:799–800.

34. Denbow ML, Cox P, Taylor M, Hammal DM, Fisk NM. Placental angioarchitecture in monochorionic twin pregnancies: relationship to fetal growth, fetofetal transfusion syndrome, and pregnancy outcome. *Am J Obstet Gynecol* 2000;182:417–26.

35. Denbow ML, Blomley MJ, Cosgrove DO, Fisk NM. Ultrasound microbubble contrast angiography in monochorionic twin fetuses. *Lancet* 1997;349:773.

36. Denbow ML, Welsh AW, Taylor MJ, Blomley MJ, Cosgrove DO, Fisk NM. Twin fetuses: intravascular microbubble US contrast agent administration – early experience. *Radiology* 2000;214:724–8.

37. Fisk NM, Borrell A, Hubinont C, Tannirandorn Y, Nicolini U, Rodeck CH. Fetofetal transfusion syndrome: do the neonatal criteria apply in utero? *Arch Dis Child* 1990;65(7 Spec No):657–61.

38. Tanaka M, Natori M, Ishimoto H, Kohno H, Kobayashi T, Nozawa S. Intravascular pancuronium bromide infusion for prenatal diagnosis of twin–twin transfusion syndrome. *Fetal Diagn Ther* 1992;7:36–40.

39. Bajoria R. Vascular anatomy of monochorionic placenta in relation to discordant growth and amniotic fluid volume. *Hum Reprod* 1998;13:2933–40.

40. Machin G, Still K, Lalani T. Correlations of placental vascular anatomy and clinical outcomes in 69 monochorionic twin pregnancies. *Am J Med Genet* 1996;61:229–36.

41. Umur A, van Gemert MJ, Nikkels PG. Monoamniotic-versus diamniotic-monochorionic twin placentas: anastomoses and twin–twin transfusion syndrome. *Am J Obstet Gynecol* 2003;189:1325–9.

42. Diehl W, Hecher K, Zikulnig L, Vetter M, Hackeloer BJ. Placental vascular anastomoses visualized during fetoscopic laser surgery in severe mid-trimester twin–twin transfusion syndrome. *Placenta* 2001;22:876–81.

43. Bermudez C, Becerra C, Bornick PW, Allen MH, Arroyo J, Quintero RA. Twin–twin transfusion syndrome with only superficial placental anastomoses: endoscopic and pathological evidence. *J Matern Fetal Neonatal Med* 2002;12:138–40.

44. Talbert DG, Bajoria R, Sepulveda W, Bower S, Fisk NM. Hydrostatic and osmotic pressure gradients produce manifestations of fetofetal transfusion syndrome in a computerized model of monochorial twin pregnancy. *Am J Obstet Gynecol* 1996;174:598–608.

45. Umur A, Van Gemert MJ, Ross MG. Amniotic fluid and hemodynamic model in monochorionic twin pregnancies and twin–twin transfusion syndrome. *Am J Physiol Regul Integr Comp Physiol* 2001;280:R1499–509.

46. Taylor MJ, Denbow ML, Tanawattanacharoen S, Gannon C, Cox PM, Fisk NM. Doppler detection of arterio-arterial anastomoses in monochorionic twins: feasibility and clinical application. *Hum Reprod* 2000;15:1632–6.

47. Fichera A, Mor E, Soregaroli M, Frusca T. Antenatal detection of arterio-arterial anastomoses by Doppler placental assessment in monochorionic twin pregnancies. *Fetal Diagn Ther* 2005;20:519–23.

48. Denbow ML, Eckersley R, Welsh AW, Taylor MJ, Carter RC, Cosgrove DO, et al. Ex vivo delineation of placental angioarchitecture with the microbubble contrast agent Levovist. *Am J Obstet Gynecol* 2000;182:966–71.

49. Tan TY, Denbow ML, Cox PM, Talbert D, Fisk NM. Occlusion of arterio-arterial anastomosis manifesting as acute twin–twin transfusion syndrome. *Placenta* 2004;25:238–42.

50. Taylor MJ, Denbow ML, Duncan KR, Overton TG, Fisk NM. Antenatal factors at diagnosis that predict outcome in twin–twin transfusion syndrome. *Am J Obstet Gynecol* 2000;183:1023–8.

51. Tan TY, Taylor MJ, Wee LY, Vanderheyden T, Wimalasundera R, Fisk NM. Doppler for artery-artery anastomosis and stage-independent survival in twin–twin transfusion. *Obstet Gynecol* 2004;103:1174–80.

52. Bajoria R, Wee LY, Anwar S, Ward S. Outcome of twin pregnancies complicated by single intrauterine death in relation to vascular anatomy of the monochorionic placenta. *Hum Reprod* 1999;14:2124–30.

53. Fusi L, McParland P, Fisk N, Nicolini U, Wigglesworth J. Acute twin–twin transfusion: a possible mechanism for brain-damaged survivors after intrauterine death of a monochorionic twin. *Obstet Gynecol* 1991;78(3 Pt 2):517–20.

54. Tanawattanacharoen S, Taylor MJ, Letsky EA, Cox PM, Cowan FM, Fisk NM. Intrauterine rescue transfusion in monochorionic multiple pregnancies with recent single intrauterine death. *Prenat Diagn* 2001;21:274–8.

55. Sebire NJ, Talbert D, Fisk NM. Twin-to-twin transfusion syndrome results from dynamic asymmetrical reduction in placental anastomoses: a hypothesis. *Placenta* 2001;22:383–91.

56. Boyd PA. Quantitative structure of the normal human placenta from 10 weeks of gestation to term. *Early Hum Dev* 1984;9:297–307.

57. Sebire NJ, Jain V, Talbert DG. Spiral artery associated restricted growth (SPAARG): a computer model of pathophysiology resulting from low intervillous pressure having fetal programming implications. *Pathophysiology* 2004;11:87–94.

58. Denbow ML, Taylor M, Cox P, Fisk NM. Derivation of rate of arterio-arterial anastomotic transfusion between monochorionic twin fetuses by Doppler waveform analysis. *Placenta* 2004;25:664–70.

59. Nakata M, Martinez JM, Diaz C, Chmait R, Quintero RA. Intra-amniotic Doppler measurement of blood flow in placental vascular anastomoses in twin–twin transfusion syndrome. *Ultrasound Obstet Gynecol* 2004;24:102–3.

60. De Paepe ME, Friedman RM, Poch M, Hansen K, Carr SR, Luks FI. Placental findings after laser ablation of communicating vessels in twin-to-twin transfusion syndrome. *Pediatr Dev Pathol* 2004;7:159–65.

61. Wee LY, Taylor MJ, Vanderheyden T, Wimalasundera R, Gardiner HM, Fisk NM. Reversal of

twin–twin transfusion syndrome: frequency, vascular anatomy, associated anomalies and outcome. *Prenat Diagn* 2004;24:104–10.

62. Rosen DJ, Rabinowitz R, Beyth Y, Fejgin MD, Nicolaides KH. Fetal urine production in normal twins and in twins with acute polyhydramnios. *Fetal Diagn Ther* 1990;5:57–60.

63. Bajoria R, Ward S, Sooranna SR. Atrial natriuretic peptide mediated polyuria: pathogenesis of polyhydramnios in the recipient twin of twin–twin transfusion syndrome. *Placenta* 2001;22:716–24.

64. Bajoria R, Ward S, Sooranna SR. Influence of vasopressin in the pathogenesis of oligohydramnios-polyhydramnios in monochorionic twins. *Eur J Obstet Gynecol Reprod Biol* 2004;113:49–55.

65. Oberg KC, Pestaner JP, Bielamowicz L, Hawkins EP. Renal tubular dysgenesis in twin–twin transfusion syndrome. *Pediatr Dev Pathol* 1999;2:25–32.

66. Bajoria R, Ward S, Chatterjee R. Brain natriuretic peptide and endothelin-1 in the pathogenesis of polyhydramnios-oligohydramnios in monochorionic twins. *Am J Obstet Gynecol* 2003;189:189–94.

67. Larrabee PB, Johnson KL, Lai C, Ordovas J, Cowan JM, Tantravahi U, et al. Global gene expression analysis of the living human fetus using cell-free messenger RNA in amniotic fluid. *JAMA* 2005;293:836–42.

68. Mahieu-Caputo D, Salomon LJ, Le Bidois J, Fermont L, Brunhes A, Jouvet P, et al. Fetal hypertension: an insight into the pathogenesis of the twin–twin transfusion syndrome. *Prenat Diagn* 2003;23:640–5.

69. Holen J, Simonsen S. Determination of pressure gradient in mitral stenosis with Doppler echocardiography. *Br Heart J* 1979;41:529–35.

70. Bajoria R, Sullivan M, Fisk NM. Endothelin concentrations in monochorionic twins with severe twin–twin transfusion syndrome. *Hum Reprod* 1999;14:1614–18.

71. Giles WB, Trudinger BJ, Cook CM, Connelly AJ. Doppler umbilical artery studies in the twin–twin transfusion syndrome. *Obstet Gynecol* 1990;76:1097–9.

72. Taylor MJ, Shalev E, Tanawattanacharoen S, Jolly M, Kumar S, Weiner E, et al. Ultrasound-guided umbilical cord occlusion using bipolar diathermy for Stage III/IV twin–twin transfusion syndrome. *Prenat Diagn* 2002;22:70–6.

73. Rizzo G, Arduini D, Romanini C. Cardiac and extracardiac flows in discordant twins. *Am J Obstet Gynecol* 1994;170(5 Pt 1):1321–7.

74. Vanderheyden TM, Fichera A, Pasquini L, Tan TY, Wee LY, Frusca T, et al. Increased latency of absent end-diastolic flow in the umbilical artery of monochorionic twin fetuses. *Ultrasound Obstet Gynecol* 2005;26:44–9.

75. Mahieu-Caputo D, Dommergues M, Delezoide AL, Lacoste M, Cai Y, Narcy F, et al. Twin-to-twin transfusion syndrome. Role of the fetal renin-angiotensin system. *Am J Pathol* 2000;156:629–36.

76. Kilby MD, Platt C, Whittle MJ, Oxley J, Lindop GB. Renin gene expression in fetal kidneys of pregnancies complicated by twin–twin transfusion syndrome. *Pediatr Dev Pathol* 2001;4:175–9.

77. Mahieu-Caputo D, Muller F, Joly D, Gubler MC, Lebidois J, Fermont L, et al. Pathogenesis of twin–twin transfusion syndrome: the renin-angiotensin system hypothesis. *Fetal Diagn Ther* 2001;16:241–4.

78. Mahieu-Caputo D, Meulemans A, Martinovic J, Gubler MC, Delezoide AL, Muller F, et al. Paradoxic activation of the renin-angiotensin system in twin–twin transfusion syndrome: an explanation for cardiovascular disturbances in the recipient. *Pediatr Res* 2005;58:685–8.

79. Cox RM, Anderson JM, Cox P. Defective embryogenesis with angiotensin II receptor antagonists in pregnancy. *BJOG* 2003;110:1038.

80. Quintero RA, Dickinson JE, Morales WJ, Bornick PW, Bermudez C, Cincotta R, et al. Stage-based treatment of twin–twin transfusion syndrome. *Am J Obstet Gynecol* 2003;188:1333–40.

81. Zikulnig L, Hecher K, Bregenzer T, Baz E, Hackeloer BJ. Prognostic factors in severe twin–twin transfusion syndrome treated by endoscopic laser surgery. *Ultrasound Obstet Gynecol* 1999;14:380–7.

82. Fisk NM, Galea P. Twin–twin transfusion – as good as it gets? *N Engl J Med* 2004;351:182–4.

83. Robyr R, Lewi L, Yamamoto M, Ortqvist L, Deprest J, Ville Y. P12.21: Permanent feto-fetal transfusion from the recipient to the donor twin. A complication of laser surgery in twin-to-twin transfusion syndrome (TTTS). *Ultrasound Obstet Gynecol* 2004;24:339.

84. Robyr R, Lewi L, Yamamoto M, Deprest J, Ville Y, Permanent feto-fetal transfusion from the recipient to the donor twin. A complication of laser surgery in twin-to-twin transfusion syndrome. 25th Annual Meeting of the Society of Maternal and Fetal Medicine; 2005, Reno, Nevada: 574.

85. Wee LY, Taylor M, Watkins N, Franke V, Parker K, Fisk NM. Characterisation of deep arterio-

venous anastomoses within monochorionic placentae by vascular casting. *Placenta* 2005;26:19–24.

86. Wee LY, Sebire NJ, Bhundia J, Sullivan M, Fisk NM. Histomorphometric characterisation of shared and non-shared cotyledonary villus territories of monochorionic placentae in relation to pregnancy complications. *Placenta* 2006;27:475–82.

Chapter 12
Twin-to-twin transfusion syndrome

Masami Yamamoto and Yves Ville

Introduction

Twin-to-twin transfusion syndrome (TTTS) may affect 15% of all monochorionic twin pregnancies and has a high perinatal mortality rate. Vascular anastomoses on the chorionic plate of the monochorionic placenta is the anatomical basis for the circulations of the twins to communicate and to create inter-twin haemodynamic imbalance. Ultrasound diagnosis of polyhydramnios/oligohydramnios has become the gold standard for the diagnosis of TTTS, irrespective of any discordance in weight or haemoglobin levels. These later, neonatal criteria are used for surviving twins but not in cases of double or single fetal demise, which are likely to be affected by the most severe forms of TTTS. Recent demonstration of the benefit of primary laser surgery over amnioreduction has highlighted the issue of optimisation of the results with laser treatment but also of the diagnosis and management of early and late complications following placental surgery.

Miscarriage, preterm prelabour rupture of membranes (PPROM) and preterm delivery account for more than 20% of perinatal mortality after treatment. Recurrence of TTTS, fetal demise or feto-fetal haemorrhage with anaemia or polycythaemia respectively are complications that have to be managed with various secondary therapeutic options such as repeat-laser, amnioreduction, intrauterine transfusion or selective cord coagulation. *Ex vivo* placental angiography has confirmed that these complications occur when anastomoses are missed.

Optimisation of laser treatment of TTTS and new insight into the follow-up of treated cases are likely to be the key to better prognosis.

Diagnosis of the pathological condition

Before the use of ultrasound, TTTS was diagnosed at birth by at least a 20% discordance in weight and at least a 5 g/dL difference in haemoglobin concentration between two twins of the same sex at birth.[1] These criteria were abandoned because they could be used for surviving twins but not in cases of double or single fetal demise, which may well have been affected by even more severe TTTS. With the development of ultrasound, new antenatal findings were correlated to the adverse outcome of TTTS. The polyhydramnios/oligohydramnios sequence has been found to be the condition associated with one of the highest perinatal mortality rates, occurring in up to 90% of cases without treatment. Understanding the mechanisms leading to complications and perinatal death is important in order to plan diagnostic and treatment strategies. With the use of Doppler and high-resolution two-dimensional imaging, new information on fetal anaemia, hypervolaemia and fetal diuresis has become available.

The mechanisms by which TTTS may lead to fetal death and sequelae are numerous (see Chapter 11). TTTS may lead to fetal demise *in utero* through cardiac overload or severe IUGR in recipients and donors, respectively. It may also lead to extreme preterm delivery as a consequence of the effect of polyhydramnios on uterine distension and cervical competence. Haemodynamic imbalance is responsible for most abnormalities developing in monochorionic twins. Studying these complications and the possibilities for treating them independently will increase the chances of survival and the overall success rate of the various treatment modalities.

Correlation with placental abnormalities

Monochorionic placentas were first described at the beginning of the twentieth century.[2] However, it was only in the late 1990s that larger series were published reviewing the evidence for their role in TTTS. All monochorionic placentas have vascular communication between the two cords, as demonstrated in all 278 such placentas in one study.[3] However, TTTS occurs in only about 15% of monochorionic pregnancies. The functional pattern of the anastomoses is therefore critical in the development of TTTS.

Anastomoses are classified into superficial artery to artery (AA), superficial vein to vein (VV) and deep artery to vein (AV). Superficial anastomoses are direct communications between two cords insertions. They are called superficial because their branches are visible and connect on the surface of the chorionic plate. The main characteristics of these is that they can compensate for the inter-twin shift of higher volumes of blood in a rapid manner and in both directions depending on the inter-twin difference in pressure in the arterial and venous systems.

Machin *et al.*[4] examined 69 placentas from monochorionic twin pregnancies. They studied the presence of vascular anastomoses, placental sharing and their correlation with perinatal mortality, growth discordance, gestational age at delivery and the presence of polyhydramnios. They used a dye injection technique but this was not performed in cases where no anastomoses could be identified by naked eye examination. They provided an interesting classification of 13 different patterns of anastomoses. In their study, the worst clinical outcomes were found in cases of unequal placental sharing with the presence of deep AV anastomoses and few or no superficial anastomoses, which were associated with TTTS in 60% of these cases. They also reported that 23% of these placentas showed no anastomoses, therefore challenging the accuracy of their technique.

Bajoria *et al.*[5] reported on ten placentas from TTTS and ten from normal monochorionic pregnancies. They also found fewer anastomoses in the TTTS group (median 1 (range 0–2) versus 6 (4–8), $P < 0.001$ Mann–Whitney). They found that TTTS placentas had fewer AA anastomoses (median 0 versus 2, $P < 0.0001$), VV anastomoses (median 0 versus 2, $P < 0.0001$) as well as deep AV anastomoses (median 1 versus 2.5, $P < 0.001$). Their conclusion was that TTTS placentas have on average one deep AV anastomoses without superficial ones. In controls, multiple anastomoses were present, with both deep and superficial ones. Denbow *et al.*[6] studied 71 placentas from monochorionic diamniotic pregnancies blinded to the perinatal outcome. They also found that TTTS placentas had fewer AA anastomoses (median 0 (range 0–1) versus 1 (0–1), $P < 0.0001$), with a similar incidence of AV and VV anastomoses. The highest incidence of TTTS was found in placentas with one AV and no AA anastomoses (78%). All TTTS placentas had deep AV anastomoses, in comparison with 84% of non-TTTS placentas. This study also introduced the interesting concept of 'rescue feto-fetal transfusion'.[6] This has been identified in fetuses with smaller placentas, but no weight discordance, in which there were deep AV anastomoses from the bigger to the smaller placental side, compensating for the difference in oxygenated blood flow to the fetuses despite the disproportion in maternal exchange surface.

Bermudez et al.[7] included placentas from 26 non-complicated monochorionic diamniotic pregnancies and from 105 TTTS cases treated by laser. They correlated the fetoscopy findings with air injection of the chorionic vessels after delivery in order to interpret the coagulated areas. This study found that deep AV anastomoses were more frequent in TTTS (4.6 ± 2.2 versus 1.4 ± 0.5, $P = 0.02$), whereas superficial vessels were equally present in both groups (1.6 ± 0.6 versus 1.7 ± 1.0 $P = 0.69$).

Even though there are technical differences in the methods used, the main conclusion of all these studies is that the presence of deep AV anastomoses and the absence of superficial anastomoses are more frequent in TTTS cases. The significant proportion of cases examined ex vivo showing no anastomoses at all should also question their validity as a gold standard for hypotheses to be built on. Ex vivo placental studies are not uniform in their selection criteria, and a greater effort should be made to select clinically valuable data. Table 12.1 summarises these data. Bajoria et al.[5] and Denbow et al.[6] disagree with the concept that an AV anastomosis is a critical condition for the occurrence of TTTS. However, all agree that the lack of AA or both AA and VV anastomoses may generate a circulatory system that favours development of hypervolaemia in one twin.[8]

Pathophysiology

Hypervolaemia and hypovolaemia in the recipient and in the donor twin, respectively, are the basis for the polyuric–polyhydramnios and oliguric–oligohydramnios sequence to develop. An interesting study was performed in 21 cases of TTTS with the death of both twins that showed striking differences in the kidneys of donors and recipients.[9] Besides a huge difference in size, most donors had renal tubular dysgenesis, characterised by the nearly complete absence of identifiable proximal tubules and by the ischaemic appearance of the glomeruli. These histological lesions have also been observed as part of a congenital autosomal recessive disorder responsible for oligohydramnios[10] as well as in fetuses exposed in utero to angiotensin-converting enzyme inhibitors.[11] This hypothesis is also supported by the observation of similar tubular changes in children with postnatal renal ischaemia. Upregulation of the renin synthesis was also demonstrated using immunohistochemistry and in situ hybridisation methods, with a strong increase in renin protein and mRNA content in the kidneys of the donors. The recipients' kidneys were larger and congestive, showing haemorrhagic infarction. No renin protein was detected in 20 of 21 recipient fetuses.[9]

Ultrasonographic evidence of this discordance is the polyhydramnios/oligohydramnios sequence. Volume overload in recipients has been demonstrated by inter-twin differences in the umbilical vein flow. Recently, umbilical vein flow has been found to be markedly different between donors and recipients,[12] and laser treatment has led to the improvement of this imbalance.[13] Absolute differences between donors and recipients were not corroborated probably because the umbilical vein flow of a donor at 26 weeks was higher than that of a recipient at 18 weeks as seen in our

Table 12.1. Twin-to-twin transfusion syndrome (TTTS) treated by laser and complicated by preterm prelabour rupture of membranes (PPROM); outcomes are organised by gestational age at PPROM; postnatal neurological development of liveborns was classified as normal or abnormal

Gestational age at rupture of the membranes (n)	Outcome of pregnancy (n)			
	Miscarriage	Fetal demise or termination before 24 weeks	Preterm delivery at 24–27 weeks	Preterm delivery at 28–34 weeks
Before 24 weeks (12)	9[a]	3[a]	0	0
At 24–27 weeks (17)	–	–	17	0
After 27 weeks (20)	–	–	–	20[b]

Gestational age at rupture of the membranes (n)	Fetal outcome		
	Fetal demise, termination or neonatal deaths (%)	Normal liveborns (%)	Abnormal liveborns (%)
Before 24 weeks (12)	100	0	0
At 24–27 weeks (17)	68	20	12
After 27 weeks (20)	33	66	2

[a] One case of TTTS in each group was treated with amnioreduction before laser
[b] One set of triplets developing normally was included

centre.[14] When the recipient to donor (R/D) index was calculated, which is the umbilical vein flow ratio between both fetuses without considering gestational age, this was found to be 3.3 on average in 50 consecutive TTTS cases before laser treatment. Favourable outcome cases, defined as double survival at birth without evidence of anaemia/polycythaemia needing intrauterine blood transfusion or recurrence of the poly/oligohydramnios sequence, presented a decrease in R/D index within 48 hours post-laser from 3.24 to 1.75 ($P = 0.006$ Wilcoxon). Unfavourable outcome cases with persistence of feto–fetal transfusion presented a non-significant decrease in R/D index from 2.32 to 2.19. We propose that a decrease in the R/D index could be an early predictor of a favourable outcome in TTTS. These data corroborate the histopathological findings on chorionic plate anastomoses and postmortem examinations of affected fetuses.

Diagnosis

First-trimester ultrasound examination is pivotal in determining chorionicity. In monochorionic pregnancies, ultrasound examinations empirically should be performed every two weeks, with assessment of amniotic fluid (AF) volume using the deepest pool measurement, fetal growth and cervical length (Figure 12.1). This should allow early diagnosis of TTTS. Actually, most TTTS cases are diagnosed at around 22 weeks of gestation, which corresponds to the routine second-trimester examination in most pregnancy care systems.

The selection criteria to qualify for percutaneous endoscopy-directed laser coagulation of placental anastomoses are: (i) gestational age of less than 26 weeks, (ii) ultrasound diagnosis of a single monochorionic placenta in the first trimester of pregnancy, (iii) polyhydramnios in the recipient's amniotic cavity with a deepest vertical pool 8 cm or more, or 10 cm or more than 10 cm before or after 20 weeks of gestation, respectively, and oligohydramnios in the donor's amniotic sac with the deepest vertical pool 2 cm or less. These selection criteria were used in the only randomised trial that showed a clear benefit of laser therapy over amnioreduction. The benefits in cases diagnosed after 26 weeks of gestation are not clear, but the high mortality of liveborns before 28 weeks of gestation should make us reconsider the value of this cut-off gestational age.

TTTS diagnosis

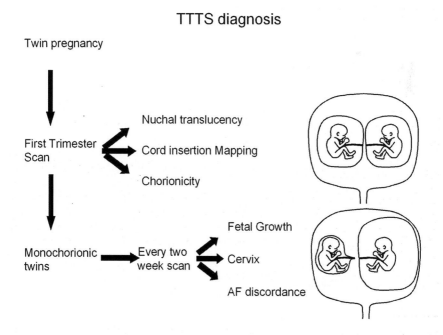

Figure 12.1. Diagnosis of twin-to-twin transfusion syndrome

Staging

Ultrasound staging of TTTS was introduced by Quintero *et al.* in 1999.[15] Stage I is characterised by the oligo/polyhydramnios sequence with the donor's bladder still visible, whereas in stage II the bladder cannot be visualised in the donor. Stage III presents with critically abnormal Doppler with absent or reversed-end diastolic flow in the umbilical artery or reverse flow in the ductus venosus in either twin. In stage IV there is hydrops and in stage V there is demise of one or both twins. The classification is very convenient for describing cases in a reproducible manner but prognosis is hardly related to staging. A prospective study of 52 cases from London[16] showed that 15% of the cases improved within the classification, with similar mortality between groups. Gestational age at presentation was 24, 20, 20, 21 and 16 weeks of gestation for stages I to V, respectively. In 175 consecutive cases treated by laser in our centre in Poissy, gestational age at presentation was similar among all groups.[17] These observations suggest that stages do not illustrate different steps in the natural progression of the disease, but rather different forms with possibly different prognoses. Quintero *et al.*[18] reported that laser photocoagulation appeared to be better than amnioreduction in stages III or IV, whereas the outcomes in stages I and II were similar in both groups. However, in the Eurofetus randomised trial,[19] survival of at least one twin was obtained in 86% and 58% of the cases treated by laser and amnioreduction, respectively, in TTTS in stages I or II, and this difference persisted in stages III and IV (66% versus 44%).

This randomised trial has demonstrated that before 26 weeks of gestation laser photocoagulation (LPC) treatment can lead to the neonatal survival of at least one surviving twin at birth and intact survival at six months of age (76% in each case), compared with 56% and 51%, respectively, of cases treated by serial amnioreduction. A systematic review[20] of Medline, Embase and the Cochrane Library for 'treatments for TTTS' led to 831 citations. From these, only four studies compared therapies such as laser versus amnioreduction (three) or amnioreduction versus septostomy (one); the rest were mainly case series. Therefore, only four series report the comparison of two treatments for TTTS: three studies were controlled[6,21,22] and one was a randomised study.[19] In this review, 240 laser photocoagulations were reported and compared with 198 cases treated with serial amnioreduction. Total survival was better in LPC cases, between 56% and 62%. Survival of one at least one twin in LPC was between 76% and 83%. With amnioreduction, total survival and survival of at least one twin ranged from 38% to 64% and 51% to 85%, respectively. All studies reported an improved overall neurological morbidity with LPC, with odds ratios ranging from 0.43 to 0.15.

Therefore, LPC treatment for TTTS will probably be more widely used as a first-line treatment in the near future. Endoscopic treatment of TTTS by LPC can also turn the disease into a different one, with newly recognised complications that need to be diagnosed and managed appropriately. Since the overall survival is probably still not optimal, improvements have to be made to the technique in order to decrease the incidence of complications and decrease further perinatal mortality as well as to improve their management.

Surgery

Preoperative evaluation consists of a detailed ultrasound examination, including morphological examination, fetal Doppler, cardiothoracic index, location of the placenta and cord insertions. Size discrepancy, Doppler and bladder discordance are not used as selection criteria. Cerclage, amnioreduction or amniocentesis should be avoided before laser because of the risk of AF contamination, unless it is necessary for transportation. Only one trocar insertion is performed. The fetoscope is inserted at right angles to the donor's longitudinal axis along an imaginary line between the two cord insertions that provides the best opportunity to visualise the anastomoses on the chorionic plate. This corresponds statistically to the highest probability of visualising the vascular equator of the placenta as well as the inter-twin membrane. Figure 12.2 shows a situation in which the donor is on the right and on the posterior uterine wall. The fetoscope is introduced from the top, close to the umbilicus. When these two criteria are met, the vascular equator of the placenta and the vascular anastomoses are more likely to be visualised in the operative field. This imaginary situation is ideal but seldom found, because the donor is stuck against the placenta far from the coagulation zone. More complex surgical situations may be found in anterior placenta, close cord insertions at the placenta or with the donor twin stuck between the cord insertions.

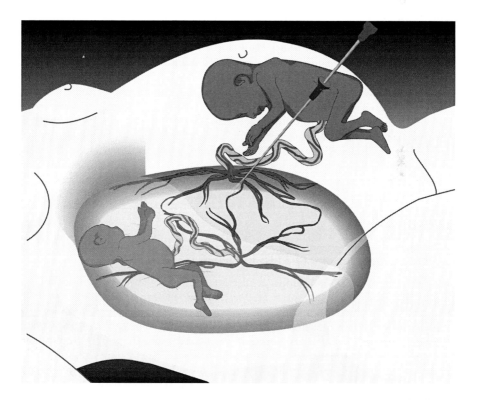

Figure 12.2.   Fetoscope insertion in the anterior uterine wall in a case of posterior placenta; the donor is stuck at the posterior wall, on the placental chorionic plate; reproduced from *Am J Obstet Gynecol* vol. 193, Yamamoto *et al*, © 2005, with permission from Elsevier.[17]

Prophylactic intravenous cefazolin (2 g) is administered routinely one hour before laser surgery. Indometacin suppository (100 mg) is administered the night before and one hour before surgery as prophylactic tocolysis. Oral flunitrazepam is given one hour before surgery and local anaesthesia with non-adrenalinised Xylocaine® (lidocaine) is injected down to the myometrium. A 10 Fr cannula loaded with a trocar is introduced percutaneously under continuous ultrasound guidance. A 2 mm 0° fetoscope (Storz 26008 AA) is used in a straight or curved sheath to operate on anterior or posterior placentas, respectively. The sheath also has a working channel carrying a 1 mm diode laser fibre that is introduced into the recipient's amniotic sac.

A systematic examination of the chorionic plate alongside the insertion of the inter-twin membrane is performed, beginning in one placental border and finishing in the other. Identification of crossing vessels and of their arterial or venous nature is possible since arteries cross over veins and show a darker red colour than veins owing to a lower oxygen saturation in the circulating blood.[23] The objective of laser coagulation is to separate the two circulations completely, in order to treat the condition and to protect one twin in the event of the death of the co-twin. A selective approach for the coagulation of anastomotic vessels is best performed with the aim of separating the monochorionic placenta into two distinct fetal–placental circulations, sparing the normal cotyledons of each placental territory. For this, each vessel that crossed the inter-twin membrane insertion in the chorionic plate should be followed up to and from both cords. The anastomotic vessels are identified as those that reach the opposite cord. The normal vessels are kept and identified as those that reach a cotyledon, penetrate the chorionic plate to perfuse the cotyledon, and are drained back towards the same cord through a venous branch.

The priority now is the optimisation of survival rates after treatment. TTTS treatment encompasses many aspects, and therefore different treatment strategies may affect the overall survival as well as morbidity in the survivors. One important problem is to stop the transfusion process by coagulating the anastomotic vessels, avoiding fetal demise and recurrence of the disease. This calls for a technique that has an appropriate balance between selectivity and coagulation efficacy. Several complications may affect the prognosis after laser surgery, such as IUGR, fetal demise, anaemia or recurrence of TTTS. Prompt diagnosis and treatment of these conditions will contribute to increasing the overall survival rate. Finally, the risk of prematurity remains high and the issues of PPROM and preterm delivery also have to be addressed.

Specific complications of TTTS following laser treatment

Besides obstetrical complications similar to those that may occur in multiple pregnancies without TTTS, cases treated by laser can develop recurrence of the polyhydramnios/oligohydramnios sequence, polycythaemia/anaemia without AF discordance[24] or death of one twin with anaemia in the survivor. These are specific complications resulting from the persistence of anastomoses. These late complications may appear one or more weeks following the first procedure (Figure 12.3).

Absent or reverse-end diastolic flow in the umbilical artery for the donor and reverse flow in the a-wave in the ductus venosus of the recipient have been identified as risks factors for fetal demise after laser treatment by three different centres.[25–27] In our series, intrauterine fetal demise (IUFD) of one twin occurred in 40 of 120 cases treated by laser.[28] These were 24 donors and 16 recipients. IUFD of both twins occurred in five cases, always within 24 hours of the death of the first twin. Death of one twin may occur as a consequence of an acute restriction of the placental territory after LPC. However, death of the survivor following its co-twin demise always occurred as the result of exsanguination into the dead fetus and its placenta through patent anastomotic vessels. In another report of 20 TTTS cases with single fetal demise before three days following treatment, anaemia was confirmed by cordocentesis in ten cases.[29] Peak systolic velocity of the middle cerebral artery (MCA-PSV)[30] was measured before and after cordocentesis in all cases. This was found to be abnormal in 11 cases and fetal anaemia was confirmed in ten by fetal blood sampling. This supports the view that MCA-PSV should be measured routinely after demise of one twin in monochorionic pregnancies. From this series, anaemia in the survivor was found in two of 11 cases after laser and in seven of eight cases after amniodrainage. These data show that LPC on inter-twin chorionic plate anastomoses has important benefits in cases with the death of one twin.

Double fetal demise is related to the persistence of vascular communications between the twins. Whether this occurs because of an incomplete coagulation of chorionic plate anastomoses after laser treatment or by the existence of intraplacental anastomoses was studied in an interesting study[31] that included dye injection and

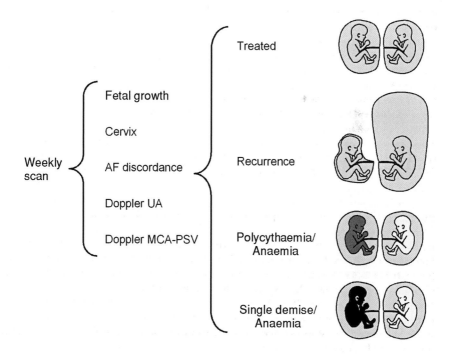

Figure 12.3. Specific complications of monochorionic pregnancies following laser treatment (AF = amniotic fluid, UA = umbilical artery, MCA-PSV = middle cerebral artery peak systolic velocity)

angiography of the same placentas. The objective was to detect missed anastomoses on the chorionic surface as well as hidden connections in the depth of the cotyledons in placentas of 43 cases with double survival and seven cases with double IUFD after laser coagulation for TTTS. Placentas with missed large AV/VA anastomoses ($n = 8$) were from cases with recurrent TTTS or double IUFD (unless compensated by a large AA anastomosis). When there were no missed anastomoses ($n = 34$), TTTS had resolved in all cases and outcome was good. Coagulation of all anastomoses visible on the chorionic surface seems adequate to solve the clinical problem of TTTS; however, the existence of hidden connections deep in some cotyledons could not be excluded except for the possibility of artefacts inherent to the perfusion technique, and might be involved in lesser degrees of inter-twin transfusion.

IUGR may occur as a consequence of placental insufficiency after laser treatment, because of necrosis of placental cotyledons. Fetal growth after laser treatment is a sign of fetal wellbeing and placental sufficiency. IUGR and IUFD may occur to any or both fetuses as a consequence of placental necrosis following LPC. Nevertheless, normal growth after laser is a feature of successful treatment, even in cases of preterm delivery without survivors. Fetal growth after laser treatment when both fetuses survived has recently been described.[32] Growth could be determined with two assessments of the twins before and after laser treatment in 47 consecutive cases of TTTS with double survivors. The main conclusion was that discrepancies between the twins' biometry decreased after laser treatment mainly because the growth rate in recipients decreased. Donors continued their growth velocity and remained with the same Z-score along the pregnancy. This study described growth patterns when two fetuses were alive after LPC in TTTS, and this may be a parameter of LPC success, despite early delivery with neonatal mortality.

Recurrence of the poly/oligohydramnios sequence occurs as a consequence of incomplete coagulation, as a sign of persistent anastomoses. This is what normally occurs after amnioreduction. In cases of anterior placenta or blood-stained AF, a second LPC may not be possible. In these cases, the persistence of placental anastomoses is the most likely explanation, and the death of one twin may lead to the death or brain damage in the survivor. This situation can be handled with amnioreduction until viability or by cord coagulation using bipolar forceps as a way to stop the TTTS in cases in which viability has not been reached because of early gestation or the agonal condition of one twin. This indication should therefore be confined to those cases in which the death of one or both twins appears imminent.

Feto-fetal blood transfusion leading to anaemia and polycythaemia, respectively, in the affected twins without recurrence of TTTS is a condition recently described that has been found in cases where the former recipient develops anaemia and the former donor develops polycythaemia without AF discordance.[24] Thirteen fetuses developed increased MCA-PSV greater than 1.5 multiples of the median (MoM) (mean 2.37 ± 0.72) 7–33 days after laser treatment. Twelve were recipient twins and one was a donor. Concomitantly, MCA-PSV values were decreased to less than 0.8 MoM (mean 0.59 ± 0.12) in all their respective co-twins without showing any other distinctive ultrasound feature but for one hydropic twin ($P < 0.0001$ between co-twins as assessed by Mann–Whitney test). Amniotic fluid volume and fetal diuresis were assessed subjectively to be normal in both twins in all cases. The fetuses were treated with intrauterine blood transfusion until viability. Transfusion was indicated when MCA-PSV increased in successive days over 2 MoM. Figure 12.4 describes the evolution of MCA-PSV in one monochorionic twin pregnancy after LPC that presented with this complication. The donor twin developed polycythaemia and the

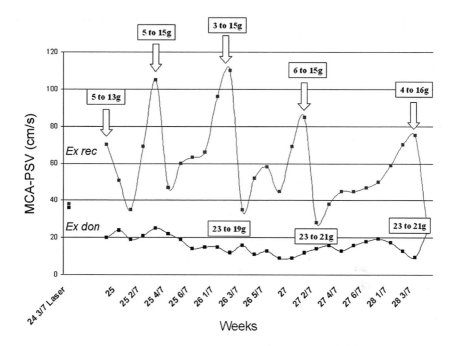

Figure 12.4. Evolution of the middle cerebral artery peak systolic velocity after laser photocoagulation in a monochorionic twin pregnancy where feto-fetal blood transfusion had led to anaemia in the recipient and polycythaemia in the donor

recipient developed anaemia. Caesarean section was performed at 28 weeks, and the children were subsequently developing well at one year of life. The placenta was studied with *ex vivo* angiography, which showed the persistence of placental anastomoses. Figure 12.3 describes specific complications of TTTS.

Miscarriage and rupture of the membranes

All invasive procedures intend to minimise the high rate of PPROM. In a series of 175 TTTS cases treated in one centre with LPC either primarily or as a rescue procedure following one or serial amnioreduction, PPROM occurred in 28% of the cases before 34 weeks of gestation.[5] Pre-viable miscarriage and prematurity itself contributed significantly to the mortality. PPROM occurred within one week of laser treatment, between eight and 21 days and after three weeks in 7%, 5% and 17% of the cases, respectively. The prognosis was uniformly poor without survivors when it occurred before 24 weeks of gestation, because of spontaneous miscarriage in all but one case where the woman requested pregnancy termination. All 17 cases with PPROM that occurred between 24 and 27 weeks delivered before 28 weeks of gestation, and the prognosis was poor with fetal demise or termination of pregnancy in five (15%), neonatal death in 18 (52%), neurodevelopmental delay in four (12%) and normal development in seven cases (21%). PPROM occurred in 20 pregnancies at 28 weeks or more of gestation. Among these, there were 13 (32%) cases with IUFD or termination of pregnancy, one neonatal death (2%) and 27 (66%) survivors including one set of triplets, who have since developed normally. Several factors play a significant role in the occurrence of PPROM; however, we could not demonstrate that PPROM would occur significantly more often following primary amnioreduction (Table 12.2).

Survival is improved by fetoscopic laser coagulation of the chorionic plate anastomotic vessels, but the risk of preterm delivery remains high.[33] There are known uterine factors that play a critical role in the duration of pregnancy, especially in cases with severe polyhydramnios. Cervical length is a predictor of preterm delivery in uncomplicated twin pregnancies[34] and it was expected to be an even stronger predictor in cases with polyhydramnios. Cervical length has been evaluated to predict preterm delivery in TTTS,[35] and a cervical length of less than 30 mm before laser treatment was found to predict spontaneous preterm delivery before 34 weeks of gestation (OR 3.53, 95% CI 1.55–8.03). In this study, cerclage was performed in nine of 137 TTTS cases, with a cervical length of less than 20 mm together with a history of cerclage or preterm delivery. Four women miscarried, three delivered before 28 weeks, one at 33 weeks and one at 34 weeks. However, the indication for cerclage remains unclear.

Conclusion

Ultrasound diagnostic criteria in cases of TTTS are universally accepted and evidence for the advantages of laser treatment has been published. Nevertheless, survival rates are far from optimal, and the condition still has high lethality after treatment. It is important to analyse the complications independently and to propose alternative management options. Prematurity and the need for cerclage are important pending issues. Late complications such as fetal demise, recurrence of TTTS and feto-fetal haemorrhage with haemoglobin difference has been diagnosed in up to 13% of double survivors, with the development of increased MCA-PSV over 1.5 MoM one to four weeks after laser treatment, mostly in the former recipient (12 of 13 cases). Concomitantly, MCA-PSV decreased to less than 0.8 MoM in all their respective co-twins without showing any other distinctive ultrasound feature of fetal anaemia except for one hydropic twin. Their management may involve repeat LPC, cord coagulation, amniodrainage or serial intrauterine transfusion in order to bring fetuses to a gestational age compatible with an elective delivery after lung maturation. We arbitrarily recommend that monochorionic pregnancies should be scanned every two weeks from 16 weeks of gestation onwards until delivery in order to detect TTTS at an early stage, and cases treated by laser need a thorough preoperative examination with cervical length measurements, umbilical artery, ductus venosus, umbilical vein flow Doppler and MCA-PSV measurements. Post-laser fetal monitoring should be frequent in the first 48 hours to monitor cervical length and to detect fetal demise promptly, which may lead to the demise of the co-twin by exsanguination. Cerclage should be considered if the cervix remains short or shortens even further after laser treatment. Ambulatory follow-up should be performed on a weekly basis, checking for growth, AF volume, cervical length and the same Doppler parameters as already mentioned.

Table 12.2. Perioperative factors and maternal complications (number of cases in brackets)

Perioperative factor	PPROM (49)	Chorioamnionitis (4)	Vaginal bleeding (7)	Miscarriage (12)	Placental abruption (3)	Perinatal survival – cases with one or two fetuses alive at 6 months (128)
Main insertion of the placenta						
Anterior (77)	24	1	5	6	2	53
Posterior, lateral, fund (98)	25	3	2	6	1	75
	$P=0.4$[a]	$P=0.31$[b]	$P=0.13$[b]	$P=0.66$[a]	$P=0.41$[b]	$P=0.25$[a]
	RR 1.22 (0.76–1.96)	0.42 (0.04–3.99)	RR 3.18 (0.63–15.95)	RR 1.27 (0.42–3.79)	RR 2.55 (0.23–27)	RR 0.9 (0.74–1.08)
Entry of the fetoscope						
Transplacental (48)	12	0	3	3	0	36
Transamniotic (127)	37	4	4	9	3	92
	$P=0.58$[b]	$P=0.27$[b]	$P=0.20$[b]	$P=0.26$[b]	$P=0.37$[b]	$P=0.11$[a]
	RR 0.86 (0.49–1.5)		RR 1.98 (0.46–8.54)	RR 0.88 (0.25–3.12)		RR 1.04 (0.85–1.25)
Intraamniotic bleeding						
Yes (14)	3	0	1	0	0	9
No (161)	46	4	6	12	3	119
	$P=0.22$[b]	$P=0.16$[b]	$P=0.34$[b]	$P=0.35$[b]	$P=0.77$[b]	$P=0.61$[a]
	RR 0.75 (0.26–2.10)		RR 1.92 (0.25–14.8)			RR 0.87 (0.58–1.29)
Cerclage before laser						
Yes (3)	1	0	0	0	0	1
No (172)	48	4	7	12	3	127
	$P=0.43$[b]	$P=0.93$[b]	$P=0.88$[b]	$P=0.8$[b]	$P=0.94$[b]	$P=0.15$[b]
	RR 0.78 (0.11–13.8)					RR 0.45 (0.09–2.24)
Cerclage after laser						
Yes (10)	6	2	1	0	0	7
No (165)	43	2	6	12	3	121
	$P=0.02$[b]	$P=0.016$[b]	$P=0.28$[b]	$P=0.48$[b]	$P=0.83$[b]	$P=0.26$[b]
	RR 2.3 (1.30–4.06)	RR 10.6 (3.24–35.1)	RR 2.75 (0.36–20.6)			RR 0.95 (0.62–1.44)
Amnioreduction before laser						
Yes (15)	3	0	1	0	0	8
No (160)	46	4	6	12	3	120
	$P=0.19$[b]	$P=0.69$[b]	$P=0.35$[b]	$P=0.32$[b]	$P=0.76$[b]	$P=0.07$[a]
	RR 0.7 (0.24–1.97)		RR 1.78 (0.22–13.8)			RR 0.7 (0.43–1.15)
Amnioreduction after laser						
Yes (10)	5	0	1	0	0	6
No (165)	44	4	6	12	3	122
	$P=0.22$[b]	$P=0.78$[b]	$P=0.289$[b]	$P=0.48$[b]	$P=0.83$[b]	$P=0.16$[b]
	RR 1.88 (0.96–3.66)		RR 2.67 (0.38–18.2)			RR 0.81 (0.48–1.35)

[a] χ^2 test
[b] Fisher exact test
All relative risk ranges are 95% confidence intervals
PPROM = preterm prelabour rupture of membranes

References

1.   Danskin FH, Neilson JP. Twin-to-twin transfusion syndrome: what are appropriate diagnostic criteria? *Am J Obstet Gynecol* 1989;161:365–9.
2.   Schatz F. *Klinische Beitrage zur Physiologie des Fotus*. Berlin: Hirschwald; 1900.
3.   Robertson EG, Neer KJ. Placental injection studies in twin gestation. *Am J Obstet Gynecol* 1983;147:170–4.
4.   Machin G, Still K, Lalani T. Correlations of placental vascular anatomy and clinical outcomes in 69 monochorionic twin pregnancies. *Am J Med Genet* 1996;61:229–36.
5.   Bajoria R, Wigglesworth J, Fisk N. Angioarchitecture of monochorionic placentas in relation to the twin–twin transfusion syndrome. *Am J Obstet Gynecol* 1995;172:856–63.
6.   Denbow ML, Cox P, Taylor M, Hammal DM, Fisk NM. Placental angioarchitecture in monochorionic twin pregnancies: relationship to fetal growth, fetofetal transfusion syndrome, and pregnancy outcome. *Am J Obstet Gynecol* 2000;182:417–26.
7.   Bermudez C, Becerra CH, Bornick PW, Allen MH, Arroyo J, Quintero RA. Placental types and twin–twin transfusion syndrome. *Am J Obstet Gynecol* 2002;187:489–94.
8.   Machin G. The monochorionic twin placenta *in vivo* is not a black box. *Ultrasound Obstet Gynecol* 2001;17:4–6.
9.   Mahieu-Caputo D, Dommergues M, Delezoide AL, Lacoste M, Cai Y, Narcy F, *et al*. Twin-to-twin transfusion syndrome. Role of the fetal renin–angiotensin system. *Am J Pathol* 2000;156:629–36.
10.   Allanson JE. Hunter AGW, Mettler GS, Jimenez C. Renal tubular dysgenesis: a not uncommon autosomal recessive syndrome. A Review *Am J Med Genet* 1992;43:811–14.
11.   Pryde PG, Sedman AB, Nugent CE, Barr M Jr. Angiotensin-converting enzyme inhibitor fetopathy. *J Am Soc Nephrol* 1993;3:1575–82.
12.   Gratacos E, van Schoubroeck D, Carreras E, Devlieger R, Roma E, Cabero L, *et al*. Impact of laser coagulation in severe twin–twin transfusion syndrome on fetal Doppler indices and venous blood flow volume. *Ultrasound Obstet Gynecol* 2002;20:125–30.
13.   Ishii K, Chmait RH, Martinez JM, Nakata M, Quintero RA. Ultrasound assessment of venous blood flow before and after laser therapy: approach to understanding the pathophysiology of twin–twin transfusion syndrome. *Ultrasound Obstet Gynecol* 2004;24:164–8.
14.   Yamamoto M, Bernard J-P, Takahashi Y, Huard F, Ville Y. Intertwin venous flow imbalance in twin to twin transfusion syndrome (TTTS). *Ultrasound Obstet Gynecol* 2005;In press.
15.   Quintero RA, Morales WJ, Allen MH. Staging twin–twin transfusion syndrome. *J Perinatol* 1999;19:550–5.
16.   Taylor MJ, Govender L, Jolly M, Wee L, Fisk NM. Validation of the Quintero Staging System for twin–twin transfusion syndrome. *Obstet Gynecol* 2002;100:1257–65.
17.   Yamamoto M, El Murr L, Robyr R, Leleu F, Takahashi Y, Ville Y. Incidence and impact of perioperative complications in 175 fetoscopy-guided laser coagulation of chorionic plate anastomoses in feto-fetal transfusion syndrome before 26 weeks of gestation. *Am J Obstet Gynecol* 2005;193(3 Pt 2):1110–16.
18.   Quintero RA, Dickinson JE, Morales WJ, Bornick PW, Bermudez C, Cincotta R, *et al*. Stage-based treatment of twin–twin transfusion syndrome. *Am J Obstet Gynecol* 2003;188:1333–40.
19.   Senat MV, Deprest J, Boulvain M, Paupe A, Winer N, Ville Y. Endoscopic laser surgery vs serial amnioreduction for severe twin-to-twin transfusion syndrome. *N Engl J Med* 2004;351:136–44.
20.   Fox C, Kilby M, Khan K. Contemporary treatments for twin–twin transfusion syndrome. *Obstet Gynecol* 2005;105:1469–77.
21.   Hecher K, Plath H, Bregenzer T, Hansmann M, Hackeloer BJ. Endoscopic laser surgery versus serial amniocentesis in the treatment of severe twin–twin transfusion syndrome. *Am J Obstet Gynecol* 1999;180:717–24.
22.   Johnson JR, Rossi KQ, O'Shaughnessy RW. Amnioreduction versus septostomy in twin–twin transfusion syndrome. *Am J Obstet Gynecol* 2001;185:1044–7.
23.   Benirschke K, Driscoll S. *The Pathology of the Human Placenta*. New York: Springer-Verlag; 1967.
24.   Robyr R, Lewi L, Salomon LJ, Yamamoto M, Bernard JP, Deprest J, Ville Y. Prevalence and management of late fetal complications following successful selective laser coagulation of chorionic plate anastomoses in twin-to-twin transfusion syndrome. *Am J Obstet Gynecol* 2006;194:796–803.
25.   Cavicchioni O, Yamamoto M, Robyr R, Ville Y. Intrauterine fetal demise (IUFD) following laser treatment in twin to twin transfusion syndrome (TTTS). *Ultrasound Obstet Gynecol* 2004;24:250.
26.   Taylor M, Denbow M, Duncan K, Overton T, Fisk N. Antenatal factors that predict outcome in twin–twin transfusion syndrome. *Am J Obstet Gynecol* 2000;183:1023–8.
27.   Martínez JM, Bermúdez C, Becerra C, López J, Morales WJ, Quintero RA. The role of Doppler

studies in predicting individual intrauterine fetal demise after laser therapy for twin–twin transfusion syndrome. *Ultrasound Obstet Gynecol* 2003;22:246–51.

28. Cavicchioni O, Yamamoto M, Robyr R, Ville Y. Prognosis of the surviving co-twin after intrauterine fetal demise (IUFD) in TTTS treated by laser. *Am J Obstet Gynecol* 2005;191:S160.

29. Senat MV, Loizeau S, Couderc S, Bernard JP, Ville Y. The value of middle cerebral artery peak systolic velocity in the diagnosis of fetal anemia after intrauterine death of one monochorionic twin. *Am J Obstet Gynecol* 2003;189:1320–4.

30. Mari G, Deter RL, Carpenter RL, Rahman F, Zimmerman R, Moise KJ Jr, *et al.* Noninvasive diagnosis by Doppler ultrasonography of fetal anemia due to maternal red-cell alloimmunization: collaborative group for Doppler assessment of the blood velocity in anemic fetuses. *N Engl J Med* 2000;342:9–14.

31. Lewi L, Jani J, Cannie M, Robyr R, Ville Y, Hecher K, *et al.* Intertwin anastomoses in monochorionic placentas after fetoscopic laser coagulation for twin-to-twin transfusion syndrome: is there more than meets the eye? *Am J Obstet Gynecol* 2006;194:790–5.

32. Moreira de Sa RA, Salomon LJ, Takahashi Y, Yamamoto M, Ville Y. Analysis of fetal growth after laser therapy in twin-to-twin transfusion syndrome. *J Ultrasound Med* 2005;24:1213–19;1220–1.

33. Ville Y, Hyett J, Hecher K, Nicolaides K. Preliminary experience with endoscopic laser surgery for severe twin–twin transfusion syndrome. *N Engl J Med* 1995;332:224–7.

34. Vayssiere C, Favre R, Audibert F, Chauvet MP, Gaucherand P, Tardif D, *et al.* Cervical length and funneling at 22 and 27 weeks to predict spontaneous birth before 32 weeks in twin pregnancies: a French prospective multicenter study. *Am J Obstet Gynecol* 2002;187:1596–604.

35. Robyr R, Boulvain M, Lewi L, Huber A, Hecher K, Deprest J, Ville Y. Cervical length as prognostic factor for preterm delivery in twin-to-twin transfusion syndrome treated by fetoscopic laser coagulation of chorionic plate anastomoses. *Ultrasound Obstet Gynecol* 2005;25:37–41.

Chapter 13

Management of twin reversed arterial perfusion (TRAP) sequence

Neil J Sebire and Waldo Sepulveda

Introduction

Acardiac anomaly, twin reversed arterial perfusion (TRAP) sequence and chorio-angiopagus parasiticus are synonymous terms referring to a rare complication unique to monochorionic multiple pregnancies in which there is an apparent lack of a well-formed cardiac structure in one fetus (the acardiac twin), which is abnormally perfused by a structurally normal co-twin (the pump twin) through a single superficial artery-to-artery placental anastomosis (Figure 13.1). This condition therefore results in arterial blood flowing in a retrograde fashion from the pump twin towards the affected fetus and this underlying pathophysiology indicates the preferred use of the clinical term TRAP sequence.[1] Pathophysiologically, the acardiac fetus acts as a parasite that can only survive *in utero* as it is haemodynamically dependent upon the pump twin. This can result in pregnancy complications, with the principal perinatal problems being pump twin congestive heart failure, polyhydramnios and severe preterm birth,[2] although intrauterine death of the pump twin has been reported even in the absence of such features.[3]

TRAP sequence affects around in 1 in 35 000–40 000 pregnancies, representing approximately 1% of monochorionic twins,[4–6] although frequencies as high as 1 in 10 000–20 000 deliveries have been recorded in some series.[7] Since the underlying pathogenesis is dependent upon the presence of placental vascular communications (see below), TRAP sequence can potentially complicate any monochorionic multiple pregnancy and, although obviously most commonly reported in twins, identical cases have also been described in higher order multiple pregnancies containing mono-chorionic sets, such as triplets or quadruplets.[8–16]

Advances in prenatal diagnosis and therapy have allowed TRAP sequence to be recognised antenatally from the first trimester and a range of *in utero* interventions has been attempted. This review summarises the current state of knowledge regarding TRAP sequence pathophysiology, diagnosis and management based on the published literature, and focuses specifically on the potential role of invasive treatment options.

Pathophysiology

Since the underlying process in TRAP sequence appears to be abnormal retrograde perfusion of the affected fetus in association with absent or abnormal cardiac

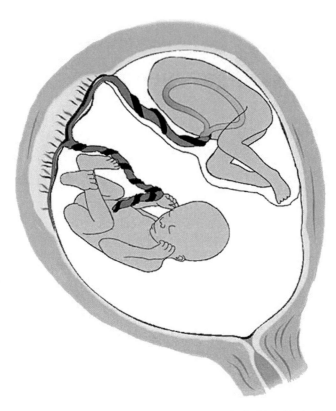

Figure 13.1.   Diagrammatic representation of the underlying pathophysiological basis of TRAP sequence demonstrating the presence of large anastomoses between the umbilical cords of the pump twin and the malformed acardiac twin; reproduced with permission from Tan and Sepulveda[92]

development, a range of structural anomalies has been reported as a presumed consequence of this abnormal perfusion pattern. The anomalies are highly variable, ranging from a relatively normal body form with well-differentiated organ structures through to an apparently amorphous structure with no recognisable normal anatomy (Figure 13.2). Similarly, the size of the acardiac mass can vary from a small incidental structure to a mass more than double that of its pump co-twin. The largest recorded acardiac fetus weighed more than 6 kg.[17] Furthermore, the heart may be completely absent (holoacardia), in a primitive state of development (pseudoacardia) or even relatively well formed. As a result of preferential perfusion of the lower body by the retrograde blood flow, acardiac twins are often acephalic with absent or extremely poorly formed upper extremities, with a trunk present in association with a recognisable spinal column. Structures that are frequently absent include the heart (fewer than 20% of fetuses have identifiable cardiac tissue), head, upper limbs, pancreas, lungs, liver and small intestines, and an abnormal two-vessel cord is found in more than two-thirds of cases.[6] Furthermore, since there is abnormal vascular development, the acardiac twin frequently develops severe subcutaneous oedema and

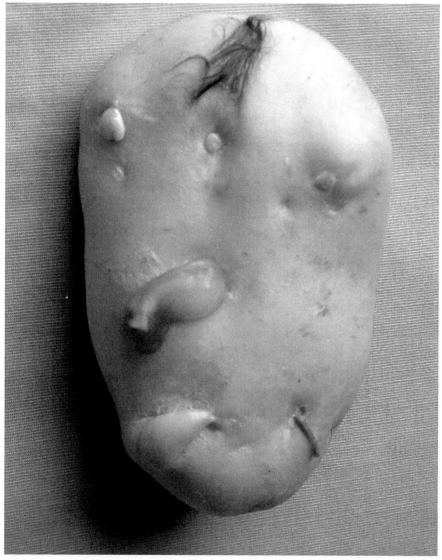

Figure 13.2. Photograph of a delivered acardiac fetus demonstrating severe malformation resulting in an amorphous mass into which the umbilical cord inserts; reproduced with permission from Tan and Sepulveda[92]

cystic hygromas, which can significantly increase the size of the fetus and distort the already abnormal anatomy.

Although the characteristic findings and associations of TRAP sequence are well described and consistent, the initiating aetiology and pathophysiology underlying its development remain incompletely understood. There are two main theories that attempt to explain the origin: the first is that the primary abnormality is aberrant placental vasculature which leads to circulatory reversal with subsequent alteration in cardiac development, and the second is that abnormal cardiac embryogenesis is the primary event with the aberrant circulatory pattern developing as a secondary consequence of pressure differentials in the context of monochorionic twin placentation. It is clear that in established cases of TRAP sequence, arterial blood flows in a retrograde manner through the umbilical artery of the acardiac fetus via artery-to-artery anastomoses with the result that the relatively poorly oxygenated and nutrient-poor blood from the pump twin bypasses the placental parenchyma directly to the acardiac twin, preferentially perfusing its caudal structures. Blood then returns to the circulation of the pump twin via a superficial vein-to-vein anastomosis. Primary umbilical cord and placental vascular anatomical abnormalities could therefore account for these findings, but are difficult to reconcile with those cases associated with three-vessel cords or complete absence of cardiac tissue. The alternative suggestion of primary defective cardiogenesis would result in the acardiac twin only surviving owing to the anastomoses that form secondarily after fetal demise. In reality it is likely that a combination of events is required in early pregnancy to result in the classic TRAP phenotype recognised as described above, with primary and secondary defects.[18,19] However, it appears that such artery-to-artery anastomoses, believed essential in the pathogenesis of TRAP sequence, may not be present in all cases since two cases with only apparent artery-to-vein anastomoses on pathological examination have now been reported.[20] In these cases, blood flow in the acardiac fetus was dorsocranial and circulated upward to the trunk rather than downward to the lower limbs, perhaps following the course of the primitive cardinal vein, yet the upper limbs remained more deformed than the lower limbs. This discordance between theory and observation suggests that retrograde flow of poorly oxygenated blood may not be the only initial cause of the phenotype.

Although the exact underlying developmental mechanism remains uncertain, it is clear that the major mechanism by which the presence of a parasitic acardiac twin threatens the survival of the co-twin is related to the vascular-steal phenomenon, resulting in continued growth of the acardiac fetus and increasing haemodynamic demands on the pump twin that lead to cardiac failure, polyhydramnios and preterm delivery. There may also be a 'hypoxic' contribution since the deoxygenated blood returning from the acardiac mass passes through vein-to-vein anastomoses into the pump twin's circulation, thus reducing the oxygen level in its circulation.[2,6] In addition, cases of monoamniotic TRAP sequence may be further complicated by cord entanglement or acute haemodynamic changes, which may be higher in the third trimester when the rate of fetal growth is the greatest.[11]

Since TRAP sequence represents an anomaly of monozygotic duplication (see Chapter 4), there is obviously a relationship with other such malformations. In one series of more than 1000 cases of conjoined twins from the literature, the association with TRAP sequence was more frequent than expected by chance alone and, in reality, these entities probably represent a continuum of abnormal conjoined twinning resulting in either an externally attached parasitic twin, an internal fetus in fetu or TRAP sequence.[21]

The pump twin is structurally normal in most cases of TRAP sequence, with complications being those noted above. However, associated pump twin structural anomalies have been reported in some cases, including prune belly with agenesis of the left ureter and kidney, dysplastic right kidney and anal atresia,[22] renal tubular dysgenesis,[23] gastroschisis[24] and pulmonary artery calcification.[25]

Anatomical features of the acardiac fetus

Several studies have reported on the detailed anatomical findings in cases of TRAP sequence. In one series of three cases, all acardiac fetuses demonstrated poorly developed skulls, limb reduction defects with phocomelia of the upper limbs and abnormal thoracic cages with or without normal development of ribs, clavicles, scapulae and vertebrae. In these cases the lower limb and pelvic anatomy was essentially normal, and consistent with the suggested vascular perfusion defect as a pathogenetic mechanism.[26] In another series of ten cases examined at autopsy, only one had a vestigial heart tube present and characteristic artery-to-artery anastomoses were demonstrated in all cases. The umbilical cords of the acardiac fetuses often consisted of only two vessels, which were attached directly to the arteries and veins of the normal co-twins on the placental surface. The vascular system of the acardiac fetuses was simplified, providing only inflow and outflow pathways through common iliac vessels and vitelline vessels and the facial area was malformed in all. The thoracic organs had abnormalities including hypoplastic lungs and tracheo-oesophageal fistulae, and the gastrointestinal tract was abnormal with absent or malformed segments.[27] In a larger series of 18 autopsy cases, numerous malformations were described. These affected especially the upper limbs and internal organs including the liver, which was abnormal in almost all cases, presumably as a consequence of its site in the circulatory route, but with malformations described involving brain, oesophagus, trachea, abdominal organs, diaphragm, vertebrae, limbs, anus and anterior abdominal wall.[28] In cases resulting in intrauterine death of the pump twin examined at autopsy, it is apparent that the pump twin may also have abnormalities including cardiomegaly, hepatomegaly and neuropathological hypoxic-ischaemic type lesions.[29]

A number of studies have also specifically examined the development of the nervous system in the acardiac fetus. In one fetus delivered at 32 weeks, there was a vertebral column with a structurally disorganised mass of neural tissue containing mature and immature neurones, glial cells and neural fibres with a focal slit-like cavity lined by ependyma and choroid plexus. The 'cerebral' mass was surrounded by a highly vascularised covering consisting of numerous thin-walled vessels but the spinal cord was relatively well organised. Such morphological features suggest that developmentally the failure probably occurred following neurulation.[30] Another study described a similarly severely disorganised cerebral cortex with cerebellar agenesis, extensive neuronal loss, gliosis and angiogenesis, suggesting effects of both developmental arrest and superimposed hypoxic-asphyxic type change,[31] and this combination of pathogeneses is supported by another case in which there were features of both developmental arrest with a holoprosencephaly-like malformation and superimposed hypoxic-type damage manifested as hydranencephaly-like areas.[32] Very rarely, the acardiac fetus may show a nearly normally developed brain and minimal reduction defects.[33,34]

Similarly, cardiac anatomy has been examined in TRAP sequence with histological evidence of cardiac tissue identified in about one-third of cases,[7] with the range of cardiac defects spanning from complete absence of cardiac tissue to malrotation of a relatively well-formed heart, with intermediate stages. This suggests that abnormalities in cardiac development may occur at different times during early embryogenesis, resulting in differing degrees of cardiac malformation.[35] Furthermore, it has been demonstrated that the aorta of acardiac fetuses is also abnormal in structure with derangement of the normal microanatomy and defective proximal to distal differences in the number of elastic lamellae and vessel calibre, presumably representing second-ary dysplastic responses to the abnormal reversed aortic flow.[36]

Classification

The simplest classification system of acardiac twins differentiates between two types: pseudoacardius, where the abnormal twin has evidence of a rudimentary cardiac structure; and holoacardius, where no such structure is present. A more detailed classification, also based entirely on the morphology of the acardiac twin, has been suggested, which separates cases into four major groups as follows:[4]

1. Acardius acephalus, in which there is a well-developed pelvis and lower limbs, but no head, usually no thoracic organs and often no arms. This is the most common form.
2. Acardius anceps, in which there is a well-developed body and extremities, but only a partially formed head and face. As the most developed form, it is likely that many of the other types begin as acardius anceps and evolve into one of the less well-differentiated forms owing to poor oxygen and nutrient supply.
3. Acardius acormus, in which only the head of the fetus is developed. This form is very rare.
4. Acardius amorphus, in which the fetus is represented by a shapeless mass of tissue containing no recognisable organs, but has some form of axial structure. This is the least differentiated form.

Although this anatomical/pathological system has been widely used, it has no direct correlation with pregnancy outcome or implications for management, since it is based on autopsy-derived anatomical data. It has therefore been suggested that prenatal classification may be more appropriately based on the size of the acardiac twin and the apparent condition of the pump twin (Table 13.1).[37] Such a system potentially provides an estimate of the 'severity' of the condition in an individual case and therefore the rationale for future management (see below). The size of the acardiac twin is best assessed using the apparent abdominal circumference, which is easy to measure and is reproducible, and correlates with both the length and girth of the fetus. Furthermore, a ratio based on abdominal circumference can be rapidly calculated to assess the relative sizes of acardiac and pump twins. A previously published formula to calculate fetal weight was based on fetal length measurements obtained at delivery[2] but this may be difficult to accurately assess prenatally for technical reasons and does not take the girth of the mass into account. According to this suggested revised classification, cases of TRAP sequence are divided into those with abdominal circumference ratio < 50% or ≥ 50% and further subdivided according to the apparent condition of the pump twin on the basis of published prenatal prognostic factors (see below).[37]

Placentation

TRAP sequence is essentially a defect of monozygotic duplication requiring the presence of vascular anastomoses, and is therefore a complication of monochorionic multiple pregnancies. In almost all cases studied, placentas demonstrate superficial artery-to-artery and vein-to-vein communications between the acardiac and pump twin's circulations. Occasionally, the umbilical cord of the acardiac fetus inserts into the cord of the pump twin, in which case the umbilical arteries and veins of the twins may be directly anastomosed and covered by Wharton's jelly (Figure 13.3). As a consequence of this vascular pattern, the acardiac twin itself lacks any functional placental

Table 13.1. Proposed prenatal classification of acardiac anomaly; adapted from Wong and Sepulveda[37]

Type	Acardiac : pump twin AC ratio	Signs of pump twin's compromise[a]	Management
Ia	< 50%	Absent	Reclassify within two weeks based on follow-up scan; consider treatment if increase in absolute size or persistence of moderate or significant vascularity of acardiac twin
Ib	< 50%	Present	Reclassify within two weeks based on follow-up scan; consider prompt intervention if increase in absolute size or persistence of moderate or significant vascularity of acardiac twin
IIa	≥ 50%	Absent	Consider intervention
IIb	≥ 50%	Present	Emergency intervention or delivery depending on gestation

[a] Defined as physical changes visualised on two-dimensional ultrasound (moderate-to-severe polyhydramnios, cardiomegaly or pericardial effusion) or abnormal Doppler signals (tricuspid regurgitation, reverse flow in the ductus venosus, pulsation in the umbilical vein, or high middle cerebral artery peak velocity)

AC = abdominal circumference

mass. In one pathological series reporting on 30 cases, about one-third were mono-chorionic-monoamniotic, with the remaining two-thirds being monochorionic-diamniotic,[8] and, similarly, in the largest published series,[6] about 25% were monoamniotic and the majority monochorionic-diamniotic. Two-vessel umbilical cords are reported in about 70% of cases.[6] There are very rare cases of pathologically confirmed dichorionic-diamniotic TRAP sequence described but all have been confirmed as monozygotic on molecular typing, although markedly skewed X-inactivation was reported in one such case.[6,38,39]

Aneuploidy

Several studies have attempted to address the role or association of fetal aneuploidy in TRAP sequence but have failed to demonstrate any consistent chromosomal abnormalities.[40] In early reports, aneuploidy was identified in the acardiac twin in multiple cases[2] and trisomy 2 has been reported on several occasions.[41,42] In the largest series, where there were 33 cases in which the acardiac fetus had been karyotyped, aneuploidy was present in 33% of cases, and in this report pump twin trisomy was also described in 8% of pregnancies.[6] However, the aetiological relationship, if any, between aneuploidy and TRAP development remains uncertain. One study using microsatellite polymorphism analysis has also demonstrated that fetuses affected by TRAP sequence are truly monozygous, thus ruling out polar body fertilisation as an underlying cause.[43]

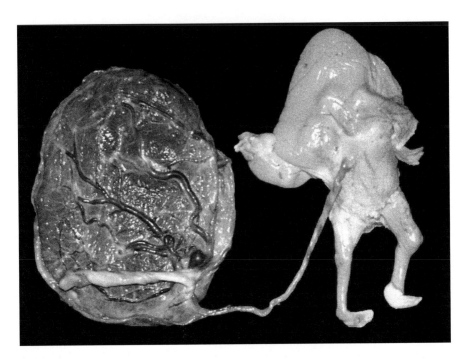

Figure 13.3. Photograph of a delivered acardiac fetus several weeks after intrauterine ablation therapy, demonstrating the presence of a malformed, macerated acardiac twin with close, marginal insertion of the two umbilical cords with large intervening anastomotic vessels

Prenatal diagnosis

Prenatal ultrasound diagnosis of TRAP sequence is now commonplace, with numerous case reports published of detection in the first and second trimesters.[44–60] Antenatal diagnosis was first described in 1978,[61] and subsequently additional techniques such as transvaginal ultrasound, pulsed and colour Doppler examination and three-dimensional ultrasound have been described for both diagnosis and assessment of pregnancies complicated by TRAP sequence.[52,62–65] The condition should be suspected when a grossly malformed fetus is seen in the setting of a monochorionic twin pregnancy,[66,67] often with marked biometric discordance between the fetuses, absence of cardiac pulsation in one twin, poor definition of the head, trunk and upper extremities, deformed lower extremities, marked and diffuse subcutaneous oedema, and abnormal cystic areas in the upper body of the affected twin (Figures 13.4–13.6).

It should be noted that the presence of some cardiac motion does not exclude the diagnosis, as it may result from pulsation of an abnormal rudimentary heart or even transmitted pulsations. Demonstration of the paradoxical circulation of blood towards the abnormal fetus along the umbilical artery with caudal-to-cranial aortic flow using Doppler ultrasound establishes the diagnosis.[68–72] The major differential diagnosis is the single intrauterine death of an abnormal monochorionic twin but the abnormal blood

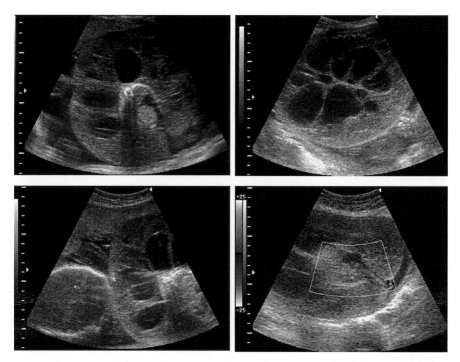

Figure 13.4.   Ultrasound images showing an acardiac fetus with marked cystic hygroma formation (top), increased size compared with the normal co-twin (bottom left) and reversed blood flow with colour Doppler imaging (bottom right)

flow pattern previously described and associated continued growth of the fetus are helpful indicators of the correct diagnosis. The documentation of blood flow within the abnormal mass on colour Doppler imaging, however, is the simplest and fastest method to confirm the presence of an acardiac twin (unpublished observations).

Doppler studies have been extensively described to delineate the umbilical cord and placental vascular anatomy, confirm reversed flow in the affected cord, and assess the cardiac status of both the acardiac and pump twin.[70–81] Umbilical cord vessel resistive index values have also been used to evaluate the haemodynamic status of the pregnancy. These studies suggest that, although no index value of the acardiac twin itself is associated with prediction of prognosis for the pump twin, a large difference in resistive index between the acardiac and pump fetuses is associated with better pump twin outcome (see below).[81] More recently, additional possible ultrasound prognostic factors have been reported even in the first trimester, with increased fetal nuchal translucency thickness and reversed ductus venosus flow in the pump fetus being anecdotally reported to be associated with poor outcome,[82] although another small case series did not support these associations.[83] The potential prognostic value of fetal nuchal translucency thickness and haemodynamic markers in the first trimester therefore remains to be established in TRAP sequence.

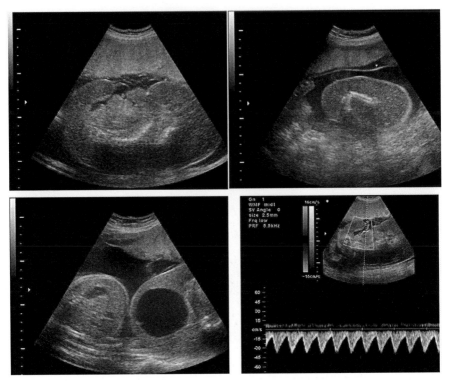

Figure 13.5.   Ultrasound images demonstrating an acardiac fetus with marked subcutaneous oedema (top), increased size compared with the normal co-twin, with cystic hygroma (bottom left) and reversed blood flow with colour Doppler imaging (bottom right)

In addition to providing diagnostic information, cases of TRAP sequence identified in the first trimester and undergoing ultrasound surveillance have allowed insights into the natural history of the disease and its possible pathogenesis. For example, several studies have now reported first-trimester identification of a monochorionic twin pregnancy with two apparently normal fetuses both demonstrating cardiac activity, followed by loss of cardiac activity in one twin and subsequent development of the classical TRAP sequence phenotype. Such reports lend support to the concept of cardiac changes secondary to haemodynamic alterations rather than primary cardiac agenesis.[84–86] Conversely, other cases diagnosed in the first trimester and managed conservatively have reported spontaneous cessation of flow to the acardiac twin with good pregnancy outcome.[87]

Outcome

None of the acardiac fetuses can survive postnatally but, as suggested above, pregnancies complicated by TRAP sequence may result in any outcome ranging from intrauterine or neonatal death of the pump twin through to spontaneous cessation of acardiac flow with a normal co-twin delivered at term. Since interventions have been attempted in more recent cases (see below), data on outcome with conservative

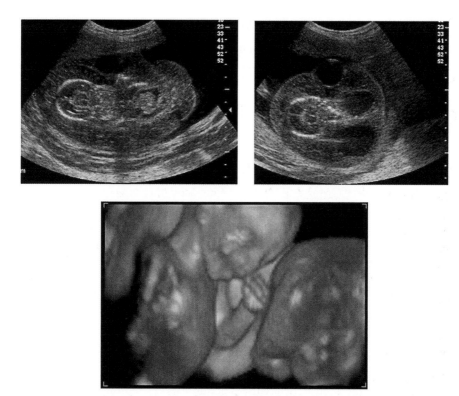

Figure 13.6.   Ultrasound images demonstrating an acardiac fetus with marked subcutaneous oedema and cystic hygromas (top), and a three-dimensional ultrasound image demonstrating the structurally normal fetus adjacent to the acardiac mass (bottom)

management is primarily based on historical data or small selected recent series, the results of which are summarised in Table 13.2.[2,6,7,16,20,27,81,88,89] There are no series reporting long-term follow-up of survivors but it should be noted that cases of developmental delay and cerebral palsy are anecdotally reported in survivors.[90] In addition to pump twin mortality, prematurity-related morbidity is also an issue since the median gestational age at delivery of pregnancies complicated by TRAP sequence with no intervention is 32 weeks.[6] Finally, other complications such as intrauterine growth restriction and hydrops may further compromise the wellbeing of the pump twin.[2,6]

Overall, with conservative management, intrauterine death of the pump twin occurs in about 25% of cases, polyhydramnios in 50% and preterm birth in 80%, all contributing to the overall perinatal loss rate. Pooled data, including 216 cases of TRAP sequence reported in the literature in which management was conservative and outcome reported, suggest that overall pump twin survival with no intervention is about 60% (Figure 13.7). However, in order to compare outcomes and interventions and aid counselling, information is required regarding the prognosis according to clinical parameters individualised to the patient (see below).

Table 13.2. Outcome of TRAP pregnancies with no interventions based on published historical series (reports of fewer than five cases are not included)

Study	Total	Survivors	Survival (%) (95% CI)
Chi (1989)[27]	8	5	63 (24–91)
Moore et al. (1990)[2]	49	22	45 (31–60)
Healey (1994)[6]	117	76	65 (56–74)
Sogaard et al. (1999)[16]	6	1	17 (4–64)
Brassard et al. (1999)[88]	9	5	56 (21–86)
Shih et al. (1999)[20]	5	3	60 (15–95)
Dashe et al. (2001)[81]	6	5	83 (36–100)
Sullivan et al. (2003)[89]	10	9	90 (55–100)
Chanoufi et al. (2004)[7]	6	1	17 (4–64)
Overall	**216**	**127**	**59 (52–65)**

It is uncertain whether any presented cases of Moore et al.[2] are included in Healey[6]

Prenatal prognostic features

Attempts to identify factors that predict pump–fetus outcome originally focused on the structure of the acardiac twin, such as acardius anceps and the presence of ears, larynx, trachea, pancreas, renal tissue and small intestine.[6] However, such features are difficult to assess prenatally and may be surrogate markers for the much more easily assessed parameter of relative size of the acardiac twin, which can be conveniently expressed as a percentage of the pump twin weight. An initial study reported that in cases associated with an acardiac:pump twin ratio > 70%, preterm delivery occurred in 90% of cases, polyhydramnios in 40% and pump twin congestive heart failure in 30%, compared with rates of 75%, 30% and 10%, respectively, when the ratio was < 70%, and with rates of 35%, 18% and 0%, respectively, when the ratio was < 50%.[2] Such data were, however, derived from postmortem measurements, and calculation of twin weight ratios prenatally is further complicated by inaccuracies in estimating acardiac fetal weight owing to its amorphous nature. The adverse prognostic value of acardiac:pump twin estimated weight ratio of > 50% has been confirmed in the antenatal setting in some studies,[7] but refuted in others.[91]

Additional prenatal prognostic markers have thus been examined, including Doppler ultrasound assessment of umbilical blood flow, for which high resistance and low flow to the acardiac fetus (expressed as different impedance indexes, ratios of umbilical artery pulsatility index values or differences in resistance index between the twins) appear to be associated with improved outcome.[81,88,91] Such data do not allow unequivocal prognostication but it appears that fetal size (by ultrasound assessment) and cardiovascular status of the pump twin are the most important factors for predicting outcome and hence guiding antenatal management. Pump twin cardiovascular status may be assessed using routine two-dimensional ultrasound to detect polyhydramnios, cardiomegaly, serous effusions or hydrops, and both colour and pulsed Doppler examination allow assessment of tricuspid regurgitation, reverse

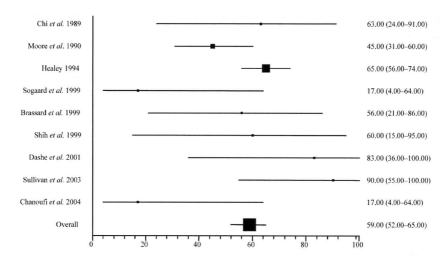

Figure 13.7. Schematic representation of series reporting outcome of pregnancies complicated by TRAP sequence managed without invasive interventions (survival percentage (95% confidence interval)[2,6,7,16,20,27,81,88,89]

flow in the ductus venosus and umbilical vein pulsatile flow, and determination of increased middle cerebral artery peak systolic velocities.

The available data would therefore suggest that cases of TRAP sequence in which the abdominal circumference ratio is < 50% with no evidence of pump twin compromise are probably associated with a low risk of adverse outcome and are best managed conservatively with ultrasound surveillance by serial assessment of the size of the acardiac twin and Doppler measurements of umbilical artery impedance and other indicators of acardiac flow, in addition to pump twin status. If there is evidence of early cardiovascular compromise of the pump twin using the parameters above, more frequent surveillance with a view to possible intervention with worsening condition may be indicated. In cases with apparently severe pump twin compromise or those with a large acardiac twin (abdominal circumference ratio > 50%), antenatal intervention should be considered. However, the optimum timing and method of any such intervention remain somewhat uncertain (see below). The role of serial assessments of acardiac growth and blood flow parameters in determining optimal management also remains unclear in the context of an apparently uncompromised pump twin, although a low pulsatility index in the acardiac fetus and rapid growth rate of the acardiac fetus were both associated with worse outcome in one study.[88] The presence of a detectable rudimentary heart does not appear to be of prognostic significance.[88]

It should, however, be noted that in a recent review of ten unselected cases of TRAP sequence managed conservatively, four demonstrated a small acardiac:pump twin weight ratio and had no complications, and in five of the remaining six cases the pump twin survived with no invasive interventions, including four of the five in which the acardiac:pump twin weight ratio was > 50%.[89] It is therefore clear that not all cases of TRAP sequence are associated with poor outcome and require intervention, even in association with factors such as large acardiac:pump twin weight ratio, which is statistically associated with worse outcome in population-based retrospective studies. Consideration of invasive treatment should therefore be restricted to those cases in which the pump twin appears to be at significant risk of prematurity from polyhydramnios or massive acardiac size, or is showing features of significant cardiac insufficiency.

Interventions

Numerous prenatal interventions have now been described in the context of TRAP sequence (Table 13.3).[92,93] Since the number of suggested treatment options for a condition is often inversely related to their effectiveness, it is clear that the optimal management of this pregnancy complication is not readily apparent. The primary issue is whether any form of intervention results in significantly better outcome than no treatment at all. There are no randomised trials to answer this question unequivocally and there are unlikely to be any in the future, since prenatal prognostic criteria are now available making randomisation to either intervention or no intervention unjustifiable (see above). The best available evidence is thus based only on small, uncontrolled series reporting outcome following interventions, compared with historical controls, but this raises significant problems for the data interpretation. In particular, the treated and control groups are not necessarily matched for disease severity, with presumably only the more severe cases having interventions attempted, which would tend to underestimate the effectiveness of any such treatments when compared with an unselected control group. Conversely, however, there is likely to be significant publication bias in the available literature, since the intervention data are based primarily on case reports and small case series, which tend to preferentially report successful outcomes, thus tending to overestimate the effectiveness of treatments. Bearing these caveats in mind, an assessment of pump twin survival following various interventions is provided in Tables 13.4 and 13.5.[94-127]

If it is accepted that intervention in a given case is indicated, there still remain issues regarding optimal timing and choice of procedure. For example, it has been suggested that early prophylactic treatment of all cases of TRAP sequence in the early second trimester is indicated if reversed blood flow is demonstrated,[117] since intervention at this gestation could reduce the technical difficulties sometimes encountered in stopping blood flow in cases with larger and sometimes hydropic acardiac twins.[96] However, since a significant proportion of cases would result in favourable outcome with conservative management and there is a risk of procedure-related complications, such a policy may not be of overall benefit and, indeed, has not been examined in any large series.

The rationale for treating TRAP sequence is to optimise outcome for the pump twin in a safe and effective manner, for which a range of prenatal interventions has been described but no single technique has been shown to be unequivocally optimal.[93] Initial interventions included the use of digoxin,[128] indometacin[129] and amniodrainage,[130] which are essentially symptomatic modifiers that attempted to prolong the pregnancy but did not address the underlying pathophysiological abnormality. Extreme interventions such as hysterotomy with selective removal of the acardiac fetus have also been described,[131-133] with six of seven (86%) pump twins surviving in initial series reporting on this technique. However, three (43%) pump twins were delivered before 30 weeks and such a procedure is associated with significant maternal risks, including pulmonary oedema due to aggressive tocolytic

Table 13.3. Minimally invasive treatment modalities for vascular occlusion of acardiac twins; adapted from Wong and Sepulveda[37]

Approach	Technique
Cord occlusion	
Ultrasound-guided	Coil
	Alcohol-suture material
	Absolute alcohol
	Ligation
	Monopolar diathermy
	Bipolar diathermy
Fetoscopy-guided	Ligation
	Laser
Intrafetal ablation	
Ultrasound-guided	Absolute alcohol
	Monopolar diathermy
	Laser
	Radiofrequency
Fetoscopy-guided	Currently not available

therapy, placental abruption, preterm labour and anaesthetic complications, and requires extensive medical resources and is therefore being largely abandoned. With advances in ultrasonography, several minimally invasive techniques have now been described and are currently the interventions of choice should *in utero* treatment be required. Such techniques may be ultrasound- or fetoscopy-guided and the target for ablation may be the umbilical cord or intra-abdominal vessels of the acardiac twin.[92]

Cord occlusion techniques

Since abnormal blood flow to the acardiac fetus is the underlying pathophysiological defect in TRAP sequence, occlusion of the umbilical cord supplying the acardiac fetus, guided by either ultrasound or fetoscopy, is a theoretically simple approach to treat this condition and was first suggested more than 20 years ago.[130] The techniques used to achieve this have included the introduction into the umbilical cord vasculature of various materials such as thrombogenic coils,[62,94,117] alcohol-soaked suture material,[109] glucose, fibrin and enbucrilate gel,[92] diathermy, both monopolar,[111,115,116] and bipolar,[104,112] and fetoscopic ligation.[95,97,98] However, although technically feasible, fetoscopy-guided ligation procedures require insertion of intrauterine trocars and there is thus a risk of preterm labour or rupture of membranes.

A review of 16 cases reported an associated perinatal mortality rate of almost 40% and delivery before 32 weeks in about 70% of cases.[92] Fetoscopy-guided coagulation of umbilical vessels using a neodymium–doped yttrium aluminium garnet (Nd:YAG) laser is now also well described and several studies have reported encouraging outcomes.[96,101,102,105] However, this technique is less effective after 24 weeks of gestation when the umbilical cord is larger or more hydropic,[96] and the trocar insertion required involves the associated risks of postoperative rupture of membranes, intra-amniotic infection and bleeding.[98,99]

Table 13.4. Studies reporting on intervention using fetoscopy- and ultrasound-guided umbilical cord occlusion methods in pregnancies complicated by TRAP sequence

Study	Number of cases	
	Intervention	Survival
Fetoscopy-guided cord occlusion		
Hamada *et al.* (1989)[94]	1 at 23 weeks	1 at 38 weeks
Donnenfeld *et al.* (1991)[74]	1 at 22 weeks	Zero
McCurdy *et al.* (1993)[95]	1 at 20 weeks	Zero
Ville *et al.* (1994)[96]	4 at 17–28 weeks	4 at 29–39 weeks
Wilcourt *et al.* (1995)[97]	1 at 24 weeks	1 at 29 weeks
Quintero *et al.* (1994)[98]	10 at 18–25 weeks	5 at 30–37 weeks
Deprest *et al.* (1996)[99] (1998)[100]	3 at 21–24 weeks	2 of 3 at 25–30 weeks
Hecher *et al.* (1997)[101]	1 at 16 weeks	1 at 41 weeks
Arias *et al.* (1998)[102]	1 at 24 weeks	1 at 35 weeks
Galankin *et al.* (2000)[103]	1 at 24 weeks	1 at 38 weeks
Deprest *et al.* (2000)[104]	1 at 19 weeks	1 at 39 weeks
Quintero *et al.* (2002)[105]	1 at 18 weeks	1 at 37 weeks
Total	**26 at 16–28 weeks**	**18 at 25–41 weeks (69%, 95% CI 48–86%)**
Ultrasound-guided cord occlusion		
Porreco (2004)[106]	1 at 24 week	1 at 39 weeks
Roberts *et al.* (1991)[107]	1 at 23 weeks	Zero
Grab *et al.* (1992)[108]	1 at 24 weeks	Zero
Holzgreve *et al.* (1994)[109]	1 at 21 weeks	1 at 37 weeks
Foley *et al.* (1995)[110]	1 at 22 weeks	1 at 35 weeks
Deprest *et al.* (2000)[104]	4 at 18–23 weeks	3 at 36–37 weeks
Holmes *et al.* (2001)[111]	3 at 18–24 weeks	3 at 32–39 weeks
Nicolini *et al.* (2001)[112]	2 at 24–27 weeks	1 at 37 weeks
Tanawattanacharoen *et al.* (2002)[113]	1 at 24 weeks	Zero
Gallot *et al.* (2003)[114]	3 at 21–23 weeks	3 at 30–38 weeks
Total	**18 at 18–27 weeks**	**13 at 30–39 weeks (72%, 95% CI 47–90%)**
Overall cord occlusion	**44 at 16–28 weeks**	**31 at 25–41 weeks (70%, 95% CI 55–83%)**

$Z = -0.23$, $P = 0.99$ for survival following fetoscopy- versus ultrasound-guided cord occlusion

Intrafetal techniques

There may be technical difficulties when attempting to occlude the umbilical cord of the acardiac fetus because the cord insertion is often close to the pump twin, with risk of inadvertent damage to the co-twin's cord. Furthermore, the close proximity of the umbilical artery and vein within the cord may hamper identification of the artery, which is necessary to avoid intravascular transfer of any ablative material into the circulation of the pump twin. In addition, the umbilical cord of the acardiac twin may be structurally abnormal, increasing the risk of rupture or bleeding and oedematous cords may cause

Table 13.5. Studies reporting on intervention using intrafetal vascular occlusion methods in pregnancies complicated by TRAP sequence.

Study	Number of cases	
	Intervention	Survival
Monopolar thermocoagulation		
Holmes *et al.* (2001)[111]	8 at 16–24 weeks	5 at 32–42 weeks
Chao *et al.* (2002)[115]	1 at 23 weeks	1 at 32 weeks
Chang *et al.* (2004)[116]	2 at 20–24 weeks	1 at 32 weeks
Interstitial laser		
Jolly *et al.* (2001)[117]	2 at 14–15 weeks	2 at 37 weeks
Soothill *et al.* (2002)[118]	2 at 19–19 weeks	2 at 38 weeks
Weisz *et al.* (2004)[91]	2 at 21–23 weeks	2 at 32–37 weeks
Sepulveda *et al.* (2004)[119]	1 at 26 weeks	1 at 36 weeks
Intrafetal alcohol injection		
Sepulveda *et al.* (1995)[120]	1 at 23 weeks	1 at 25 weeks
Tongsong *et al.* (2002)[121]	1 at 25 weeks	1 at 34 weeks
Ozeren *et al.* (2004)[122]	1 at 16/24 weeks	Zero
Porreco (2004)[106]	1 at 17 weeks	1 at 39 weeks
Sepulveda *et al.* (2004)[123] a	8 at 20–32 weeks	5 at 23–38 weeks
Gul *et al.* (2005)[125]	1 at 27 weeks	1 at 36 weeks
Radiofrequency ablation		
Tsao *et al.* (2002)[126]	13 at 17–23 weeks	12 at 26–40 weeks
Hirose *et al.* (2004)[127]	1 at 27 weeks	1 at 32 weeks
Total intrafetal occlusion	**45 at 14–32 weeks**	**35 at 26–40 weeks (78%, 95% CI 63–89%)**
Total intervention group	**89 at 14–32 weeks**	**66 at 25–41 weeks (74%, 95% CI 64–83%)**

a Includes Heredia and Quiroz 2002[124]

difficulties in achieving cord occlusion by laser ablation or coagulation.[96] Many of these difficulties may be avoided by using an intrafetal approach that targets the abdominal aorta or pelvic vessels of the acardiac twin, which are easily identified by the use of colour Doppler ultrasound. Intrafetal vascular ablation has been reported using injection of sclerosants such as alcohol,[120–125] or by use of monopolar thermocoagulation,[111,136,115,116] ultrasound-guided Nd:YAG laser[117–119] and radiofrequency ablation.[126,127] In all such techniques, colour Doppler ultrasound examination is required to monitor the procedure and confirm obliteration of blood flow.

Alcohol chemosclerosis

Alcohol injection into the intrafetal vessels has the potential to be the most widely available technique for TRAP ablation, since it is minimally invasive, can be performed as an outpatient procedure, and requires expertise that is similar to other intrauterine needling procedures. The major potential disadvantages of any such injection technique are failed sclerosis and passage of sclerosant into the circulation of the pump twin. In one recent multicentre series of eight cases, there were three procedure-related pump twin deaths, possibly as a consequence of vascular migration of alcohol.[92] In one case of attempted chemosclerosis (with fibrin polymer rather than alcohol), there was pump twin death and postmortem examination revealed chorionic artery thrombosis of the pump twin, presumably as a consequence of material injected into the circulation of the acardiac fetus passing to the circulation of the pump twin via the superficial placental anastomoses previously described.[19]

Diathermy

Intrafetal vascular coagulation by diathermy may also be performed under ultrasound guidance, usually using an 18G needle, as an outpatient procedure under local anaesthesia. Diathermy allows effective vascular occlusion with no risk of transfer of sclerosant agents but carries a potential risk of thermal injury along the path of the needle.

Laser coagulation

In addition to laser ablation of umbilical vessels under fetoscopic guidance, interstitial intrafetal laser ablation has also been described, also using an 18G needle and standard Nd:YAG laser fibre with ultrasound guidance to place the tip into the abdomen or pelvis of the acardiac twin close to the target vessel.[117–119] With such a technique there is no risk of needle-tract cautery burns but only specialist laser-approved centres have access to such equipment.

Radiofrequency ablation

The most recently described technique for intrafetal vascular occlusion is radio-frequency ablation using a 14G needle with a radiofrequency generator. In a similar way to laser ablation, energy is selectively applied only to the tip, thus minimising injury to surrounding tissues. Although the device has a large diameter and therefore has the theoretical risk of increasing rates of rupture of membranes, no postoperative rupture of membranes occurred in these reported series. Based on the data from two published reports, radiofrequency ablation appears to be a relatively safe and effective technique for the treatment of acardiac anomaly.[126,127]

Summary of intrauterine interventions

No randomised controlled trials to assess either outcome following intervention versus no intervention or different types of interventions are available, and no data are available to allow matching of historical control and intervention groups by disease severity. Therefore, all available data regarding outcome of TRAP sequence according to management is based on relatively low-quality grade III or IV evidence, from case series with either historical or no controls. However, since the best available evidence is likely to be better than no evidence at all, the following paragraph summarises the pooled data. It is not possible to account for potential differences in clinical characteristics or disease severity between the no-intervention 'control' groups and the intervention groups, which presumably recruited only the more severe cases of

TRAP sequence (although this is not necessarily the case and certainly not always apparent from the published reports). However, since such bias would tend to underestimate the advantage of intervention, the fact that much of the intervention data is based on small case series or individual case reports, with inherent publication bias which would tend to overestimate the effects of interventions, results in overall reduced net directional bias of the intervention effect. Nevertheless, it should be remembered that the data presented below, having such inherent problems with assessment, should be regarded as a best estimate only. Accurate quantitative comparative evaluations will be only available in future should prospective studies be carried out, or detailed registry data be collected on all cases regardless of management, to allow severity-matched comparisons of outcome to be performed.

In pregnancies complicated by TRAP sequence with no invasive intervention, about 60% of pump twins will survive (Table 13.2, Figure 13.8) compared with about 75% of pump twins in those managed by invasive vascular occlusion techniques (Tables 13.4 and 13.5; $Z=2.60$, $P<0.01$). The available data therefore suggest that such intervention is associated with a 16% (95% CI 4–26%) improvement in survival, the relative risk of death in the treatment group being 0.62 (95% CI 0.42–0.90), and treatment would be required in seven (95% CI 4–26) pregnancies to prevent one pump twin death. There is no significant difference in pump twin outcome between cord occlusion and intrafetal techniques ($Z=0.85$, $P=0.35$) but intrafetal ablation techniques tend to a slightly improved survival and are technically easier and more widely available, and should therefore probably be the strategy of choice if invasive intervention is attempted. There is no significant difference in pump twin survival between those cases with interventions carried out before or after 20 weeks of gestation ($Z=0.42$, $P=0.64$). No data are available on long-term morbidity or outcome of pump twin survivors according to antenatal management.

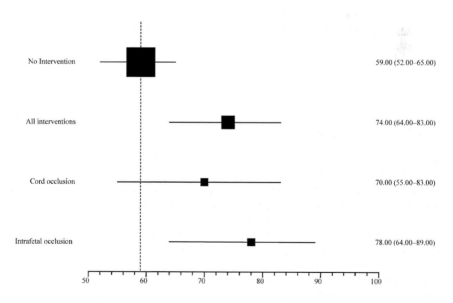

Figure 13.8.   Summary data for pregnancy outcome of TRAP sequence by management strategy on the basis of published data

Acknowledgements

Dr Sepulveda was supported for this work in part by the Sociedad Profesional de Medicina Fetal 'Fetalmed' Limitada and a grant from the Direccion Academica, Clínica Las Condes, Chile. We are grateful to Dr Oscar Atobe and Dr Jorge Gutierrez for some of the pictures used in this review.

References

1. Van Allen MI, Smith DW, Shepard TH. Twin reversed arterial perfusion (TRAP) sequence: a study of 14 twin pregnancies with acardius. *Semin Perinatol* 1983;7:285–93.
2. Moore TR, Gale S, Benirschke K. Perinatal outcome of forty nine pregnancies complicated by acardiac twinning. *Am J Obstet Gynecol* 1990;163:907–12.
3. Fusi L, Fisk N, Talbert D, Gau G, Rodeck C. When does death occur in an acardiac twin? Ultrasound diagnostic difficulties. *J Perinat Med* 1990;18:223–7.
4. Napolitani FD, Schreiber I. The acardiac monster. A review of the world literature and presentation of 2 cases. *Am J Obstet Gynecol* 1960;80:582–9.
5. James WH. A note on the epidemiology of acardiac monsters. *Teratology* 1977;16:211–16.
6. Healey MG. Acardia: predictive risk factors for the co-twin's survival. *Teratology* 1994;50:205–13.
7. Chanoufi MB, Ben Temime R, Masmoudi A, Ounaissa K, Jebnoun S, Abid W, Nsiri R, Chelli H, Khrouf N, Siala-Gaigi S. Clinical and anatomic features of acardiac twins. *Med Princ Pract* 2004;13:375–9.
8. Benirschke K, Kaufmann P. *Pathology of the Human Placenta*, 2nd edn. New York: Springer; 2000. p. 702–10.
9. Abboud P, Garnier R, Mansour G, Gabriel R, Gaillard D, Quereux C. Acardiac fetus in a triplet pregnancy: ultrasound pitfalls. A case report. *Eur J Obstet Gynecol Reprod Biol* 2000;89:75–80.
10. Bolaji II, Mortimer G, Meehan FP, England S, Greally M. Acardius in a triplet pregnancy: cytogenetic and morphological profile. *Acta Genet Med Gemellol* 1992;41:27–32.
11. Chang DY, Chang RY, Chen RJ, Chen CK, Chen WF, Huang SC. Triplet pregnancy complicated by intrauterine fetal death of conjoined twins from an umbilical cord accident of an acardius. A case report. *J Reprod Med* 1996;41:459–62.
12. Dahiya P, Agarwal U, Sangwan K, Sen J. Antenatal diagnosis of twin-reversed arterial perfusion sequence (acardiac amorphous) in a triplet pregnancy: case report. *Arch Gynecol Obstet* 2004;269:147–8.
13. Landy HJ, Larsen JW, Schoen M, Larsen ME, Kent SG, Weingold AB. Acardiac fetus in a triplet pregnancy. *Teratology* 1988;37:1–6.
14. Loh SF, Tee CS, Chew SY. Acardiac anomaly. *Int J Gynaecol Obstet* 1994;45:153–7.
15. Sanjaghsaz H, Bayram MO, Qureshi F. Twin reversed arterial perfusion sequence in conjoined, acardiac, acephalic twins associated with a normal triplet. A case report. *J Reprod Med* 1998;43:1046–50.
16. Sogaard K, Skibsted L, Brocks V. Acardiac twins: pathophysiology, diagnosis, outcome and treatment. *Fetal Diagn Ther* 1999;14:53–9.
17. Sato T, Kaneko K, Konuma S, Sato I, Tamada T. Acardiac anomalies: review of 88 cases in Japan. *Asia Oceania J Obstet Gynaecol* 1984;10:45–52.
18. Severn CB, Holyoke EA. Human acardiac anomalies. *Am J Obstet Gynecol* 1973;116:358–65.
19. Baldwin VJ. *Pathology of Multiple Pregnancy*. Springer-Verlag: New York; 1994. p.277–349.
20. Shih JC, Shyu MK, Hunag SF, Jou HJ, Su YN, Hsieh FJ. Doppler waveform analysis of the intertwin blood flow in acardiac pregnancy: implications for pathogenesis. *Ultrasound Obstet Gynecol* 1994;14:375–9.
21. Spencer R. Parasitic conjoined twins: external, internal (fetuses in fetu and teratomas), and detached (acardiacs). *Clin Anat* 2001;14:428–44.
22. Buntinx IM, Bourgeois N, Buytaert PM, Dumon JE. Acardiac amorphous twin with prune belly sequence in the co-twin. *Am J Med Genet* 1991;39:453–7.
23. Genest DR, Lage JM. Absence of normal-appearing proximal tubules in the fetal and neonatal kidney: prevalence and significance. *Hum Pathol* 1991;22:147–53.
24. Habbal OA, Kenue RK, Venugopalan P. Acardia syndrome coexisting with gastroschisis in the co-twin. *Clin Dysmorphol* 2005;14:45–7.
25. Popek EJ, Strain JD, Neumann A, Wilson H. *In utero* development of pulmonary artery calcification in monochorionic twins: a report of three cases and discussion of the possible etiology. *Pediatr Pathol* 1993;13:597–611.

26. Chen CP, Shih SL, Liu FF, Jan SW, Lin YN, Lan CC. Skeletal deformities of acardius anceps: the gross and imaging features. *Pediatr Radiol* 1997;27:221–5.

27. Chi JG. Acardiac twins – an analysis of 10 cases. *J Korean Med Sci* 1989;4:203–16.

28. Gimenez-Scherer JA, Davies BR. Malformations in acardiac twins are consistent with reversed blood flow: liver as a clue to their pathogenesis. *Pediatr Dev Pathol* 2003;6:520–30.

29. Kosno-Kruszewska E, Deregowski K, Schmidt-Sidor B, Wierzba-Bobrowicz T, Pawlowska B, Lechowicz W, *et al*. Neuropathological and anatomopathological analyses of acardiac and "normal" siblings in an acardiac-twin pregnancy. *Folia Neuropathol* 2003;41:103–9.

30. Laure-Kamionowska M, Maslinska D, Deregowski K, Piekarski P, Raczkowska B. Effects of ischaemia and hypoxia on the development of the nervous system in acardiac foetus. *Folia Neuropathol* 2004;42:227–33.

31. Morizane M, Ohara N, Mori T, Murao S. Neuropathological features of the brain in acardius acormus. *J Perinat Med* 2002;30:269–72.

32. Sergi C, Schmitt HP. Central nervous system in twin reversed arterial perfusion sequence with special reference to examination of the brain in acardius anceps. *Teratology* 2000;61:284–90.

33. Petersen BL, Broholm H, Skibsted L, Graem N. Acardiac twin with preserved brain. *Fetal Diagn Ther* 2001;16:231–3.

34. Ersch J, Stallmach T. Cardiac regression sequence: reversal of blood flow is diagnostic but not causative in an acardiac fetus. *Early Hum Dev* 1998;52:81–5.

35. Nerlich A, Wisser J, Draeger A, Nathrath W, Remberger K. Human acardiac anomaly: a report of three cases. *Eur J Obstet Gynecol Reprod Biol* 1991;38:79–85.

36. Park HW, Kapur RP, Shepard TH. Reversed circulation in acardiac fetuses is associated with anatomic inversions in the aortic wall. *Teratology* 1994;49:267–72.

37. Wong AE, Sepulveda W. Acardiac anomaly: current issues in prenatal assessment and treatment. *Prenat Diagn* 2005;24:796–806.

38. French CA, Bieber FR, Bing DH, Genest DR. Twins, placentas, and genetics: acardiac twinning in a dichorionic, diamniotic, monozygotic twin gestation. *Hum Pathol* 1998;29:1028–31.

39. Masuzaki H, Miura K, Yoshimura S, Yoshiura K, Ishimaru T. A monozygotic twin pregnancy discordant for acardia and X-inactivation pattern. *Eur J Obstet Gynecol Reprod Biol* 2004;117:102–4.

40. Moore CA, Buehler BA, McManus BM, Harmon JP, Mirkin LD, Goldstein DJ. Acephalus–acardia in twins with aneuploidy. *Am J Med Genet* 1987;3:139–43.

41. Blaicher W, Repa C, Schaller A. Acardiac twin pregnancy: associated with trisomy 2: case report. *Hum Reprod* 2000;15:474–5.

42. Chaliha C, Schwarzler P, Booker M, Battash MA, Ville, Y. Trisomy 2 in an acardiac twin in a triplet in-vitro fertilization pregnancy. *Hum Reprod* 1999;14:1378–80.

43. Fisk NM, Ware M, Stanier P, Moore G, Bennett P. Molecular genetic etiology of twin reversed arterial perfusion sequence. *Am J Obstet Gynecol* 1996;174:891–4.

44. Aggarwal N, Suri V, Saxena S, Malhotra S, Vasishta K, Saxena AK. Acardiac acephalus twins: a case report and review of literature. *Acta Obstet Gynecol Scand* 2002;81:983–4.

45. Borrell A, Pesarrodona A, Puerto B, Deulofeu P, Fuster JJ, Fortuny A. Ultrasound diagnostic features of twin reversed arterial perfusion sequence. *Prenat Diagn* 1990;10:443–8.

46. Cardwell MS. The acardiac twin. A case report. *J Reprod Med* 1988;33:320–2.

47. Chandra S, Crane JM, Young DC, Shah S. Acardiac twin pregnancy with neonatal resolution of donor twin cardiomyopathy. *Obstet Gynecol* 2000;96:820–1.

48. Chmait R, Hull A. Placental pathology casebook. Unusually large acardiac twin pregnancy at term. *J Perinatol* 2001;21:150–2.

49. Comerford JA. An acardiac twin. *Aust N Z J Obstet Gynaecol* 1991;31:184–6.

50. Erkaya S, Kutlay B, Kara F, Uygur D, Bebitoglu I. Acardiac twinning where the pump twin dies *in utero* due to thrombosis in the umbilical arteries. *Eur J Obstet Gynecol Reprod Biol* 2000;90:51–4.

51. Imai A, Hirose R, Kawabata I, Tamaya T. Acardiac acephalic person extremely larger than its co-twin. A case report. *Gynecol Obstet Invest* 1991;32:62–4.

52. Langlotz H, Sauerbrei E, Murray S. Transvaginal Doppler sonographic diagnosis of an acardiac twin at 12 weeks gestation. *J Ultrasound Med* 1991;10:175–9.

53. Ozuysal S, Yerci O, Uncu G, Filiz G. Acardiac fetus: a case report. *Clin Exp Obstet Gynecol* 1999;24:169–70.

54. Pratibha D, Sagar DV, Suvarchala P. Acardiac acephalic twin causing obstructed labour. *J Indian Med Assoc* 1995;93:210.

55. Rajangam S, Mohan C, Thomas IM. Acardiac anceps. *Indian Heart J* 1999;51:86–7.

56. Rajesh B, Mahadhevan B, Rao S, Bhat VB. Acephalus acardiac fetus. *Indian J Pediatr* 2004;71:948.

57. Sohi I, Chacko B, Masih K, Choudhary S. A case of TRAP sequence: acardiac twin. *Indian J*

Pathol Microbiol 2003;46:664–5.

58. Stiller RJ, Romero R, Pace S, Hobbins JC. Prenatal identification of twin reversed arterial perfusion syndrome in the first trimester. *Am J Obstet Gynecol* 1989;160:1194–6.

59. Veridiano NP, Fresko O, Chervenak FA. Antenatal diagnosis of acardiac, acephalic twin. *Int J Gynaecol Obstet* 1989;30:179–83.

60. Wenstrom KD. Midtrimester selective delivery of an acardiac twin. *Am J Obstet Gynecol* 1993;168:1647.

61. Lehr C, Dire J. Rare occurrence of a holoacardious acephalic monster: sonographic and pathologic findings. *J Clin Ultrasound* 1978;6:259–61.

62. Porreco RP, Barton SM, Haverkamp AD. Occlusion of umbilical artery in acardiac, acephalic twin. *Lancet* 1991;337:326–7.

63. Shalev E, Zalel Y, Ben-Ami M, Weiner E. First-trimester ultrasonic diagnosis of twin reversed arterial perfusion sequence. *Prenat Diagn* 1992;12:219–22.

64. Zucchini S, Borghesani F, Soffriti G, Chirico C, Vultaggio E, Di Donato P. Transvaginal ultrasound diagnosis of twin reversed arterial perfusion syndrome at 9 weeks' gestation. *Ultrasound Obstet Gynecol* 1993;3:209–11.

65. Bonilla-Musoles F, Machado LE, Raga F, Osborne NG. Fetus acardius: two- and three-dimensional ultrasonographic diagnoses *J Ultrasound Med* 2001;20:1117–27.

66. Sepulveda WH, Quiroz VH, Giuliano A, Henriquez R. Prenatal ultrasonographic diagnosis of acardiac twin. *J Perinat Med* 1993;21:241–6.

67. Sebire NJ, Sepulveda W, Jeanty P, Nyberg DA, Nicolaides KH. Multiple gestations. In: Nyberg DA, McGahan JP, Pretorius DH, Pilu G, editors. *Diagnostic Imaging of Fetal Anomalies.* Philadelphia: Lippincott William & Wilkins; 2003. p. 777–813.

68. Pretorius DH, Leopold GR, Moore TR, Benirschke K, Sivo JJ. Acardiac twin. Report of Doppler sonography. *J Ultrasound Med* 1988;7:413–16.

69. Benson CB, Bieber FR, Genest DR, Doubilet PM. Doppler demonstration of reversed umbilical blood flow in an acardiac twin. *J Clin Ultrasound* 1989;17:291–5.

70. Sherer DM, Armstrong B, Shah YG, Metlay LA, Woods JR. Prenatal sonographic diagnosis, Doppler velocimetric umbilical cord studies, and subsequent management of an acardiac twin pregnancy. *Obstet Gynecol* 1989;74:472–5.

71. Crade M, Nageotte MP, MacKenzie ML. The acardiac twin: a case report using color Doppler ultrasonography. *Ultrasound Obstet Gynecol* 1992;2:364–5.

72. Fouron JC, Leduc L, Grigon A, Maragnes P, Lessard M, Drblik SP. Importance of meticulous ultrasonographic investigation of the acardiac twin. *J Ultrasound Med* 1994;13:1001–4.

73. Al Malt A, Ashmead G, Judge N, Mann L, Ashmead J, Stepanchak W. Color-flow and Doppler velocimetry in prenatal diagnosis of acardiac triplet. *J Ultrasound Med* 1991;10:341–5.

74. Donnenfeld AE, van de Woestijne J, Craparo F, Smith CS, Ludomirsky A, Weiner S. The normal fetus of an acardiac twin pregnancy: perinatal management based on echocardiographic and sonographic evaluation. *Prenat Diagn* 1991;11:235–44.

75. Hecher K, Ville Y, Nicolaides KH. Color Doppler ultrasonography in the identification of communicating vessels in twin–twin transfusion syndrome and acardiac twins. *J Ultrasound Med* 1995;14:37–40.

76. Ishimatsu J, Nakanami H, Hamada T, Yakushiji M. Color and pulsed Doppler ultrasonography of reversed umbilical blood flow in an acardiac twin. *Asia Oceania J Obstet Gynaecol* 1993;19:271–5.

77. Kirkinen P, Herva R, Rasanen J, Airaksinen J, Ikaheimo M. Documentation of paradoxical umbilical blood supply of an acardiac twin in the antepartum state. *J Perinat Med* 1989;17:63–5.

78. Osborn P, Gross TL, Shah JJ, Ma L. Prenatal diagnosis of fetal heart failure in twin reversed arterial perfusion syndrome. *Prenat Diagn* 2000;20:615–7.

79. Papa T, Dao A, Bruner JP. Pathognomonic sign of twin reversed arterial perfusion using color Doppler sonography. *J Ultrasound Med* 1997;16:501–3.

80. Schwarzler P, Ville Y, Moscoso G, Tennstedt C, Bollmann R, Chaoui R. Diagnosis of twin reversed arterial perfusion sequence in the first trimester by transvaginal color Doppler ultrasound. *Ultrasound Obstet Gynecol* 1999;13:143–6.

81. Dashe JS, Fernandez CO, Twickler DM. Utility of Doppler velocimetry in predicting outcome in twin reversed-arterial perfusion sequence. *Am J Obstet Gynecol* 2001;185:135–9.

82. Meyberg H, Gross C. Increased nuchal translucency and pathological ductus venosus flow: two cases of TRAP sequence with different outcomes. *Ultrasound Obstet Gynecol* 2002;20:72–4.

83. Labadie G, David N, Herveau C. Prognostic value of nuchal translucency and ductus venosus Doppler in TRAP sequence. *Ultrasound Obstet Gynecol* 2003;21:306–7.

84. Coulam CB, Wright G. First trimester diagnosis of acardiac twins. *Early Pregnancy* 2000;4:261–70.

85. Gembruch U, Viski S, Bagamery K, Berg C, Germer U. Twin reversed arterial perfusion sequence

in twin-to-twin transfusion syndrome after the death of the donor co-twin in the second trimester. *Ultrasound Obstet Gynecol* 2001;17:153–6.

86. Kamitomo M, Kouno S, Ibuka K, Oku S, Sueyoshi K, Maeda T, *et al*. First-trimester findings associated with twin reversed arterial perfusion sequence. *Fetal Diagn Ther* 2004;19:187–90.

87. Cox M, Murphy K, Ryan G, Kingdom J, Whittle M, McNay M. Spontaneous cessation of umbilical blood flow in the acardiac fetus of a twin pregnancy. *Prenat Diagn* 1992;12:689–93.

88. Brassard M, Fouron JC, Leduc L, Grignon A, Proulx F. Prognostic markers in twin pregnancies with an acardiac fetus. *Obstet Gynecol* 1999;94:409–14.

89. Sullivan AE, Varner MW, Ball RH, Jackson M, Silver RM. The management of acardiac twins: a conservative approach. *Am J Obstet Gynecol* 2003;189:1310–13.

90. Goh A, Loke HL, Tan KW. The 'TRAP' sequence – life threatening consequences to the pump twin. *Singapore Med J* 1994;35:329–31.

91. Weisz B, Peltz R, Chayen B, Oren M, Zalel Y, Achiron R, *et al*. Tailored management of twin reversed arterial perfusion (TRAP) sequence. *Ultrasound Obstet Gynecol* 2004;23:451–5.

92. Tan TYT, Sepulveda W. Acardiac twin: a systematic review of minimally invasive treatment modalities. *Ultrasound Obstet Gynecol* 2003;22:409–19.

93. Sepulveda W, Sebire NJ. Acardiac twin: too many invasive treatment options – the problem and not the solution. *Ultrasound Obstet Gynecol* 2004;24:387–9.

94. Hamada H, Okane M, Koresawa M, Kubo T, Iwasaki H. Fetal therapy *in utero* by blockage of the umbilical blood flow of acardiac monster in twin pregnancy. *Nippon Sanka Fujinka Gakkai Zasshi* 1989;41:1803–9.

95. McCurdy CM, Childers JM, Seeds JW. Ligation of the umbilical cord of an acardiac-acephalus twin with an endoscopic intrauterine technique. *Obstet Gynecol* 1993;82:708–11.

96. Ville Y, Hyett JA, Vandenbussche FP, Nicolaides KH. Endoscopic laser coagulation of umbilical cord vessels in twin reversed arterial perfusion sequence. *Ultrasound Obstet Gynecol* 1994;4:396–8.

97. Willcourt RJ, Naughton MJ, Knutzen VK, Fitzpatrick C. Laparoscopic ligation of the umbilical cord of an acardiac fetus. *J Am Assoc Gynecol Laparosc* 1995;2:319–21.

98. Quintero RA, Reich H, Puder KS, Bardicef M, Evans MI, Cotton DB, *et al*. Brief report: umbilical-cord ligation of an acardiac twin by fetoscopy at 19 weeks of gestation. *N Engl J Med* 1994;330:469–71.

99. Deprest JA, Evrard VA, Van Schoubroeck D, Vandenberghe K. Endoscopic cord ligation in selective feticide. *Lancet* 1996;348:890–1.

100. Deprest JA, Van Ballaer PP, Evrard VA, Peers KH, Spitz B, Steegers EA, *et al*. Experience with fetoscopic cord ligation. *Eur J Obstet Gynecol Reprod Biol* 1998;81:157–64.

101. Hecher K, Hackeloer BJ, Ville Y. Umbilical cord coagulation by operative microendoscopy at 16 weeks' gestation in an acardiac twin. *Ultrasound Obstet Gynecol* 1997;10:130–2.

102. Arias F, Sunderji S, Gimpelson R, Colton E. Treatment of acardiac twinning. *Obstet Gynecol* 1998;91:818–21.

103. Galinkin JL, Gaiser RR, Cohen DE, Crombleholme TM, Johnson M, Kurth CD. Anesthesia for fetoscopic fetal surgery: twin reversed arterial perfusion sequence and twin–twin transfusions syndrome. *Anesth Analg* 2000;91:1394–7.

104. Deprest JA, Audibert F, Van Schoubroeck D, Hecher K, Mahieu-Caputo D. Bipolar coagulation of the umbilical cord in complicated monochorionic twin pregnancy. *Am J Obstet Gynecol* 2000;182:340–5.

105. Quintero RA, Munoz H, Pommer R, Diaz C, Bornick PW, Allen MH. Operative fetoscopy via telesurgery. *Ultrasound Obstet Gynecol* 2002;20:390–1.

106. Porreco RP. Percutaneous ultrasonographically guided ablation of an acardiac twin. *Am J Obstet Gynecol* 2004;190:572–4.

107. Roberts RM, Shah DM, Jeanty P, Beattie JF. Twin, acardiac, ultrasound-guided embolization. 1991 [www.thefetus.net/page.php?id=307].

108. Grab D, Schneider V, Keckstein J, Terinde R. Twin, acardiac, outcome. 1992 [www.thefetus.net/page.php?id=312].

109. Holzgreve W, Tercanli S, Krings W, Schuierer G. A simpler technique for umbilical-cord blockade of an acardiac twin. *N Engl J Med* 1994;331:56–7.

110. Foley MR, Clewell WH, Finberg HJ, Mills MD. Use of the Foley Cordostat grasping device for selective ligation of the umbilical cord of an acardiac twin: a case report. *Am J Obstet Gynecol* 1995;172:212–14.

111. Holmes A, Jauniaux E, Rodeck C. Monopolar thermocoagulation in acardiac twinning. *BJOG* 2001;108:1000–2.

112. Nicolini U, Poblete A, Boschetto C, Bonati F, Roberts A. Complicated monochorionic twin pregnancies: experience with bipolar cord coagulation. *Am J Obstet Gynecol* 2001;185:703–7.

113. Tanawattanacharoen S, Tantivatana J, Charoenvidhya D, Wisawasukmongchol W, Uerpairojkit B, Wacharaprechanont T, et al. Occlusion of umbilical artery using a Guglielmi detachable coil for the treatment of TRAP sequence. *Ultrasound Obstet Gynecol* 2002;19:313–5.

114. Gallot D, Laurichesse H, Lemery D. Selective feticide in monochorionic twin pregnancies by ultrasound-guided umbilical cord occlusion. *Ultrasound Obstet Gynecol* 2003;22:484–8.

115. Chao AS, Hsieh CC, Liou JD, Soong YK. Application of monopolar thermocoagulation in an acardiac fetus. *Prenat Diagn* 2002;22:499–500.

116. Chang PJ, Liou JD, Hsieh CC, Chao AS, Soong YK. Monopolar thermocoagulation in the management of acardiac twins. *Fetal Diagn Ther* 2004;19:271–4.

117. Jolly M, Taylor M, Rose G, Govender L, Fisk NM. Interstitial laser: a new surgical technique for twin reversed arterial perfusion sequence in early pregnancy. *BJOG* 2001;108:1098–102.

118. Soothill P, Sohan K, Carroll S, Kyle P. Ultrasound-guided, intra-abdominal laser to treat acardiac pregnancies. *BJOG* 2002;109:352–4.

119. Sepulveda W, Hasbun J, Dezerega V, Devoto JC, Alcalde JL. Successful sonographically guided laser ablation of a large acardiac twin at 26 weeks' gestation. *J Ultrasound Med* 2004;23:1663–6.

120. Sepulveda W, Bower S, Hassan J, Fisk NM. Ablation of acardiac twin by alcohol injection into the intra-abdominal umbilical artery. *Obstet Gynecol* 1995;86:680–1.

121. Tongsong T, Wanapirak C, Sirichotiyakul S, Chanprapaph P. Intrauterine treatment for an acardiac twin with alcohol injection into the umbilical artery. *J Obstet Gynaecol Res* 2002;28:76–9.

122. Ozeren S, Caliskan E, Corakci A, Ozkan S. Unsuccessful management of acardiac fetus with intrafetal alcohol injection. *Ultrasound Obstet Gynecol* 2004;24:473–4.

123. Sepulveda W, Corral E, Aiello H, Otano L, Paredes R, Escobar MF, et al. Intrafetal alcohol chemosclerosis of acardiac twins: a multicenter experience. *Fetal Diagn Ther* 2004;19:448–52.

124. Heredia F, Quiroz V. TRAP sequence, embolization. 2002 [www.thefetus.net/page.php?id=1000].

125. Gul A, Cebeci A, Yildirim G, Aslan H, Ceylan Y. Successful intrauterine treatment with alcohol ablation in a case of acardiac twin pregnancy. *J Perinatol* 2005;25:352–5.

126. Tsao K, Feldstein VA, Albanese CT, Sandberg PL, Lee H, Harrison MR, et al. Selective reduction of acardiac twin by radiofrequency ablation. *Am J Obstet Gynecol* 2002;187:635–40.

127. Hirose M, Murata A, Kita N, Aotani H, Takebayashi K, Noda Y. Successful intrauterine treatment with radiofrequency ablation in a case of acardiac twin pregnancy complicated with a hydropic pump twin. *Ultrasound Obstet Gynecol* 2004;23:509–12.

128. Simpson PC, Trudinger BJ, Walker A, Baird PJ. The intrauterine treatment of fetal cardiac failure in a twin pregnancy with an acardiac, acephalic monster. *Am J Obstet Gynecol* 1983;147:842–4.

129. Ash K, Harman CR, Gritter H. TRAP sequence – successful outcome with indomethacin treatment. *Obstet Gynecol* 1990;76:960–2.

130. Platt LD, DeVore GR, Bieniarz A, Benner P, Rao R. Antenatal diagnosis of acephalus acardia: a proposed management scheme. *Am J Obstet Gynecol* 1983;146:857–9.

131. Robie GF, Payne GG, Morgan MA. Selective delivery of an acardiac, acephalic twin. *N Engl J Med* 1989;320:512–3.

132. Fries MH, Goldberg JD, Golbus MS. Treatment of acardiac-acephalus twin gestations by hysterotomy and selective delivery. *Obstet Gynecol* 1992;79:601–4.

133. Ginsberg NA, Applebaum M, Rabin SA, Caffarelli MA, Kuuspalu M, Daskal JL, et al. Term birth after midtrimester hysterotomy and selective delivery of an acardiac twin. *Am J Obstet Gynecol* 1992;167:33–7.

Chapter 14

Management of labour in multiple pregnancies

Jon FR Barrett

Introduction

The incidence of twins worldwide continues to increase.[1] Attempts to reduce the incidence of higher order multiples such as triplets or more have met with some success in countries that have legislated against multiple-embryo re-implantation during *in vitro* fertilisation cycles. However, even in these tightly controlled cycles, twin pregnancies occur at a rate ten-fold that of normal-cycle conception.[2] It is unfortunate that many countries, including the author's (Canada), still do not have effective control of or even accurate information on the practices within fertility centres and significant numbers of higher order multiples are still conceived. Although not without some controversy and ethical considerations, these higher order multiples are often reduced. However, the final number following reduction is usually two,[3] thus further increasing a population of twins that will ultimately need to be delivered.

In Western countries the number of spontaneously conceived twins is increasing as a consequence of the population's choosing to conceive at a later maternal age.[4] The end result of all of this is reflected in the author's hospital, a university centre in Toronto, Canada, in which 6% of all deliveries were twins in 2001–02, compared with 2.3% just four years previously.

In twin fetuses with birthweights of more than 2500 g there is a higher risk of death than among singletons of the same birthweight. Kiely[5] reviewed the data on 16 831 multiple births from the New York City Department of Health's computerised records for the period 1978–84. The neonatal mortality rate for twins versus singletons with birthweights of 2501–3000 g and 3001 g or more was 4.3/1000 versus 3.8/1000 (RR 1.12) and 7.4/1000 versus 2.2/1000 (RR 3.32), respectively. Of even more cause for alarm is the fact that the intrapartum fetal death rate for twins is higher than singletons. In the same study Kiely[5] reported that the intrapartum death rate for twins with birthweights of 2501 g or more was 1.22/1000 versus 0.34/1000 in singletons (RR 3.54, 95% CI 1.82–6.88). Other studies have confirmed this higher risk of fetal and neonatal death in twins versus singletons if the pregnancy is at or near term or above 2500 g in birthweight.[6–9] Neonatal seizures, respiratory morbidity and low Apgar scores at one and five minutes have also been shown to be higher for twins versus singleton infants with birthweights of more than 1500 g and more than 3000 g.[10–13]

One of the possible explanations for these data is an increase in the risk of labour and delivery in twins, which is the focus of this chapter.

Who should not labour? Indications for elective lower segment caesarean section

There are few absolute indications for elective caesarean section (CS) and certainly no good clinical studies on which to base strong recommendations. It seems that CS without a trial of labour should be performed in cases of conjoined twins and monoamniotic twins. There are case reports and even some older series of mono-amniotic twins being delivered vaginally without complication.[14] This author has had one personal experience of a set of undiagnosed monoamniotic twins delivering vaginally with only the occasional variable deceleration noted through the labour despite intense intertwining of both umbilical cords. However, most authorities now agree that elective CS is the preferred route for monoamniotic twins although the timing of delivery is still in question.[15-17]

The other indications for elective CS are not dissimilar to those for a singleton pregnancy and include placenta praevia and antenatal evidence of significant fetal compromise likely to be exacerbated during labour.

Caesarean section is generally the recommended method of delivery in twin gestations when twin A is non-vertex.[18-25] In a study in which 31% of the twins were breech/breech and 36% were breech/vertex the investigators found excessive morbidity in vaginally delivered breeches, which caused them to suggest CS for non-vertex first twins.[21]

Pregnancies in which the first twin presents as a breech have, for a long time, been regarded as representing a relative contraindication for vaginal delivery. One of the major concerns with breech/vertex twins, which occurs in about 20% of all twins in labour, is the risk of locked twins.[26] This complication is uncommon, with an estimated frequency of 1/645 twin births, and only 147 cases reported in the world literature between 1958 and 1987. However, the mortality associated with fetal entanglement is extremely high at between 30% and 43%.[27,28]

Two recent studies have challenged the need to perform a CS for all twins where the first fetus is in a breech presentation.[28] In a total of 141 twin pairs, all of whom had a non-vertex twin A, there was no difference in neonatal mortality or morbidity. These studies, although small, have indicated the need for further study. However, the recent randomised controlled trial (RCT) on singleton term breech delivery found that in developed countries the chance of an infant dying as a result of a policy of planned vaginal birth (VB) is 1/300 and the chance of significant handicap is 1/20.[29] This well-conducted study provided grade A evidence that a policy of planned lower segment CS would reduce morbidity and mortality without a significant increase in immediate maternal complications. It seems difficult, therefore, to recommend VB in the twin circumstance, which has the additional risks discussed above and in the rest of this chapter. With consensus attained with respect to the appropriate delivery route for a singleton breech gestation, CS for a twin gestation with twin A in a non-vertex presentation seems to be the appropriate recommendation.

When and how should a twin delivery be conducted?

When?

The majority of twin pregnancies will labour spontaneously by 37 weeks of gestation. However, there are overwhelming cohort and epidemiological data demonstrating the increased risk of stillbirth in twins at more than 37–38 weeks compared with singletons.[30–34] In the absence of an RCT, but extrapolating from the RCT addressing the management of post-term singletons, many authorities including the International Society for Twin Studies and the Society of Obstetricians and Gynaecologists of Canada (SOGC) now recommend delivery before the end of the 38th week of gestation.[35] Failing that, very close fetal surveillance such as twice-weekly biophysical profile (BPP) tests should be undertaken. A word of caution: one should not extrapolate these data to delivery by CS too early. There is evidence that the risk of neonatal respiratory problems increases if elective CS is undertaken prior to 38 weeks.[36] Thus, the ideal time to schedule an elective CS is at 38 weeks of gestation.

If there is uncertainty about the gestational age, consideration may be given to confirming fetal maturity by checking the amniotic fluid lecithin/sphingomyelin (L/S) ratio or managing the pregnancy expectantly using serial fetal monitoring (twice-weekly non-stress and/or BPP tests) until one is confident that the fetuses are mature.

How?

Twin A vertex, twin B vertex

Vertex/vertex twins occur in about 41% of twins in labour. There is still widespread consensus that attempted vaginal delivery is appropriate for vertex/vertex twins, unless other obstetric circumstances militate against it. Most series reveal a 17–25% rate of CS in planned vertex/vertex deliveries.[19,21,35] While these data are encouraging it should not lull the attendants into a false sense of security. Several pitfalls await the unwary and all readers are urged to follow the labour and delivery guidelines deliberated over by the SOGC Consensus Group that are given below.

1. Timely attendance by a physician competent to manage a twin birth.
2. The presence of additional antenatal risk factors should be reviewed at the onset of labour. Intrapartum risk factors should be assessed on an ongoing basis and changes attended to appropriately.
3. When participating in a call system, the replacing physician should be of similar competence and informed of all facts pertaining to a case when care is transferred.
4. The diagnosis of twins is usually antenatal. Therefore, arrangements for delivery and/or transfer should be set in place. This may include antenatal consultation with a high-risk centre.
5. The assessment of lie and presentation of each fetus on admission in labour, preferably by ultrasound.
6. Intravenous access should be secured and blood sent for group and antibody screen.
7. Oxytocin augmentation may be used before the delivery of the first twin and/or between twins for hypotonic contractions.

8. For either twin, the indication(s) for any intervention should be convincing, compelling and documented at the time of the event(s). However, for the cephalic second twin, vaginal delivery should be expedited should fetal distress occur.
9. Documentation of all aspects of labour and delivery should be clear, contemporaneous and consistent among all involved healthcare providers.
10. Progress of labour should emerge clearly from the documentation.
11. Continuous electronic fetal heart-rate monitoring of twins A and B should ensure that both twins are being monitored individually. The presence of an ultrasound machine in the delivery room may be advantageous.
12. For attempted delivery by mid-forceps, for vaginal breech delivery and for multiple pregnancies, CS should be available immediately. Immediate availability means the presence in the hospital of an anaesthetist and nursing staff trained in CS. A note should be dictated describing all operative deliveries and complicated labour and delivery events. The time difference between the delivery of each baby should be noted.
13. Cord blood samples should be taken at the time of delivery.
14. The third stage of labour should be managed actively, with oxytocin being administered with the delivery of the second twin.
15. Placentas should be sent for pathological examination.

The recommendation for continuous electronic monitoring is not evidence-based. There have been no good studies on the use of intermittent monitoring in twin gestations. However, practical experience, common sense and unfortunately several medico-legal cases illustrate that intermittent auscultation does not ensure that each fetus is separately auscultated. Twin monitors are widely available and ideal and, to increase maternal comfort, the author prefers a fetal scalp electrode on the leading twin in order to reduce the number of straps on the maternal abdomen.

Ultrasonographic examination is a useful adjunct after delivery of the first twin in order to establish the fetal lie and presentation of the second twin. Depending on the gestational age, up to 20% of second twins will spontaneously change presentation once the first twin is delivered.[35] In the case of vertex/vertex births, breech extraction will be required in between 0.8% and 3.9% of cases and intrapartum CS for fetal distress/cord prolapse or failure of engagement in up to 10% of cases.[13,30] This emphasises the need for all the precautions listed above as the situation can change rapidly from a relatively low-risk delivery to one fraught with complications for mother and baby should the practitioner be unprepared.

Twin A vertex, twin B non-vertex

The optimal mode of delivery of vertex/non-vertex twins continues to be widely disputed in obstetrics. Both caesarean delivery and vaginal delivery are options which have been debated in the literature. Even as recently as 1986, certain reports advocated caesarean delivery if the second twin is non-vertex, suggesting increased perinatal morbidity and mortality in non-vertex twins delivered vaginally.[37–48]

The results of numerous subsequent reports have emphasised the fetal safety of vaginal delivery when compared with the abdominal route if limited to infants with birthweights of greater than 1500–2000 g.[38,42,43,48] Rabinovici et al.[45] published the only RCT investigating this issue. Vertex/non-vertex twins after the 35th gestational week were randomly allocated to vaginal or abdominal delivery according to a protocol.

Twenty-seven women were delivered by CS and 27 were delivered vaginally (14 assisted breech extractions, five total breech extractions and eight internal podalic versions and total breech extractions). There were no statistically significant differences in fetal outcomes. Maternal febrile morbidity was significantly higher in the CS group than in the vaginal delivery group (40.7% versus 11.1%, $P < 0.05$).[45]

Barrett *et al.*[49] found that breech-extracted second twins with birthweights of less than 1500 g had lower Apgar scores and increased neonatal morbidity when compared as a group with their first-born siblings. This difference was not found among the twins delivered by CS. Comparisons between the second twins delivered vaginally and by CS were not made. The authors, however, recommended routine CS for second non-vertex twins expected to weigh less than 1500 g. Chervenak *et al.*[42] reported 76 breech-extracted second twins of whom 16 weighed less than 1500 g[42] Although delivery mode was not associated with any difference in outcome, they recommended routine caesarean delivery for non-vertex second twins with birthweights of less than 1500 g.

External cephalic version versus breech extraction

In 1983 Chervenak *et al.*[44] advocated an alternative approach of external cephalic version (ECV) of the second non-vertex twin after delivery of the first in order to achieve delivery of the second as a vertex presentation. ECV was attempted in 25 sets of twins after successful delivery of the first vertex twin. This was successful in 18 of the cases (72%) and was not associated with increased perinatal complications.[10,44] On the basis of this report, the American College of Obstetricians and Gynecologists recommended ECV as a reasonable option for delivery of the second non-vertex twin.[42] Subsequent to Chervenak's report, numerous other investigators have published similar findings.[43,47]

In an effort to examine this controversy, four retrospective studies have been published reporting the success rates and CS rates in the second non-vertex twins delivered by ECV versus breech extraction. Overall, breech extraction was associated with higher success rates and lower CS rates than ECV. There was also significantly less intrapartum fetal distress attributed to breech extractions than ECVs. Analysis of neonatal and maternal outcomes concluded that there were no significant differences between the two groups.[50-57]

Our group reviewed the management of 206 vertex/non-vertex twin deliveries in major obstetrical units in Toronto in order to compare the different methods of delivering the second non-vertex twin following vaginal delivery of the first. Delivery was attempted by primary breech extraction with or without internal podalic version in 183 patients. This was successful in all but two patients (98.9%) who were delivered by CS for failed breech extraction. External cephalic version was attempted in 23 second twins. This was successful in six (26.1%) resulting in vertex vaginal delivery. In 12 patients, secondary breech extraction was performed and successful in all but one patient who required delivery by CS.

Intrapartum complications including placental abruption, fetal distress and cord prolapse occurred more frequently in the ECV group (30.4% versus 6.0%, $P = 0.001$). Despite the fact that there were no differences in the five minute Apgar scores and incidence of neonatal trauma, there were more neonatal intensive care unit admissions and a greater incidence of respiratory distress syndrome and intraventricular haemorrhages in the ECV group. There were no significant differences in maternal outcomes including postpartum haemorrhage or infection.

The following guidelines for the performance of ECV of the second twin are recommended:

1.   Ultrasonographic assessment of estimated fetal weights of both fetuses should be performed. If twin B is larger than twin A and a great disparity exists, ECV with attempted vaginal delivery should be avoided.
2.   Epidural anaesthesia is advisable prior to delivery to provide abdominal wall relaxation.
3.   The procedure should be performed only if immediate access to CS is possible.
4.   The fetal heart rate should be monitored throughout delivery.
5.   A real-time ultrasound machine should be present in the delivery room to ascertain accurately the fetal presentation of twin B after delivery of the first twin. Gentle pressure with the ultrasound transducer is used to guide the infant in the vertex presentation into the birth canal. If this fails, forward or backward rolls are used to convert the malpresenting fetus to the vertex presentation. The shortest arc between the vertex and the pelvic inlet should be attempted first.
6.   If ECV is successful, amniotomy should be performed and oxytocin augmentation may be used as necessary.
7.   If version is unsuccessful, if the fetal heart rate of twin B reveals a non-reassuring fetal heart rate, or if twin B fails to descend after a successful ECV, secondary breech extraction or CS is necessary.[43]

Time interval between delivery of twins

It was previously believed that the time interval between twin deliveries should be no longer than 30 minutes, as a prolonged interval placed the second twin at risk of asphyxia from decreased placental circulation.[58–61] This time limit was considered to be appropriate when electronic fetal monitoring and ultrasound were not routinely available. More recent studies have shown no correlation between five minute Apgar scores and the time interval between twin deliveries. Rayburn *et al.*[58] found that perinatal morbidity was lowest with expectant therapy and subsequent spontaneous delivery regardless of fetal presentation. One study based on a small sample size reported a six-fold increase in the risk of CS for the second twin with a delivery interval greater than 15 minutes.[61]

What is the evidence that a policy of planned caesarean section might be beneficial for twins at or near term?

Now that the reader is familiar with the standard, I would like to draw his or her attention to the crucial question in this field. Should vaginal delivery be attempted at all?

In a recent study of 1305 twin pairs delivered between 1988 and 1999 in Nova Scotia in which second-born twins were compared with first-born twins with birthweights of 1500 g or more, the risk of adverse perinatal outcome (intrapartum fetal death, neonatal death, moderate–severe respiratory distress syndrome, asphyxia, trauma and complications of prematurity) was significantly increased (RR 2.1, 95% CI 1.4–3.1) for second-born twins.[11] There is also evidence that the second twin is at greater risk of adverse perinatal outcome compared with the first twin if delivery is vaginal, but the same has not been shown if delivery is by CS. Arnold et al.[10] undertook a matched case–control study of preterm twin pairs. The risk of respiratory distress syndrome was increased for the second twin compared with the first if delivery was vaginal (OR 14.2, 95% CI 2.5–81.1) but not if delivery was by CS (OR 0.90, 95% CI 0.0–17.8).

In the Kiely review,[5] for twins in vertex presentation weighing more than 3000 g at birth the neonatal mortality rate was 12.3/1000 versus 2.9/1000 (RR 4.22) if delivery was vaginal versus by CS. These data are possibly strongly affected by selection bias and therefore the best approach is to compare outcomes for twins delivered by planned VB (actual VB plus emergency CS) versus planned CS.

As mentioned earlier, there has been only one RCT of planned CS versus planned VB for twins, in which 60 pairs of twins were enrolled.[45] There were no perinatal deaths or cases of serious neonatal morbidity in either group. The sample size was too small to answer the question of the better approach to delivery. A Cochrane review,[62] incorporating this one trial, has recommended that a larger RCT be undertaken.

Because of the limited information from RCTs, we undertook a systematic review of studies that compared the policies of planned VB and planned CS for the delivery of twins weighing at least 1500 g or reaching at least 32 weeks of gestation.[63] The meta-analysis did not find significant differences between the two approaches to delivery in terms of mortality or neonatal morbidity, although low Apgar score at five minutes was reduced with a policy of CS. This finding, however, was confined to the twins in which twin A presented as a breech. Since that analysis was undertaken, a further cohort study of 2890 pairs of twins of at least 36 weeks of gestation found that, in those delivered by planned CS ($n = 454$) there were no deaths of either twin; however, in those undergoing planned VB ($n = 2436$) there were no deaths of the first twin but nine second-twin deaths.[64]

Clinical equipoise – time for a trial?

It seems that many physicians are in equipoise on this most fundamental of all aspects of twins research. What is the best way to deliver twins?

In 2001, Hutton undertook a survey of Canadian practitioners to determine their views of the various delivery options for twins.[65] Most respondents indicated that for twins at 32 or more weeks of gestation in which twin A was vertex, they would usually recommend a planned VB, with the recommendation of planned VB being as high as 100% for the vertex/vertex combination at term and as low as 78% for the vertex/footling breech combination at 32–36 weeks. However, the respondents were not convinced that planned VB was the best approach to delivery, as 64% indicated they would be willing to enrol their patients with twin pregnancies in a well-designed RCT comparing planned VB with planned CS. The interest in a large twin delivery trial was greatest for twins at term (55%) and for twins presenting vertex/non-vertex (58%). However, 48% were willing to enrol women with twins at 32–36 weeks of gestation, and 42% were willing to enrol twins presenting vertex/vertex.

The high number of physicians willing to enrol vertex/vertex twins[22] probably reflects the following. Firstly, up to 20% of vertex second twins will change presentation spontaneously after twin A is delivered.[66] Secondly, it was for the twin in vertex presentation that Kiely found better outcomes if delivery was by caesarean versus vaginal delivery.[5] Thirdly, it is the view of practitioners experienced in the management of labour and the delivery of twins that a substantial number of those presenting vertex/vertex will present with serious acute intrapartum problems following the delivery of twin A (e.g. conversion to transverse lie, cord prolapse, prolonged interval delivery of twin B), which may lead to emergency CS, perinatal death and neonatal morbidity. Lastly, if there are benefits to avoiding labour, both twins, regardless of presentation, should benefit.

Many policies in obstetrics have been accepted as the standard of care without adequate evidence to support them. Once a policy of clinical management has been accepted and implemented into practice, it is very difficult to undertake research that is designed to determine the effectiveness of the practice. Although the Term Breech Trial[29] emphasised the relative safety of a policy of planned CS for the mother, the recently updated Cochrane review[67] has found a higher risk of serious maternal morbidity following a policy of planned CS if the fetus is a singleton breech, and the longer-term impact of a policy of planned CS for the mother is not known.

The focus among practitioners has moved away from keeping CS rates low and more towards supporting maternal choice for method of delivery. When the Term Breech Trial was conducted, practice had already shifted towards planned CS. Recruitment to this study was therefore confined to a minority of practitioners who had maintained their skills and confidence in vaginal breech delivery. We believed that a large RCT of planned CS for twins should be conducted soon before practice changes.

Thankfully, the Canadian Institutes of Health Research agreed and in the spring of 2003 the Twin Birth Study was funded to the value of 8.6 million $CAN.

The Twin Birth Study

This Twin Birth Study is a multicentre international RCT of planned CS versus planned VB for twins of at least 32 weeks of gestation in which twin A is presenting vertex. Proposed inclusion criteria are: twins at 32 weeks or more of gestation in which twin A is presenting vertex, both twins are alive and the estimated fetal birthweight is expected to be between 1500 and 4000 g. Monoamniotic twins, lethal anomaly of either twin, or other contraindications to labour or VB are exclusion criteria. Women with a twin pregnancy at 32–35 weeks of gestation, who meet the selection criteria and consent to participate in the trial, will be randomised from 32 weeks of gestation onwards. Because of the data mentioned earlier showing an increase in stillbirth rate at 38 weeks of gestation, trial participants will be delivered at 38–39 weeks of gestation. Vaginal delivery will be conducted, in accordance with the SOGC guidelines as discussed above, by experienced personnel. If twin B is non-vertex, the options for delivery will be spontaneous or assisted vaginal breech delivery (if breech), total breech extraction with or without internal podalic version, ECV and vaginal delivery of the fetus as a vertex or CS.

The proposed primary outcome is a composite of perinatal/neonatal mortality and/or serious neonatal morbidity (excluding lethal congenital anomalies) that has a prevalence of 4% from retrospective data. The proposed secondary outcome is problematic urinary or faecal/flatal incontinence at three months and at two years. Other outcomes that will be evaluated will be death or serious maternal morbidity within 28 days of delivery, maternal satisfaction with method of delivery (three months), maternal quality of life (three months and two years) and death or poor neurodevelopmental outcome of the children at two years of age (corrected for gestational age at birth). The sample size of 2400 women is designed to detect a difference in the primary outcome of 2%.

There are currently 55 active centres in 17 countries. To date, 350 patients have been randomised with the first interim analysis scheduled after 1000 patients. There are currently four active and 12 interested centres in the UK; we are hoping that the UK centres will play a major role in this trial. Interested centres are asked to contact tbs@sw.ca.

It is the author's bias that a properly conducted vaginal twin delivery is safe for both mothers and babies. By the time that this chapter is in print, we hope to be well on the way to defining the optimal method of twin delivery.

References

1. Barrett J, Bocking A. The SOGC consensus statement: Management of twin pregnancies Part 2. *SOGC* 2000;22:623.
2. Wimalasundera RC, Trew G, Fisk NM. Reducing the incidence of twins and triplets. *Best Pract Res Clin Obstet Gynaecol* 2003;17:309–29.
3. Evans MI, Berkowitz RL, Wapner RJ, Carpenter RJ, Goldberg JD, Ayoub MA, *et al.* Improvement in outcomes of multifetal pregnancy reduction with increased experience. *Am J Obstet Gynecol* 2001;184:97–103.
4. Martin JA, Park M. *Trends in Twin and Triplet Births: 1980–97.* vol. 47, no. 20. PHS: Chicago; 1999. p. 99–1120.
5. Kiely JL. The epidemiology of perinatal mortality in multiple births. *Bull NY Acad Med* 1990;66:618–37.
6. Cheung YB, Yip P, Karlberg J. Mortality of twins and singletons by gestational age: a varying-coefficient approach. *Am J Epidemiol* 2000;152:1107–16.
7. Lie RT. Invited commentary: Intersecting perinatal mortality curves by gestational age – are appearances deceiving? *Am J Epidemiol* 2000;152:1117–19.
8. Ghai V, Vidyasagar D. Morbidity and mortality factors in twins, an epidemiologic approach. *Clin Perinatol* 1988;15:123–40.
9. Fabre E, de Agüero R, de Augustin JL, Pérez-Hiraldo MP, Bescos JL. Perinatal mortality in twin pregnancy: an analysis of birth weight-specific mortality rates and adjusted mortality rates for birth weight distributions. *J Perinat Med* 1988;16:85–91.
10. Arnold C, McLean F, Kramer M, Usher R. Respiratory distress syndrome in second-born versus first-born twins. A matched case–control analysis. *N Engl J Med* 1987;317:1121–5.
11. Persad V, Young D, Armson A, Joseph KS, Baskett T. Determinants of perinatal morbidity and death among the second of twins. *Am J Obstet Gynecol* 2001;184:S188 (abstract 0647).
12. Joseph KS, Marcoux S, Ohlsson A, Liu S, Allen AC, Kramer MS, *et al.* Changes in stillbirth and infant mortality associated with increases in preterm birth among twins. *Pediatrics* 2001;108:1055–61.
13. Cheung YB, Yip P, Karlberg J. Mortality of twins and singletons by gestational age: a varying-coefficient approach. *Am J Epidemiol* 2000;152:1107–16.
14. Dubecq F, Dufour P, Vinatier D, Thibault D, Lefebvre C, Tordjeman N, *et al.* Monoamniotic twin pregnancies, review of the literature, and a case report with vaginal delivery. *Eur J Obstet Gynecol Reprod Biol* 1996;66:183–6.
15. Griffith HB. Monoamniotic twin pregnancy. *Br J Clin Pract* 1986;40:294–7.
16. Tessen JA, Zlatnik FJ. Monoamniotic twins: A retrospective controlled study. *Obstet Gynecol* 1991;77:832–4.
17. Carr SR, Aronson MP, Coustan DR. Survival rates of monoamniotic twins do not decrease after 30 weeks' gestation. *Am J Obstet Gynecol* 1990;163:719–22.
18. Chervenak FA, Johnson RE, Berkowitz RL, Hobbins JC. Intrapartum external version of the second twin. *Obstet Gynecol* 1983;62:160–5.
19. Adams DM, Chervenak FA. Intrapartum management of twin gestation. *Clin Obstet Gynecol* 1990;33:52–60.
20. Ismajovich B, Confino E, Sherzer A, Lidor A, David MP. Optimal delivery of nonvertex twins. *Mt Sinai J Med* 1985;52:106–9.
21. Chervenak FA, Johnson RE, Youcha S, Hobbins JC, Berkowitz RL. Intrapartum management of twin gestation. *Obstet Gynecol* 1985;65:119–24.
22. Laros RK, Dattel BJ. Management of twin pregnancy; the vaginal route is still safe. *Am J Obstet Gynecol* 1998;158:1330–8.

23. Caspersen LS. A discussant to paper by Laros RK, Dattel BJ. *Am J Obstet Gynecol* 1988;158:1334–6.

24. Kelsick F, Minkoff H. Management of the breech second twin. *Am J Obstet Gynecol* 1982;144:783–6.

25. Farooqui MO, Grossman JH, Shannon RA. A review of twin pregnancy and perinatal mortality. *Obstet Gynecol Surv* 1973;28:144–53.

26. Nissen ED. Twins: collision, impaction, compaction, and interlocking. *Obstet Gynecol* 1958;11:514–26.

27. Kahunda S. Locked twins. *Obstet Gynecol* 1972;39:453–9.

28. Rydhstrom H, Cullberg G. Pregnancies with growth-retarded twins in breech–vertex presentation at increased risk for entanglement during delivery. *J Perinat Med* 1990;18:45–50.

29. Hannah ME, Hannah WJ, Hewson SA, Hodnett ED, Saigal S, Willan AR. Planned caesarean section versus planned vaginal birth for breech presentation at term: A randomised multicentre trial. Term Breech Trial Collaborative Group. *Lancet* 2000;356;1375–83.

30. Hartley RS, Emanuel I, Hitti J. Perinatal mortality and neonatal morbidity rates among twin pairs at different gestational ages: Optimal delivery timing at 37 to 38 weeks' gestation. *Am J Obstet Gynecol* 2001;184:451–8.

31. Puissant F, Leroy F. A reappraisal of perinatal mortality factors in twins. *Acta Genet Med Gemellol* 1982;31:213–19.

32. Imaizumi Y. Perinatal mortality in twins and factors influencing mortality in Japan, 1980–98. *Paediatr Perinat Epidemiol* 2001;15:298–305.

33. Minakami H, Sato I. Reestimating date of delivery in multifetal pregnancies. *JAMA* 1996;275:1432–4.

34. Thompson SA, Lyons TJ, Makowski EL. Outcomes of twin gestation at the University of Colorado Health Sciences Centre. *J Reprod Med* 1987;32:328–39.

35. Barrett J, Bocking A. The SOGC consensus statement on management of twin pregnancies (part I). *JSOGC* 2000;22:519–29.

36. Chasen ST, Madden A, Chervenak FA. Cesarean delivery of twins and neonatal respiratory disorders. *Am J Obstet Gynecol* 1999;181:1052–6.

37. Kelsick F, Minkoff H. Management of the breech second twin. *Am J Obstet Gynecol* 1982;144:783–6.

38. Cetrulo CL. The controversy of mode of delivery in twins: The intrapartum management of twin gestation (part I). *Semin Perinatol* 1986;10:39–43.

39. Ware HH. The second twin. *Am J Obstet Gynecol* 1971;110:865–73.

40. Ho SK, Wu PYK. Perinatal factors and neonatal morbidity in twin pregnancy. *Am J Obstet Gynecol* 1975;122:979–87.

41. Taylor ES. Editorial. *Obstet Gynecol Surv* 1976;31:535–6.

42. Chervenak FA, Johnson RE, Berkowitz RL, Grannum P, Hobbins JC. Is routine cesarean section necessary for vertex–breech and vertex–transverse twin gestations? *Am J Obstet Gynecol* 1984;148:1–5.

43. Acker D, Lieberman M, Holbrook H, James O, Phillipe M, Edelin KC. Delivery of the second twin. *Obstet Gynecol* 1982;59:710–11.

44. Chervenak FA, Johnson RE, Berkowitz RL, Hobbins JC. Intrapartum external version of the second twin. *Obstet Gynecol* 1983;62:160–5.

45. Rabinovici J, Barkai G, Reichman B, Serr DM, Mashiach S. Randomized management of the second nonvertex twin: Vaginal delivery or cesarean section. *Am J Obstet Gynecol* 1987;156:52–6.

46. Rabinovici J, Barkai G, Reichman B, Serr DM, Mashiach S. Internal podalic version with unruptured membranes for the second twin in transverse lie. *Obstet Gynecol* 1988;71:428–30.

47. Adam C, Allen AC, Baskett TF. Twin delivery: Influence of the presentation and method of delivery on the second twin. *Am J Obstet Gynecol* 1991;165:23–7.

48. Fishman A, Grubb DK, Kovacs BW. Vaginal delivery of the nonvertex second twin. *Am J Obstet Gynecol* 1993;168:861–4.

49. Barrett JM, Staggs SM, Van Hooydonk JE, Growdon JH, Killam AP, Boehm FH. The effect of type of delivery upon neonatal outcome in premature twins. *Am J Obstet Gynecol* 1982;143:360–7.

50. American College of Obstetricians and Gynecologists. *Multiple Gestation.* ACOG Technical Bulletin 131. Washington DC: ACOG: 1988.

51. Tchabo JG, Tomai T. Selected intrapartum external cephalic version of the second twin. *Obstet Gynecol* 1992;79:421–3.

52. Kaplan B, Peled Y, Rabinerson D, Goldman GA, Nitzan Z, Neri A. Successful external version of B-twin after the birth of A-twin for vertex-non-vertex twins. *Eur J Obstet Gynecol Reprod Biol*

1995;58:157–60.

53. Gocke SE, Nageotte MP, Garite T, Towers CV, Dorcester W. Management of the nonvertex second twin: Primary cesarean section, external version, or primary breech extraction. *Am J Obstet Gynecol* 1989;161:111–14.

54. Wells SR, Thorp JM, Bowes WZ. Management of the nonvertex second twin. *Surg Gynecol Obstet* 1991;172:383–5.

55. Chauhan SP, Roberts WE, McLaren RA, Roach H, Morrison JC, Martin JN. Delivery of the nonvertex second twin: Breech extraction versus external cephalic version. *Am J Obstet Gynecol* 1995;173:1015–20.

56. Smith SJ, Zebrowitz J, Latta RA. Method of delivery of the nonvertex second twin: A community hospital experience. *J Matern Fetal Med* 1997;6:146–50.

57. Rydhstrom H. Prognosis for twins with birth weight less than 1500 gm: The impact of cesarean section in relation to fetal presentation. *Am J Obstet Gynecol* 1990;163:528–33.

58. Rayburn WF, Lavin JP, Miodovnik M, Varner MW. Multiple gestation: Time interval between delivery of the first and second twins. *Obstet Gynecol* 1984;63:502.

59. Bartnicki J, Meyenburg M, Saling E. Time interval in twin delivery: The second twin need not always be born shortly after the first. *Gynecol Obstet Invest* 1992;33:19–20.

60. Poeschmann PP, Van Oppen CAC, Bruinse HW. Delayed interval delivery in multiple pregnancies: Report of three cases and review of the literature. *Obstet Gynecol Surv* 1992;47:139–47.

61. Rydhstrom H, Ingemarsson I. Interval between birth of the first and the second twin and its impact on second twin perinatal mortality. *J Perinat Med* 1990;18:449.

62. Crowther CA. Caesarean delivery for the second twin. *Cochrane Database Syst Rev* 2000;(2):CD000047.

63. Hogle KL, Hutton EK, McBrien KA, Barrett JF, Hannah ME. Delivery for twins: a systematic review and meta-analysis. *Am J Obstet Gynecol* 2003;188:220–7.

64. Smith GC, Pell JP, Dobbie R. Birth order, gestational age, and risk of delivery related perinatal death in twins: Retrospective cohort study. *BMJ* 2002;325:1004.

65. Hutton EK, Hannah ME, Barrett J. Use of external cephalic version for breech pregnancy and mode of delivery for breech and twin pregnancy: a survey of Canadian practitioners. *J Obstet Gynaecol Can* 2002;24:804–10.

66. Houlihan C, Knuppel RA. Intrapartum management of multiple gestations. Complicated labor and delivery II. *Clin Perinatol* 1996;23:91–116.

67. Hofmeyr GJ, Hannah ME. Planned caesarean section for term breech delivery. *Cochrane Database Syst Rev* 2001;(1):CD000166. Update in: *Cochrane Database Syst Rev* 2003;(3):CD000166.

Chapter 15

Does neonatal and infant neurodevelopment of twins and singletons differ?

Neil Marlow

Introduction

There is much anxiety about the burden of health and social care that has accompanied the rise in multiple pregnancy rates over the past 15 years. Twin pregnancies have considerably greater pregnancy loss, perinatal mortality and neonatal mortality. Twin pregnancies deliver on average two weeks earlier and more are delivered after short gestations or with very low birthweight (VLBW). Associated with this is a six-fold rise in the rate of cerebral palsy, which is discussed further in Chapter 16. All of these adverse outcomes are more common in higher order multiples, their prevalence being proportional to the number of fetuses in the pregnancy.

Twinning provides a natural experiment in which to study developmental disorders and normal development within a nature–nurture context. The variance in outcome due to genetic and environmental factors is minimised when studying such a dyad. Many studies, however, have used relatively small and highly selected samples, which makes their conclusions difficult to extrapolate from. Nevertheless, there are many studies using such cohorts that have contributed greatly to the literature. There are also some important large epidemiology studies that have contributed to our under-standing of the genetic factors relating to language in particular, for example the Twins and Early Development Study (TEDS). Most of these studies simply examine twins; comparative studies of twins and singletons for the question of later development in childhood are rare. There appear to be few consistent cognitive and learning differences between twins and singletons at school age. However, this statement hides a range of perinatal and early childhood issues that may alter early developmental processes and the phenomenon of twinning may be associated with differences in behaviour that are not reflected in cognitive scores.[1]

Given the high risk of preterm birth and the known association of prematurity and later disability, it is appropriate to question whether the developmental progress of twins differs in any systematic way from that of singletons. In particular, this chapter will concentrate on those studies that have tried to identify the influence of particular factors on such outcomes.

Why might one expect neurodevelopment to differ between twins and singletons?

Many factors leading to developmental disadvantage in the population are related to social disadvantage. Twinning rates appear to be independent of social status and, if anything, with the increase in the use of assisted reproductive technologies (ART) and consequent multiple pregnancies, some decrease in the frequency of social disadvantage among multiple births might be expected. This may offset some of the biological and environmental risks described below.

The possible causes of developmental disadvantage in twins are as follows:

■ **biological factors during pregnancy and the neonatal period:**
  – increased rate of very preterm birth
  – increased risk of fetal and neonatal brain injury
  – fetal growth restriction (FGR)
  – twin-specific disorders (differential fetal growth and twin-to-twin transfusion)

■ **environmental issues:**
  – maternal psychological health
  – increased 'stress' at home
  – decreased frequency of breastfeeding
  – reduced attention in the home environment

■ **twinning issues:**
  – role models
  – inter-twin communication (private language)
  – shared experience/shared identity.

Biological factors operative in the pregnancy/neonatal period

Very preterm birth

The modal delivery time of twin pregnancies is approximately 38 weeks, compared with 40 weeks in term babies. However, the median gestation is considerably lower than this – approximately 35 weeks – indicating that there is an increased risk of very preterm birth. The relative effects of twinning itself need to be separated out from the effects of prematurity, although this is rarely done.[2]

The increased risk of very preterm birth must therefore increase the number of disabilities within a population of twins, simply from the effect of prematurity itself. The frequency of disability in the population increases with decreasing gestation, as does perinatal and neonatal mortality, as well as a range of other short- and long-term morbidities. A multiple pregnancy is usually considered a significant risk factor in most areas of neonatal care.

At the margins of viability, twins and triplets comprise a higher proportion of neonatal admissions than expected: of the babies admitted for intensive care in the UK and Ireland during 1995 at between 22 and 25 weeks of gestation, 23% were from twin pregnancies (84% of twin live births at these gestations) and a further 5% were from triplet pregnancies,[3] compared with a multiple birth rate of around 2% of all pregnancies.

One further question is whether being the product of a multiple pregnancy by itself increases the risk of neonatal morbidity. At low gestations, multiple births also have a higher mortality: on multivariate analysis of factors present at birth between 22 and 25 weeks of gestation, the odds ratio for neonatal death was 1.55 (95% CI 1.08–2.22) for babies from multiple pregnancies compared with singletons. This became nonsignificant when condition at birth was added into the statistical model, implying that babies of multiple pregnancies may be in poorer condition when born at extremely low gestations. Considering important neonatal morbidities, twins were not significantly more likely to have a serious cerebral ultrasound abnormality (OR 0.85; 95% CI 0.42–1.69) or treatment for retinopathy (OR 0.51; 95% CI 0.21–1.18) but tended to have chronic lung disease more frequently (OR 1.45; 95% CI 0.87–2.44).[3] It would thus appear that, from this study, relative to singletons and independently of other risk factors, children from multiple births have higher risks of death and possibly chronic lung disease but not of brain injury or eye disease.

The data reported above were derived from a total population (the UK and Ireland) and based on gestational age. Other studies of neonatal morbidity have been based on populations in which there was selection bias. In one large study of neonatal admissions reported to the US National Institute of Child Health and Human Development (NICHD) Neonatal Research Network of over 9000 babies under 1501 g birthweight, twins were not more likely to die or have chronic lung disease or severe intraventricular haemorrhage after adjustment in multiple regression: the subgroup of children born at less than 28 weeks of gestation showed similar findings.[4] Clearly the bias of simply reporting admissions may have hidden excess mortality risk (given poorer delivery room condition) and the birthweight-based analyses were confounded by the excess of births following fetal growth restriction (FGR) (see below).

However, because of the higher proportion of twins who are of low gestation at birth it is not surprising that the prevalence of cerebral palsy and other neuromotor disabilities is higher in the general populations of twins than singletons. For example, in the Mersey Regional Register between 1982 and 1989 the crude prevalence of cerebral palsy was 2.3 per 1000 singleton survivors, 12.6 in twins and 44.8 in triplets, and rose as birthweight decreased. The birthweight-specific prevalence among those of low birthweight below 2500 g was not significantly different in singleton compared with multiple births. Among infants weighing at least 2500 g, there was a significantly higher risk in multiple than in singleton births.[5] Thus, the higher rate of neuromorbidity in multiple pregnancies is partly due to the excess of small babies with their attendant higher risk and partly due to an increased risk in normal birthweight children.

This latter is an important point, as any small effect of twinning on developmental progress may be swamped by the serious sequelae of very preterm birth[6] and, as many studies have done, simply examining a preterm cohort may hide differences in outcome for more mature children.

To illustrate these difficulties, in a matched cohort study, the outcome at 18–22 months was compared between 101 twins and singletons born after 24–30 weeks of gestation from 1997 to 1999.[7] Twin pregnancies were less likely to be complicated by hypertension or prelabour rupture of membranes. The prevalence of death or disability as a combined outcome was similar in the two groups (30% versus 23%). Poor developmental scores ('disability') was the most common problem at follow-up in both groups. Among the twins, 36% were monochorionic (MC), and of them 7% had twin-to-twin transfusion syndrome (TTTS), a known risk factor for poor outcome (see below). Discordant growth was more prevalent in MC twins and they were more immature and had higher rates of neonatal morbidity than dichorionic (DC) twins. The combined outcome variable differed between MC and DC twins –

39% versus 25% – but the cohort was small and the difference not statistically significant. The authors did not correct for gestation or birthweight differences.

Cognitive outcome may be correlated with gestation at birth.[8,9] In the systematic review by Bhutta et al.[8] the relationship was assumed to be linear as they reviewed comparator studies between VLBW and normal birthweight children and not those in between. That this may be fallacious is demonstrated by the results of cognitive testing in the Bavarian low birthweight study where a full population was studied.[9] In this group the relationship between gestational age and later IQ at five years was weak between 33 and 43 weeks gestational age (approximately +0.7 points per week of gestation). Below this gestational age, IQ fell off at a more rapid rate: 2.5 points per week for each week below 33 weeks. This is consistent with the IQ data reported in the UK and Ireland EPICure study.[10,11] Hence a population with a high proportion of very preterm children is likely to have lower IQ scores than one with few very preterm children. These effects persist even after making an age correction for gestation at birth. There is reasonable correlation in preterm populations between low IQ and other psychological morbidity, such as behaviour and attention deficit hyperactivity disorder (ADHD). Within the EPICure population there was also significant comorbidity between cognitive and language scores, such that differences in language scores were no longer significant after correction for IQ.[12] It thus follows that performance in other related areas will segregate in mixed populations in the same manner as IQ.

If the cognitive scores of children recruited into the EPICure study by sex and plurality are examined, it becomes clear that there are no consistent differences that can be attributed to multiple birth (Table 15.1) and multiple birth does not have any independent effect on growth or development, after correction for other factors.[13,14]

Table 15.1. Results of cognitive testing of singleton and multiple births for extremely preterm (< 25 weeks of gestation) boys and girls at 2.5 years and 6 years of age; data from the EPICure study[10,42]

Mean	Boys				Girls			
	Singleton		Multiple		Singleton		Multiple	
	Mean SEM		SEM Mean		Mean SEM		SEM	
2.5 year assessment								
Bayley mental development index (MDI)	75.4	1.9	83.4	2.2	84.3	1.4	88.2	2.7
Bayley psychomotor development index (PDI)	75.6	2.2	84.4	2.1	87.7	1.5	92.7	3.5
6 year assessment								
Overall cognitive score (Kaufman ABC/GQ)	75.3	2.2	81.7	2.6	88.3	1.7	83.7	4.1
NEPSY sensorimotor	75.2	2.0	71.4	1.9	83.3	1.8	80.6	3.4
Visuospatial	84.6	1.7	81.6	1.6	88.5	1.5	85.3	2.9
Attention/executive	100.2	1.3	97.2	1.9	104.1	1.2	104.9	2.5

SEM = standard error of the mean

Fetal growth restriction

The growth of preterm twin fetuses begins to tail off after 30 weeks compared with singletons, presumably because of competition for nutrients. Twin pregnancies are also more likely to be complicated by pre-eclampsia and other hypertensive disorders and by conditions associated with poor fetal growth. Furthermore, growth restriction in one twin is not an uncommon finding. Among cohorts of children with FGR defined by antenatal assessment (absent end diastolic flow velocity (EDFV)[15,16] or cerebral blood flow redistribution[17]) there is evidence that worse fetal condition markers are associated with cognitive and motor deficits at follow-up. It would thus be logical that twin pregnancies, being more commonly complicated by FGR, may be associated with poor longer term outcomes, at least in those with FGR. In particular, the two conditions peculiar to twins discussed below may be informative.

Differential fetal growth

A priori, the situation where one twin has a significantly lower birthweight than the other would seem to offer an ideal natural experiment to evaluate the effect of FGR on later development. However, studies have shown very different outcomes.[18-23] Most recently, the three year outcome of 21 VLBW discordant twin pairs (defined as > 15% discrepancy in birthweight) and of 24 non-discordant twin pairs was examined.[18] None had cerebral palsy. For the discordant twins at three years the smaller twin was lighter, shorter, had a smaller head circumference and on developmental testing had lower overall Griffiths quotients, particularly in locomotor functioning. When the subgroup of 12 pairs with > 30% weight discrepancy was evaluated, the differences were a little more obvious: 9 points in locomotor function and 7 points overall. These differences were independent of social factors. Interestingly, when the non-discordant group was examined the values obtained were intermediate between the larger and smaller of the discordant group. The non-discordant group also contained several twin pairs with large intra-twin differences in scores. This raises the question as to whether there is any disadvantage to the smaller of the discordant twins.

Zygosity was not evaluated, which may be of relevance as monochorionic monozygous twins are thought to be at particular risk of developmental problems.[22] In a family study of sextuplets with mixed zygosity, no relationship was observed between fetal growth and a range of outcomes at school age, but tendencies were noted for genetic groupings to account for some of the variance in outcome.[24] It would thus seem that the clinically based studies are inconclusive as to the differential effect of fetal growth, per se, in twinships.

Twin-to-twin transfusion

The management of TTTS is described in Chapter 12. Four studies have evaluated outcome after TTTS, two after conservative management with amnioreduction[25,26] and two following laser ablation.[27,28] The Eurofetus study[29] is currently comparing outcome in early infancy following conservative management or laser ablation. Making generalisable observations from the small published studies is difficult. TTTS clearly carries with it a huge fetal risk of death and cerebral palsy in survivors but these survivors are often very preterm at birth making comparison with other twin populations difficult. Cincotta et al.[25] compared the outcome of TTTS to gestational-age-matched twin pairs and observed the anticipated excess risk of death and cerebral palsy. Developmental studies following laser ablation[27,28] imply normal development in those that survive free of cerebral palsy. The results of the Eurofetus study in this regard are awaited.

Environmental issues

The rearing environment has significant implications for child development. A substantial body of research has attempted to tease out the effects that various influences might have on twin development. Most clinical groups are difficult to study because of the comorbidity that derives from social disadvantage. Multiple pregnancies, however, do not appear to be socially distributed and thus these investigations are relatively protected from such bias.

The rearing environment of young infant twins differs in important ways from the environment in which a singleton is raised. Having two infants of the same age at home increases the time spent in physical activity related to child care, the time available for adult–infant interaction, the stress and noise in the home environment and the social isolation of parents. Some of these issues will be less evident with the support of an extended family but others will be more evident with increasing sibship size, both in terms of higher order multiple gestations and other siblings at home.

Maternal psychological health and the home environment

The quality of experience at home may differ between twins and singletons and lead to developmental differences. The presence of twins in the home may lead to exceptional stresses on family life, which may affect the wellbeing of the mother.[30] Such psychological stress may reduce the quality of the interaction with her children. There is a large body of work which indicates that maternal depression and depressive symptoms have important influences on child development.[31] For mothers of singletons who are depressed, there is evidence that they are less responsive and provide a less structured environment for their children.[2] This may result in cognitive impairment, although the studies are to some extent inconsistent.[32] There are few studies evaluating the same influences on twins but there is evidence that mothers of twins have higher rates of depressive symptoms than mothers of singletons,[33] and a suggestion that adjustment to twins may be challenged by a history of infertility.[34]

In the home setting a mother must divide her attention between two children of the same age. The time for interaction may be reduced further because of interruptions, which occur more frequently in families with twins as compared with singletons. Mothers may speak to both twins at once and use more directive language, for example instructions and direct comments,[35] again reducing the richness of interaction and their opportunity to learn language in particular, which is the most studied area of twin development (see below).

A twin is less likely to be fully breastfed until weaning than a singleton.[36] This may result from the difficulty many women encounter in feeding two children and/or from the stress of raising twins and the easy availability of formula milk that can be given by the father or other family members. Again, this is likely to compromise the quality of attachment and interaction. Formula feeding itself may be associated with lower developmental scores but the difficulty of separating out social class effects from the effect of breastfeeding makes this very difficult to assess. By comparing twins with closely spaced sibling dyads, Thorpe et al.[37] demonstrated that there was no advantage conferred by breastfeeding after allowance for mothers' verbal scores.

A twin also has much greater interaction with a child of the same age than would a singleton and thus also reduced time for interaction with adults. Children raised in large families have less well-developed language[38] and may have lower early developmental scores[39] than children raised in smaller families or as only children. Given that there is likely to be reduced exposure to adult and complex language, poorer language scores might be expected. In singleton infants language development is considered to be closely allied with cognitive development, hence twins may be expected to do less well in developmental testing.

Thus, a priori, it would seem likely that twins are more likely to develop early developmental problems secondary to a less facilitative home environment and differing relationships compared with singletons.

Influence of the twinship on development

The increased interaction of twins with each other is likely to reduce the quality of experience or exposure to a role model for language and development. For many years, there has been fascination with autonomous language, which frequently evolves in twinships. It is commonly considered to be the privilege of twins to evolve such 'twin-speak', a feature that emphasises the bond between twins.

There are many forms of such language, ranging from a few idiosyncratic words only understood by the other twin to a more exclusive and comprehensive system of communication, or 'jargon', not understood outside the twinship.[36,40] Using a strict definition of a language used by twins not understood by others, the prevalence may be as high as 43%, with a mean age of onset of 21 months and duration of 16 months. It is not clear whether autonomous language is a unique feature of twinning or simply associated with poorer conventional language development.

In a group of twins (76 pairs) born at greater than 32 weeks of gestation, at 20 months 39% were classed as having a 'shared verbal understanding', defined as 'language understood within the twinship, not understood by others, [that] did not sound abnormal nor was it particularly directed exclusively towards the other sibling', and 7.1% were considered to have a 'private language', one 'used and spoken exclusively within the twinship'.[37] The group were compared with a further group of singleton pairs from families with an inter-child interval of less than 30 months, some of whom did demonstrate autonomous language but at a much lower frequency. Twins with autonomous language at 20 months had a vocabulary age of 16–17 months and where the autonomous language persisted to 36 months the mean 20 month language level was 13–14 months.

At 20 months, the quality of verbal interaction in singleton pairs was better than in twins.[38] Although this may be expected as one sibling is clearly older and has more complex language, it does emphasise the relative paucity of verbal environment for twins.

There is a suggestion that monozygotic twins may have more delayed language than dizygotic twins[41] and that autonomous language may be more prevalent in monozygotic as opposed to dizygotic twinships,[42] implying that this may be an inherent feature of twin development. However, such twin languages may indicate a lower level of conventional language development and that the shared experience of adult language is actually poorer in these twins, necessitating the development of ad hoc communication methods.

Summary

The incidence of twins in the general population has risen dramatically over the past two decades, with the increase in use of ART. This has resulted in an increase in neonatal intensive care admissions around the world as the proportion of very preterm babies born from multiple pregnancies is higher.

Allowing for this, it would appear that the risks of neonatal death and of major neonatal morbidities such as chronic lung disease and intraventricular haemorrhage are not dissimilar in twins compared with singletons.

The effects of preterm birth are considerably more important than the differences, if any, between twins and singletons. Studies of twins must control carefully for differences in gestational age and fetal growth.

Although there is evidence that monozygotic twins are at particular risk of neurodevelopmental problems, in those that escape focal brain injury there is little evidence of impaired developmental outcome.

Development in twins over the first two to three years may follow a different trajectory to that of singletons, related to differences in the rearing environment in terms of family interaction and the quality of the verbal environment. However, these differences do not seem to be related to later cognitive or learning difficulties.

References

1. Akerman BA, Suurvee E. The cognitive and identity development of twins at 16 years of age: a follow-up study of 32 twin pairs. *Twin Res* 2003;6: 328–33.

2. Rutter M, Thorpe K, Greenwood R, Northstone K, Golding J. Twins as a natural experiment to study the causes of mild language delay: I: Design; twin–singleton differences in language, and obstetric risks. *J Child Psychol Psychiatry* 2003;44:326–41.

3. Costeloe K, Hennessy E, Gibson AT, Marlow N, Wilkinson AR. The EPICure study: outcomes to discharge from hospital for infants born at the threshold of viability. *Pediatrics* 2000;106:659–71.

4. Donovan EF, Ehrenkranz RA, Shankaran S, Stevenson DK, Wright LL, Younes N, et al. Outcomes of very low birth weight twins cared for in the National Institute of Child Health and Human Development Neonatal Research Network's intensive care units. *Am J Obstet Gynecol* 1998;179:742–9.

5. Pharoah PO, Platt MJ, Cooke T. The changing epidemiology of cerebral palsy. *Arch Dis Child Fetal Neonatal Ed* 1996; 75: F169–73.

6. Miyahara M, Jongmans MJ, Mercuri E, de Vries LS, Henderson L, Henderson SE. Multiple birth versus neonatal brain lesions in children born prematurely as predictors of perceptuo-motor impairment at age 6. *Dev Neuropsychol* 2003;24:435–59.

7. Asztalos E, Barrett JF, Lacy M, Luther M. Evaluating 2 year outcome in twins < or = 30 weeks gestation at birth: a regional perinatal unit's experience. *Twin Res* 2001;4:431–8.

8. Bhutta AT, Cleves MA, Casey PH, Cradock MM, Anand KJ. Cognitive and behavioral outcomes of school-aged children who were born preterm: a meta-analysis. *JAMA* 2002;288:728–37.

9. Wolke D, Schulz J, Meyer R. Entwicklungslangzeitfolgen bei ehemaligen, sehr unreifen Frühgeborenen. *Monatsschr Kinderheilkd* 2001;149 (Suppl 1):53–61.

10. Marlow N, Wolke D, Bracewell MA, Samara M. Neurologic and developmental disability at six years of age after extremely preterm birth. *N Engl J Med* 2005;352:9–19.

11. Marlow N. Outcome following preterm birth. In: Rennie J, editor. *Robertson's Textbook of Neonatology*. Edinburgh: Churchill Livingstone; 2005.

12. Marlow N. Unpublished data.

13. Wood NS, Costeloe K, Gibson AT, Hennessy E, Marlow N, Wilkinson AR. The EPICure Study: Growth and associated problems in children born at 25 weeks or less gestational age. *Arch Dis Child* 2003;88:F492–500.

14. Wood NS, Costeloe K, Gibson AT, Hennessy EM, Marlow N, Wilkinson AR. The EPICure study: associations and antecedents of neurological and developmental disability at 30 months of age following extremely preterm birth. *Arch Dis Child Fetal Neonatal Ed* 2005;90:F134–40.

15. Ley D, Laurin J, Bjerre I, Marsal K. Abnormal fetal aortic velocity waveform and minor

neurological dysfunction at 7 years of age. *Ultrasound Obstet Gynecol* 1996;8:152–9.

16. Ley D, Tideman E, Laurin J, Bjerre I, Marsal K. Abnormal fetal aortic velocity waveform and intellectual function at 7 years of age. *Ultrasound Obstet Gynecol* 1996;8:160–5.

17. Scherjon S, Briet J, Oosting H, Kok J. The discrepancy between maturation of visual-evoked potentials and cognitive outcome at five years in very preterm infants with and without hemodynamic signs of fetal brain-sparing. *Pediatrics* 2000;105:385–91.

18. Goyen TA, Veddovi M, Lui K. Developmental outcome of discordant premature twins at 3 years. *Early Hum Dev* 2003;73:27–37.

19. Fujikura T, Froehlich LA. Mental and motor development in monozygotic co-twins with dissimilar birth weights. *Pediatrics* 1974;53:884–9.

20. Stauffer A, Burns WJ, Burns KA, Melamed J, Herman CE. Early developmental progress of preterm twins discordant for birthweight and risk. *Acta Genet Med Gemellol (Roma)* 1988;37:81–7.

21. Babson SG, Phillips DS. Growth and development of twins dissimilar in size at birth. *N Engl J Med* 1973;289:937–40.

22. O'Brien PJ, Hay DA. Birthweight differences, the transfusion syndrome and the cognitive development of monozygotic twins. *Acta Genet Med Gemellol (Roma)* 1987;36:181–96.

23. Ylitalo V, Kero P, Erkkola R. Neurological outcome of twins dissimilar in size at birth. *Early Hum Dev* 1988;17:245–55.

24. Marlow N, Ellis AM, Roberts BL, Cooke RW. Five year outcome of preterm sextuplets related to size at birth. *Arch Dis Child* 1990;65:451–2.

25. Cincotta RB, Gray PH, Phythian G, Rogers YM, Chan FY. Long term outcome of twin–twin transfusion syndrome. *Arch Dis Child Fetal Neonatal Ed* 2000;83:F171–7.

26. Lopriore E, Nagel HT, Vandenbussche FP, Walther FJ. Long-term neurodevelopmental outcome in twin-to-twin transfusion syndrome. *Am J Obstet Gynecol* 2003;189:1314–19.

27. De Lia JE, Worthington D. Long-term neurodevelopmental outcome after intrauterine laser treatment for twin–twin transfusion syndrome (TTTS). *Am J Obstet Gynecol* 2004;190:1170–1.

28. Sutcliffe AG, Sebire NJ, Pigott AJ, Taylor B, Edwards PR, Nicolaides KH. Outcome for children born after *in utero* laser ablation therapy for severe twin-to-twin transfusion syndrome. *BJOG* 2001;108:1246–50.

29. Eurofoetus. *Endoscopic Access to the Fetoplacental Unit.* 2005. [www.eurofetus.org/tts.htm].

30. Thorpe K, Golding J, MacGillivray I, Greenwood R. Comparison of prevalence of depression in mothers of twins and mothers of singletons. *BMJ* 1991;302:875–8.

31. Murray L, Cooper PJ. Postpartum depression and child development. *Psychol Med* 1997;27:253–60.

32. Murray L, Cooper P. Effects of postnatal depression on infant development. *Arch Dis Child* 1997;77:99–101.

33. Damato EG. Prenatal attachment and other correlates of postnatal maternal attachment to twins. *Adv Neonatal Care* 2004;4:274–91.

34. Klock SC. Psychological adjustment to twins after infertility. *Best Pract Res Clin Obstet Gynaecol.* 2004;18:645–56.

35. Barton ME, Strosberg R. Conversational patterns of two-year-old twins in mother–twin–twin triads. *J Child Lang* 1997;24:257–69.

36. Thorpe K, Greenwood R, Eivers A, Rutter M. Prevalence and developmental course of 'secret language'. *Int J Lang Commun Disord* 2001;36:43–62.

37. Thorpe K, Rutter M, Greenwood R. Twins as a natural experiment to study the causes of mild language delay: II: Family interaction risk factors. *J Child Psychol Psychiatry* 2003;44:342–55.

38. Rutter M, Madge N. *Cycles of Disadvantage.* London: Heinemann Educational; 1976.

39. Anonymous. A randomised trial of parental support for families with very preterm children. The Avon Premature Infant Project. *Arch Dis Child* 1998;79:F4–11.

40. Bishop DVM, Bishop SJ. Twin language. A risk factor for language impairment? *J Speech Lang Hear Res* 1998;41:150–60.

41. Mittler P. Biological and social aspects of language development in twins. *Dev Med Child Neurol* 1970;12:741–57.

42. Wood NS, Marlow N, Costeloe K, Gibson AT, Wilkinson AR. Neurologic and developmental disability after extremely preterm birth. EPICure Study Group. *N Engl J Med* 2000;343:378–84.

Chapter 16

Epidemiology of cerebral palsy in multiple pregnancies

Isaac Blickstein

Introduction

The term cerebral palsy (CP) describes a heterogeneous set of functional conditions caused by lesions to the brain that occur during pregnancy, intrapartum, or during the neonatal period. This kind of brain damage results in a disorder of movement and posture, and is, by definition, nonprogressive.

Historically, CP was considered to be related to birth asphyxia – the so-called Little's disease, after the English surgeon William John Little who in 1843 described a 'spasmodic tetanus-like rigidity and distortion of the limbs of new-born infants'. Little correlated the condition to asphyxia at birth, preterm birth and direct mechanical injury. Sigmund Freud was apparently the first who questioned the relationship between CP and an intrapartum event in commenting that, in some instances, difficult birth might be a result of brain damage rather than its cause. However, it was not until the 1980s that it became clear that intrapartum events are associated with fewer than 10% of CP cases. A set of strict criteria has now been defined by both obstetricians and paediatricians that should be met before such an association in an individual case can be established.[1,2]

The relationship between an alleged cause and subsequent CP is quite difficult to establish in an individual case because the diagnosis is often reached months or years postpartum. Furthermore, when an individual case is reviewed in retrospect, antenatal aetiologies are almost impossible to discern. Clinical measures to assess or monitor fetal brain function are not yet available.

Despite these shortcomings, the most important observation relating to the epidemiology of CP is a reiteration of one of the seminal observations of Little almost 150 years ago, namely that a correlation exists between CP and preterm birth: the more preterm the infant the higher the risk of brain damage.

As recently as the early 1980s, most, if not all, multiples were naturally conceived and were thus a rare occurrence in daily practice. This has changed dramatically since then, primarily because of the use of assisted reproductive technologies (ART).[3] Data published by the UK-based Twins and Multiple Births Association (TAMBA)[4] show that during the period 1982–98 in England and Wales twin births increased by 40%, from around 10 to around 14 per 1000 births and the rate for the same period for triplet births increased by 400%, from around 0.1 to 0.5 per 1000 births. Importantly, between 1998 and 2003, the rate for twins increased further to 15 per 1000 births (i.e. 50% higher than in 1982) but the rate for triplets gradually declined to 0.2 per 1000 births (i.e. twice as high as that in 1982). In simple terms, the data indicate an addition of 10 twin pairs concomitant with a reduction of three sets of triplets since 1998. Despite this encouraging reduction in the number of triplet births, the total number of multiples is still increasing – the overall rate in the UK in 2003 was 14.9 per 1000 maternities, i.e. one in every 67 births is a multiple birth. The net result is that the 'epidemic' of multiple births is not yet over.[5]

US data for the year 2003 showed that 11.9% of twins and 36.1% of triplets were born very preterm (less than 32 completed weeks of gestation) and that 10.2% of twins and 34.5% of triplets weighed less than 1500 g at birth.[6] These figures represent 7.4- and 9.3-fold increases for twins and 22.6- and 31.4-fold increases for triplets compared with the respective figures in singletons. Because CP rates are higher in preterm and low birthweight (LBW) infants, and because multiples are undoubtedly over-represented among these infants, it is not surprising that CP is more common in twins and higher order multiples. However, twins and higher order multiples also have additional and unique causes that may increase CP rates. This chapter discusses the epidemiology and various circumstances that may explain the increased prevalence of CP among multiples.

Cerebral palsy prevalence in multiples

The association of CP and multiples has been reported from all over the world and, somewhat surprisingly, with a similar prevalence in the various reports.[7-11] The data indicate a 7.4% average prevalence of twins among CP cases, and a six- to eight-fold increased prevalence of CP in twins compared with singletons.[12,13]

Not surprising, however, were the reports showing a significant exponential relationship between CP prevalence and plurality, reflecting the over-representation of multiples among very preterm and LBW infants.[14] Specifically, the prevalence of CP in triplets exceeds that of twins and of singletons: 28 versus 7.3 versus 1.6 per 1000 survivors to one year[15] and 44.8 versus 12.6 versus 2.3 per 1000 survivors.[16] Observations from Japan confirmed this trend in quadruplets as well: 9, 31 and 111 per 1000 for twins, triplets and quadruplets, respectively.[17]

Admittedly, most of these CP registries compiled data preceding the 'epidemic' of multiple births or limited to its early stages. Since the data come from countries where assisted conceptions are abundant, it is expected that, with the increasing proportions of multiple births, the prevalence of CP will also increase. For example, a more recent study[18] described demographic and clinical factors associated with CP in over 25 000 twins using vital statistics from five populations in the USA and Australia. Overall, twins were at an approximately four-fold increased risk of CP compared with singletons. However, even this recent large dataset, spanning a ten year period, only covered the period until 1989, well before the peak of the 'epidemic' of multiple births.

Effect of birthweight and gestational age

It is important to bear in mind that the major contributors to the increased prevalence of CP among multiples are the seven- and 23-fold increased incidence of deliveries at less than 32 weeks of gestation for twins and triplets, respectively, compared with singleton pregnancies. For this reason, a cause and effect relationship between CP and the multiple pregnancy or multiple birth, per se, may be questioned. To show such a relationship it is necessary to stratify the prevalence of CP in multiples and singletons according to birthweight and gestational age. Such data, however, exist for twins only. Several authors have found that the risk of CP was higher in twins weighing more than 2499 g than in singletons of a similar weight[8,9,16] whereas the risk was comparable among very low birthweight (VLBW) twins and singletons.[9,16] One potential explanation for these observations is that the lower CP prevalence among small multiples is a result of a higher mortality rate among multiples compared with singletons.[10] In contrast, normal birthweight multiples have similar mortality rates and thus more survivors to demonstrate a higher prevalence of CP than in singletons. This explanation is in contrast to the observations of Scher *et al.*,[18] who found that at birthweights of less than 2500 g, twins generally did better than singletons, with respect to both mortality and CP rates.

Similar findings have been observed regarding gestational age. Yokoyama *et al.*[17] found that the risk of CP among multiples was 20 times higher in births before 32 weeks of gestation than at 36 weeks or more. Williams *et al.*[8] also presented a strong correlation between the risk of CP in twins and gestational age. However, the comparison with singleton births showed that the relative risk of CP was greatest, and significant, only for twins delivered at more than 36 weeks.

Taken together, the data indicate that multiple and singleton pregnancies have similar risks for CP until near term, with a possible advantage for the former. Although low birthweight and preterm birth are apparently the most significant risk factors for CP among multiples, the disadvantage (at least for twins) becomes evident near term. Support for this statement comes from Shinwell *et al.*,[19] who recently studied the Israel National VLBW Infant Database and compared 3717 singletons and all complete sets of twins (*n* = 1394) and triplets (*n* = 483). Plurality did not influence the risk of adverse neurological outcome among infants weighing less than 1500 g (OR 1.29, 95% CI 0.91–1.85).

The excess risk for CP beyond 36 weeks of gestation may suggest that 'term' occurs earlier in twins compared with singletons. This view is in accordance with observations that twins experience increased morbidity compared with singletons[20] and are at increased risk of death[21] and severe handicap[22] after reaching 38 weeks of gestation. This also constitutes a strong argument in favour of delivering twins by 38 weeks[23] despite the lack of a large-scale randomised trial to prove this set of circumstantial evidence.

Contribution of ART to cerebral palsy in multiple pregnancies

In current obstetrics, a significant proportion of multiple pregnancies results from ovulation induction or ART and these are rightfully termed iatrogenic multiple pregnancies.[24] These ART babies are remarkably over-represented among the cohort of VLBW infants. For example, only 10% of singletons in the Israel National VLBW Infant Database were conceived by ART compared with 60% of the twins and 90% of the triplets.[19] Thus, iatrogenic conceptions are undoubtedly associated with increased risk of perinatal complications, including CP, merely because of their risk of being born prematurely. This fact is even more disappointing because a significant proportion of iatrogenic multiples could have been avoided by reducing the number of transferred embryos where *in vitro* fertilisation-embryo transfer (IVF-ET) methods were employed.[25]

To estimate the risk of CP among IVF babies following three-embryo transfers, we integrated the excess risk of multifetal pregnancies after three-embryo transfers with the excess risk of CP among multiples.[26] Estimated rates of CP after the transfer of three embryos were 16.86 per 1000 neonates, 8.77 per 1000 following the transfer of two embryos, and 10.31 per 1000 neonates after the transfer of three embryos with a reduction of all triplets to twins. These figures were significantly higher than the rate of 2.7 per 1000 neonates in spontaneous conceptions. Using a similar extrapolation method, Kiely et al.[27] estimated that in the USA there might be an 8% increase in the prevalence of CP due solely to the rise in iatrogenic multiple births.

The increased risk of CP among iatrogenic multiples might be even more striking given the recent systematic review of controlled studies published in the period 1985–2002, which found that in twins the perinatal mortality was about 40% (OR 0.58, 95% CI 0.44–0.77) lower after assisted conception compared with natural conception.[28] In simple terms, this means that more premature twin infants survive to manifest CP. It has been emphasised, however, that the type of IVF procedure (i.e. with or without intracytoplasmic sperm injection) probably does not affect the risk of neurological sequelae.[29]

Effect of fetal death and zygosity/chorionicity

It is well known that brain damage is more common in the surviving fetus after demise of a co-fetus in a multifetal pregnancy. Pharoah and Adi[30] evaluated data for all twin births in England and Wales in which one twin was registered as having died *in utero*. The authors confirmed that the gestational age specific prevalence of CP after single fetal death was much higher than that reported for the general twin population. This study clearly showed that the survivor was at an overall 20% risk of cerebral impairment. Scher et al.[18] also confirmed that twins whose co-twins died were at increased risk of both mortality and CP. The highest rates of CP were in surviving twins whose co-twin was stillborn (4.7%), had died shortly after birth (6.3%) or had survived to have CP (11.8%).

Most clinicians, however, would agree that adverse neurological outcome is almost exclusively seen in the subset of monochorionic (MC) twins that comprises about two-thirds of monozygotic (MZ) twins. MC placentation is thus expected in about 20% and 3% of spontaneous and iatrogenic twins, respectively.[31] Practically all MC twins have inter-twin transplacental vascular connections. However, in 10–15% of MC placentas, an unbalanced inter-twin shunt occurs via the vascular connection and results in various degrees of twin-to-twin transfusion syndrome (TTTS).[32]

It has been postulated that following death of one twin thromboplastin-like material is shunted through the vascular connection(s) into the survivor's circulation, causing end-organ damage. This circumstance established the 'embolic' theory and the so-called twin embolisation syndrome. However, failure to identify such emboli and signs of ischaemic injury in meticulous postmortem studies led to the alternative 'ischaemic' theory, in which blood is assumed to drain via an open anastomosis into the low-resistance vascular system of the dead fetus, resulting in acute hypovolaemia, ischaemia and end-organ injury in the survivor.

Despite the accepted relationship between CP rates and MZ twinning, large-scale data sets are not available. This limitation comes from the inability of clinical measures (ultrasound and placental examination) to differentiate same-sex dichorionic (DC)-dizygotic (DZ) twins (half of all DZ twins) from DC-MZ twins (one-third of all MZ twins).[31] Instead, researchers use the proxy of same-sex versus opposite-sex twins to extrapolate to the risk of CP in MZ twins.

Pharoah[33] compared, in same-sex and opposite-sex twins, the birthweight-specific neonatal death rate and CP prevalence in the surviving twin when the co-twin had died in infancy. The author found that the prevalence of CP in the extremely LBW group (less than 1000 g) was marginally higher in same-sex than in opposite-sex twin survivors whereas it was significantly higher in the 1000–1999 g birthweight group. The author concluded that preterm birth per se predisposes to cerebral damage but same-sex twins may have cerebral damage in excess of that due to immaturity.

In a more recent analysis, Pharoah[34] compared the prevalence of CP among same-sex and opposite-sex twins. In the case of single fetal death, the prevalence of CP among same-sex twins was 103.9 per 1000 survivors compared with 37.6 per 1000 survivors from opposite-sex pairs. When both twins were born alive and one twin died during infancy, the prevalence of CP was 132.0 compared with 74.1 per 1000 survivors in same-sex and opposite-sex twins, respectively. When both twins survived infancy, the figures were still higher among same-sex twins: 8.1 versus 4.8 per 1000 survivors. When the data were stratified by birthweight below or above 1500 g, the differences seemed to be clearer among the heavier twins, supporting the idea that twinning per se increases the risk of CP beyond the effect of premature birth. These findings are supported by the compilation of cases performed by Javier Laplaza et al.[7] but not by the studies of Petterson et al.[15] and Nelson and Ellenberg,[35] who found similar prevalence of CP in same-sex and opposite-sex pairs. In addition, by using the Hardy–Weinberg rule to estimate zygosity, similar risks of CP were found in MZ and DZ twins.[36]

In the absence of population-based information regarding chorionicity, data from hospital-based studies should be interpreted with caution because of small sample sizes and the case mix of MC twins with and without TTTS or those delivered at or before term. Adegbite et al.[37] determined the incidence of neurological morbidity in 76 MC and 78 DC twins born between 24 and 34 weeks of gestation. Overall, neurological morbidity in these preterm MC infants was seven-fold higher than in DC infants because of chronic TTTS, discordant birthweight and co-twin death *in utero*. MC infants had a higher incidence of CP (8% versus 1%) and neurological morbidity (15% versus 3%) than DC infants. Minakami et al.[38] examined the effects of chorionicity on infant outcome at one year of age in a cohort study of 44 MC and 164 DC twin pregnancies and concluded that MC twins had an increased risk of adverse outcomes compared with DC twins, mainly because of TTTS. Finally, MC placentation constituted the highest risk (six-fold increased) for CP and severe disability in a group of prospectively examined preterm infants.[39]

Effect of twin-to-twin transfusion syndrome

TTTS is a relatively rare condition that has been known for centuries. It is expected to occur spontaneously in 10–15% of MC twins, i.e. 2–4 per 10 000 births. It is not known exactly how many MC twins occur among iatrogenic twins but this is, logically, much lower. The condition has attracted the attention of researchers for nearly two decades, mainly because the availability of ultrasound has made prenatal diagnosis possible and thus allowed selective treatment of this complex condition.[32]

Unfortunately, information about CP among treated and untreated cases of TTTS is available mainly from small, almost anecdotal, series. There are a few studies from referral centres, but these have inevitable selection bias. Furthermore, comparing the available studies is made difficult by the different diagnostic criteria and different treatment protocols. Nevertheless, it is generally accepted that the vascular shunt in

MC placentas neatly explains the mechanism of neurological handicap in cases of TTTS irrespective of fetal death. A few examples of the discrepant data follow.

In a case–control study of 17 cases, Cincotta et al.[40] found periventricular leucomalacia and cerebral atrophy in 17% of the TTTS group but none in the controls. Among survivors of the syndrome, 22% had CP and global developmental delay. The authors concluded that long-term neurodevelopmental morbidity in survivors of TTTS is high. In contrast, Mari et al.[41] evaluated the long-term outcomes of 33 pregnancies complicated by TTTS treated with one or more amnioreductions. The authors concluded that in the group of fetuses where both twins had been delivered alive after 27 weeks of gestation without congenital malformations and survived the neonatal period, no major neurological handicaps developed in any of the infants. Dickinson et al.[42] recently assessed the long-term outcomes of 49 children from pregnancies complicated by TTTS in comparison with a contemporaneous regional cohort of preterm infants. The authors found that TTTS was associated with a significant reduction in IQ score in very preterm survivors, but there seemed to be no increase in the prevalence of CP and no difference in the overall behaviour and adaptive behaviour scale scores. Lopriore et al.[43] assessed the long-term neurodevelopmental outcomes in children after TTTS treated conservatively (amnioreduction or no intervention). Abnormal cranial ultrasound findings were reported in 41% of the 29 surviving neonates and the incidence of CP was high at 21%. This was especially true after intrauterine fetal demise of a co-twin, as was also noted by Seng et al.[44] in their series of 18 pairs of twins with TTTS. The largest compilation of severe TTTS cases at mid-gestation comes from the Eurofetus randomised trial to compare the efficacy and safety of either serial amnioreduction ($n = 70$) or selective fetoscopic laser coagulation ($n = 72$) of the communicating vessels on the chorionic plate.[45] The study was concluded earlier than expected because a planned interim analysis demonstrated a significant benefit in the laser treatment arm. Compared with amnioreduction, the laser group had (among other advantages) a lower incidence of cystic periventricular leucomalacia and infants in this group were more likely to be free of neurological complications at six months of age.

In summary, it appears that neurological damage in TTTS is primarily gestational age dependent and associated with TTTS-related death of one of the twins. The more severe the TTTS, the more likely it is that one twin will die *in utero* or that pregnancy will end at an earlier gestational age. The risk of CP is therefore reduced when (any) treatment can prolong pregnancy and/or increase the chances of avoiding fetal death.

Effect of fetal growth

In nearly 99% of human pregnancies the female carries only one fetus and it is thus logical to assume that the uterine environment is frequently unable to provide for two (or more) fetuses to the same extent as in singleton gestations.[46] This limitation increases with increasing gestational age and becomes evident in the third trimester, when birthweight curves of infants from multiple gestations begin to lag behind that of singletons. In addition, absolute intrauterine or relative (discordant) growth restriction is common. At lower levels, birthweight discordance may indicate an adaptive measure to promote an advanced gestational age at birth, whereas higher levels of birthweight discordance often imply genuine growth restriction.[47] Williams and O'Brien[48] found that phenotypic markers of asymmetric growth restriction were better correlates of both mortality and CP. A Swedish population-based study,[49] however, found no significant difference between the distributions of birthweight discordance when the twins with disability were compared with the population of all liveborn twins weighing less than 2500 g. Disabled twins had a significantly lower birthweight for gestational age, but only 8.7% of the twins were considered small for gestational age. Rydhstrøm concluded that birthweight discordance does not seem to be related to neurological disability later in life.

These conflicting opinions may result from considering all discordant twins as growth-restricted, a misconception that was disproved recently by the finding that even in severely (more than 25%) discordant twins, as many as 40% of the smaller twins are, in fact, appropriately grown.[50] Where there is a lesser degree of discordance, the likelihood that both twins are appropriate for gestational age is considerably higher.

There is virtually no information available related to genuine growth restriction in twins and the association with CP. However, Scher et al.[18] found that twins from growth-discordant pairs were at increased risk of both mortality and CP. This finding is indirectly supported by the observations of Yinon et al.[51] who found that growth restriction in preterm discordant twins was associated with a 7.7-fold increased risk for major neonatal morbidity, including intraventricular haemorrhage.

It follows that common growth aberrations such as growth discordance are unlikely to contribute significantly to neurological damage unless growth restriction is present.

Embryonic and early fetal loss

Embryonic loss is frequently seen in multiple gestations, creating the so-called vanishing twin syndrome.[52] It has been hypothesised[53] that the mechanism involved in brain damage in the survivor following single fetal demise in advanced pregnancies might also be implicated in the aetiology of spastic CP in singleton survivors of the vanishing twin syndrome. However, the 'classical' sonographic image of the vanishing twin syndrome is suggestive of DC placentas that usually lack inter-twin anastomoses.[54] Furthermore, a strong argument against the relationship between early fetal demise and CP is based on the lack of reported affected infants following multifetal pregnancy reduction – the iatrogenic equivalent of the vanishing twin syndrome. Opponents of this view suggest that this argument may be misleading because CP would probably be attributed to other factors such as preterm birth or low birthweight. In one small study, Geva et al.[55] found that in a cohort of premature infants who developed periventricular leucomalacia, 28.6% were exposed to multifetal pregnancy reduction, compared with 1.9% of the controls (OR 20.9, 95% CI 5.5–79.4). The results suggested that multifetal pregnancy reduction may be an additional risk factor for brain lesions among premature infants.

It is apparent that many early fetal deaths are overlooked. Pharoah[56] noted that in 58 fetal deaths that were registered as being of indeterminate sex, 56 were coded as males and two as females. A fetus papyraceous was registered as male in 19 and as female in 19 cases. Other fetal deaths weighing more than 100 g, with no mention of papyraceous on the death certificate, and likely to be of indeterminate sex, were registered as male in 26 and as female in 23 cases. In 13 maternities, the number of infants registered at birth was less than the number mentioned on the registration certificate. The author concluded that, given the miscoding and inconsistency in recording fetal sex, it is difficult to assume that multiple births of different registered sex are, in fact, DZ. At the same time, the findings point to the need for meticulous recording of lost embryos/fetuses.

In summary, the association of embryonic and early fetal loss and CP cannot be proved or disproved unless further research on this intriguing subject is done.

Mode of delivery

Multiple births might be associated with increased intrapartum risks mainly because of fetal size and malpresentation leading to potentially traumatic delivery. It has been known for many years that, irrespective of the mode of delivery, the second-born has a worse prognosis in terms of immediate neonatal outcome.[18] The epidemiological studies of Rydhstrøm[57] focused on the effect of caesarean section on CP and mental retardation in twins weighing less than 1500 g. The analysis failed to reveal any significant impact of abdominal birth on the CP rates for LBW twins, even when fetal presentation was taken into consideration. Rydhstrøm[58] also evaluated the effect of caesarean section on delivery of twins whose birthweight was discordant by 1.0 kg or more. In this cohort, no correlation was found between mode of delivery and CP and/or mental retardation at the age of eight years or more. Shinwell et al.[19] also reported a lack of effect of mode of delivery on adverse neurological findings among VLBW twins and triplets.

Summary

The prevalence of CP among multiples seems to be plurality-dependent, with the prevalence in quadruplets greater than that in triplets, and that in triplets greater than that in twins or singletons. Because multiples are over-represented among preterm births and LBW infants, prematurity is apparently the most significant risk factor for CP among multiples. However, the CP risk for singletons decreases near term and the risk for multiples persists after 36 weeks of gestation and in infants weighing more than 2500 g. Because fertility treatment contributes significantly to the increased incidence of multiple pregnancies and births, such treatment can be considered to be an associated risk for CP.

There is a close relationship between fetal death and CP in the survivor, especially in the subset of same-sex pairs, which includes the more risky group of MZ-MC twins. Overall, CP rates in surviving twins whose co-twins were stillborn are high, they are higher when the co-twin died shortly after birth, and they are highest when the co-twin survived to have CP. In MC pairs affected by TTTS, the neurological damage seems to be primarily age-dependent and associated with TTTS-related death of one of the twins. The more severe the TTTS the more likely it is that one twin will die in utero or pregnancy will end at an earlier gestational age, and thus the survivor is more likely to suffer brain damage.

Common growth aberrations such as growth discordance are unlikely to contribute significantly to neurological damage unless growth restriction is present. The same seems to be true for the mode of delivery.

References

1. MacLennan A. A template for defining a causal relation between acute intrapartum events and cerebral palsy: international consensus statement. BMJ 1999;319:1054–9.
2. Hankins GD, Speer M. Defining the pathogenesis and pathophysiology of neonatal encephalopathy and cerebral palsy. Obstet Gynecol 2003;102:628–36.
3. Fauser BCJM, Devroey P, Macklon NS. Multiple birth resulting from ovarian stimulation for subfertility treatment. Lancet 2005;365:1807–16.

4. The Twins and Multiple Births Association [www.tamba.org.uk].
5. Blickstein I, Keith LG. The decreased rates of triplet birth: temporal trends and biologic speculations. *Am J Obstet Gynecol* 2005;193:327–31.
6. Martin JA, Hamilton BE, Sutton PD, Ventura SJ, Menacker F, Munson ML. Births: final data for 2002. *Natl Vital Stat Rep* 2003;52:1–113.
7. Javier Laplaza F, Root L, Tassanawipas A, Cervera P. Cerebral palsy in twins. *Dev Med Child Neurol* 1992;34:1053–63.
8. Williams K, Hennessy E, Alberman B. Cerebral palsy: effects of twinning, birthweight, and gestational age. *Arch Dis Child* 1996;75:F178–82.
9. Grether JK, Nelson KB, Cummins SK. Twinning and cerebral palsy: experience in four northern California counties, births 1983 through 1985. *Pediatrics* 1993;92:854–8.
10. Liu J, Li Z, Lin Q, Zhao P, Zhao F, Hong S, et al. Cerebral palsy and multiple births in China. *Int J Epidemiol* 2000;29:292–9.
11. Touyama M, Ochiai Y, Touyama J. Cerebral palsy in twins in Okinawa. *No To Hattatsu* 2000;32:35–8.
12. Blickstein I. Cerebral palsy in multifoetal pregnancies. *Dev Med Child Neurol* 2002;44:352–5.
13. Blickstein I. Do multiple gestations raise the risk of cerebral palsy? *Clin Perinatol* 2004;31:395–408.
14. Blickstein I. Cerebral palsy in multifetal pregnancies: facts and hypotheses. In: Chervenak FA, Kurjak A, editors. *Fetal Medicine: The Clinical Care of the Fetus as a Patient*. London: Parthenon Publishing; 1999. p. 368–73.
15. Petterson B, Nelson KB, Watson L, Stanley F. Twins, triplets, and cerebral palsy in births in Western Australia in the 1980s. *BMJ* 1993;307:1239–43.
16. Pharoah POD, Cooke T. Cerebral palsy and multiple births. *Arch Dis Child* 1996;75:F174–7.
17. Yokoyama Y, Shimizu T, Hayakawa K. Prevalence of cerebral palsy in twins, triplets and quadruplets. *Int J Epidemiol* 1995;24:943–8.
18. Scher AI, Petterson B, Blair E, Ellenberg JH, Grether JK, Haan E, et al. The risk of mortality or cerebral palsy in twins: a collaborative population-based study. *Pediatr Res* 2002;52:671–81.
19. Shinwell ES, Blickstein I, Lusky A, Reichman B. Excess risk of mortality in very low birthweight triplets: a national, population based study. *Arch Dis Child Fetal Neonatal Ed* 2003;88:F36–40.
20. Luke B, Bigger HR, Leurgans S, Sietsema D. The cost of prematurity: a case–control study of twins vs singletons. *Am J Public Health* 1996;86:809–14.
21. Minakami H, Sato I. Reestimating date of delivery in multifetal pregnancies. *JAMA* 1996;275:1432–4.
22. Luke B, Keith LG. The contribution of singletons, twins and triplets to low birth weight, infant mortality and handicap in the United States. *J Reprod Med* 1992;37:661–6.
23. Luke B, Brown MB, Alexandre PK, Kinoshi T, O'Sullivan MJ, Martin D, et al. The cost of twin pregnancy: maternal and neonatal factors. *Am J Obstet Gynecol* 2005;192:909–15.
24. Blickstein I, Keith LG. The spectrum of iatrogenic multiple pregnancy. In: Blickstein I, Keith LG, editors. *Iatrogenic Multiple Pregnancy: Clinical Implications*. London: Parthenon Publishing; 2001. p. 1–7.
25. Templeton A, Morris JK. Reducing the risk of multiple births by transfer of two embryos after *in vitro* fertilization. *N Engl J Med* 1998;339:573–7.
26. Blickstein I, Weissman A. Estimating the risk of cerebral palsy following assisted conceptions. *N Engl J Med* 1999;341:1313–14.
27. Kiely JL, Kiely M, Blickstein I. Contribution of the rise in multiple births to a potential increase in cerebral palsy *Pediatr Res* 2000:47, 314A.
28. Helmerhorst FM, Perquin DA, Donker D, Keirse MJ. Perinatal outcome of singletons and twins after assisted conception: a systematic review of controlled studies. *BMJ* 2004;328:261–5.
29. Pinborg A, Loft A, Schmidt L, Greisen G, Rasmussen S, Andersen AN. Neurological sequelae in twins born after assisted conception: controlled national cohort study. *BMJ* 2004;329:311–16.
30. Pharoah PO, Adi Y. Consequences of in-utero death in a twin pregnancy. *Lancet* 2000;355:1597–602.
31. Blickstein I. Estimation of iatrogenic monozygotic twinning rate following assisted reproduction: pitfalls and caveats. *Am J Obstet Gynecol* 2005;192:365–8.
32. Blickstein I. The twin–twin transfusion syndrome. *Obstet Gynecol* 1990;76:714–22.
33. Pharoah PO. Cerebral palsy in the surviving twin associated with infant death of the co-twin. *Arch Dis Child Fetal Neonatal Ed* 2001; 84: F111–16.
34. Pharoah PO. Risk of cerebral palsy in multiple pregnancies. *Obstet Gynecol Clin North Am* 2005;32:55–67.
35. Nelson KB, Ellenberg JH. Childhood neurological disorders in twins. *Paediatr Perinat Epidemiol* 1995;9:135–45.

36. Petterson B, Stanley F, Henderson D. Cerebral palsy in multiple births in Western Australia: genetic aspects. *Am J Med Genet* 1990;37:346–51.

37. Adegbite AL, Castille S, Ward S, Bajoria R. Neuromorbidity in preterm twins in relation to chorionicity and discordant birth weight. *Am J Obstet Gynecol* 2004;190:156–63.

38. Minakami H, Honma Y, Matsubara S, Uchida A, Shiraishi H, Sato I. Effects of placental chorionicity on outcome in twin pregnancies. A cohort study. *J Reprod Med* 1999;44:595–600.

39. Burguet A, Monnet E, Pauchard JY, Roth P, Fromentin C, Dalphin ML, *et al*. Some risk factors for cerebral palsy in very premature infants: importance of premature rupture of membranes and monochorionic twin placentation. *Biol Neonate* 1999;75:177–86.

40. Cincotta RB, Gray PH, Phythian G, Rogers YM, Chan FY. Long term outcome of twin–twin transfusion syndrome. *Arch Dis Child Fetal Neonatal Ed* 2000;83:F171–6.

41. Mari G, Detti L, Oz U, Abuhamad AZ. Long-term outcome in twin–twin transfusion syndrome treated with serial aggressive amnioreduction. *Am J Obstet Gynecol* 2001;183:211–17.

42. Dickinson JE, Duncombe GJ, Evans SF, French NP, Hagan R. The long term neurologic outcome of children from pregnancies complicated by twin-to-twin transfusion syndrome. *BJOG* 2005;112:63–8.

43. Lopriore E, Nagel HT, Vandenbussche FP, Walther FJ. Long-term neurodevelopmental outcome in twin-to-twin transfusion syndrome. *Am J Obstet Gynecol* 2003;189:1314–19.

44. Seng YC, Rajadurai VS. Twin–twin transfusion syndrome: a five year review. *Arch Dis Child Fetal Neonatal Ed* 2000;83:F168–70.

45. Senat MV, Deprest J, Boulvain M, Paupe A, Winer N, Ville Y. Endoscopic laser surgery versus serial amnioreduction for severe twin-to-twin transfusion syndrome. *N Engl J Med* 2004;351:136–44.

46. Blickstein I. Growth aberration in multiple pregnancy. *Obstet Gynecol Clin North Am* 2005;32:39–54.

47. Blickstein I, Goldman RD, Mazkereth R. Adaptive growth restriction as a pattern of birth weight discordance in twin gestations. *Obstet Gynecol* 2000;96:986–90.

48. Williams MC, O'Brien WF. Low weight/length ratio to assess risk of cerebral palsy and perinatal mortality in twins. *Am J Perinatol* 1998;15:225–8.

49. Rydhstroem H. The relationship of birth weight and birth weight discordance to cerebral palsy or mental retardation later in life for twins weighing less than 2500 grams. *Am J Obstet Gynecol* 1995;173:680–6.

50. Blickstein I, Keith LG. Neonatal mortality rates among growth-discordant twins, classified according to the birth weight of the smaller twin. *Am J Obstet Gynecol* 2004;190:170–4.

51. Yinon Y, Mazkereth R, Rosentzweig N, Jarus-Hakak A, Schiff E, Simchen MJ. Growth restriction as a determinant of outcome in preterm discordant twins. *Obstet Gynecol* 2005;105:80–4.

52. Landy HJ, Keith LG. The vanishing twin: a review. *Hum Reprod Update* 1998;4:177–83.

53. Pharoah PO, Cooke RW. A hypothesis for the aetiology of spastic cerebral palsy – the vanishing twin. *Dev Med Child Neurol* 1997;39:292–6.

54. Blickstein I. Reflections on the hypothesis for the etiology of spastic cerebral palsy caused by the "vanishing twin" syndrome. *Dev Med Child Neurol* 1998;40:358.

55. Geva E, Lerner-Geva L, Stavorovsky Z, Modan B, Freedman L, Amit A, *et al*. Multifetal pregnancy reduction: a possible risk factor for periventricular leukomalacia in premature newborns. *Fertil Steril* 1998;69:845–50.

56. Pharoah PO. Errors in birth registrations and coding of twins and higher order multiples. *Twin Res* 2002;5:270–2.

57. Rydhstrom H. Prognosis for twins with birth weight less than 1500 gm: the impact of cesarean section in relation to fetal presentation. *Am J Obstet Gynecol* 1990;163:528–33.

58. Rydhstrom H. Prognosis for twins discordant in birth weight of 1.0 kg or more: the impact of cesarean section. *J Perinat Med* 1990;18:31–7.

Chapter 17

Systematic reviews of research on multiple pregnancy: an overview of their quality and a guide to methods

Khalid S Khan, Pradeep M Jayaram, Caroline Fox and Mark D Kilby

Introduction

Clinicians providing care to women with multiple pregnancies need evidence about efficient diagnostic strategies, about prognostic information concerning outcomes and about effectiveness of therapeutic interventions.[1,2] Remaining well-informed about these issues is the cornerstone of high-quality healthcare provision. However, individual pieces of research concerning multiple pregnancy are scattered across the literature in such a way that they are not easily accessible. This problem is solved by using literature reviews to underpin practice.[3] In recent years systematic reviews and meta-analyses have been accepted as an integral part of evidence-based decision making. Reviewers new to this method, when planning to write a review, might ask: how should some studies be selected and others rejected? How should the results be collated? Should insignificant results from individual studies be combined in meta-analysis? This chapter will attempt to demystify these and other intrigues surrounding systematic reviews.

Systematic reviews are robust pieces of research that, based on a clearly formulated question, identify relevant studies, appraise their quality and summarise their evidence using a scientific and explicit method. It is the use of an explicit and systematic approach that differentiates such reviews from traditional reviews, opinions and commentaries. Whenever we use the term 'review' in this chapter it will mean a systematic review. Figure 17.1 provides a step-by-step explanation of the methods behind reviews – there are just five steps.[4] As multiple pregnancies are fewer than singleton pregnancies, research papers on them are limited in numbers, reducing the statistical power. This problem in particular may be addressed by collating results in a review. Nevertheless, there are few studies of robust and valid designs including randomised controlled trials (RCTs). This means that reviewers have to be vigilant about the quality of evidence reviewed. Multiple pregnancies are often reported as a subgroup of published studies of pregnant women. They are also often evaluated in observational research designs without any control groups. Methods for reviews of observational data[5] are not as widespread as those for reviews of randomised trials.[6]

Step 1: Framing questions

The review should be a protocol-driven project with the problem to be addressed specified up front in the form of clear, unambiguous and structured questions. Once the review questions have been set, modifications to the protocol should only be considered if alternative ways of defining the populations, interventions, outcomes or study designs become apparent.

Step 2: Identifying relevant literature

The search for studies should be extensive, as publication bias is likely to be a bigger problem than in reviews based solely on randomised controlled trials. Multiple resources should be searched without language restrictions. The study selection criteria should flow directly from the review questions and be specified a priori. It is likely that the study design criterion will include a range of designs. Reasons for inclusion and exclusion of citations and papers should be recorded. The risk of publication and related biases may be explored statistically.

Step 3: Assessing the quality of the literature

The minimum acceptable level of quality can be crudely defined by study design during question formulation (Step 1) and study selection (Step 2). Selected studies should then be subjected to a more refined quality assessment (Step 3). These detailed assessments can be used to explore heterogeneity, to inform decisions regarding suitability of meta-analysis (Step 4), to examine strength of inferences, and to make recommendations for future research (Step 5)

Step 4: Summarising the evidence

Study characteristics, quality and results should be tabulated first. Data synthesis may then use statistical methods for exploring differences between studies (heterogeneity) and combining the results (meta-analysis) appropriately. If an overall meta-analysis is not feasible, subgroup meta-analysis may be feasible and may provide clinically useful answers. In many reviews where meta-analysis is not feasible, diagrammatic representation of their results helps understand their meaning.

Step 5: Interpreting the findings

For the findings of a review to have validity, the issues highlighted in each of the four steps above should be satisfied first. Exploration of the reasons behind heterogeneity should help determine whether any practical inferences can be generated. Any recommendations, whether for practice or research, should take into account the strengths and weaknesses of the evidence reviewed.

Figure 17.1.   Steps involved in a systematic review of studies of multiple pregnancy; adapted from Khan *et al.*[3,4]

Reviewers of multiple pregnancy literature thus face significant challenges in generating strong influences. Their readership also faces difficulties in critically appraising reviews.

In this chapter we will illustrate the five steps of a review using a published review concerning the effectiveness of interventions for twin-to-twin transfusion syndrome (TTTS).[7] To explore the extent to which reviews of this research are systematic and unbiased, we will also assess the quality of systematic reviews done on any aspect of care for multiple pregnancies. We hope to highlight the challenges in conducting reviews robustly and to encourage researchers and experts to adopt this approach.

Scenario: twin-to-twin transfusion syndrome

You are the lead obstetrician in your hospital for multiple pregnancies. TTTS complicates approximately one in five of all monochorionic diamniotic twin pregnancies. When the onset of this condition occurs before 26 weeks of gestation, there is a significant associated risk of fetal loss, perinatal death and subsequent disability in survivors.[1] If untreated, early-onset severe TTTS is associated with a dismal prognosis, with high rates of perinatal mortality and neurodevelopmental morbidity among survivors. You recently came across a patient with this condition. Serial, aggressive amnioreduction is what you have been using with a view to preventing preterm labour related to polyhydramnios and improving fetal haemodynamics by decreasing pressure on the placental surface vasculature. Fetoscopic laser photocoagulation of the chorionic plate vascular anastomoses at the inter-twin membrane has been introduced in a specialist centre near you. You are considering whether this would be an effective option for affected twin pregnancies in your unit. You have come across a systematic review that examines its value[7] and wish to use it to assist you in decision making.

Step 1: framing the question

The research question may initially be stated as a query in free form using simple language but reviewers prefer to pose it in a structured and explicit way. The relationship between various components of the question and the research design is shown in Figure 17.2.

Free-form question

Which among the two modalities, serial amnioreduction and laser photocoagulation, is better for the treatment of TTTS?

It is obvious that the target population is pregnant women with a twin gestation having features of TTTS. The question has a narrow focus on interventions for treatment of TTTS with a testable hypothesis that one intervention (laser photocoagulation) could be better or worse than another (amnioreduction). Although the original review includes comparison of various treatment modalities, for simplicity we have considered only the two procedures, i.e. laser photocoagulation and serial amnioreduction, relevant to the scenario above. The review examines perinatal survival, neurological morbidity and complications as outcomes of interventions for TTTS. Appropriate study design for this type of research would be RCTs[3,7–9] but it is obvious that, owing to the small number of TTTS cases, observational studies are more likely to be present in the literature, a situation applicable to most of the reviews on multiple pregnancy.

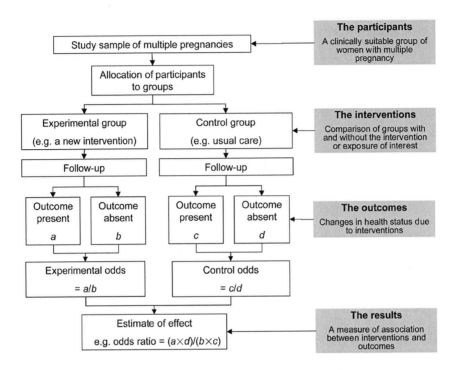

Figure 17.2. Structured questions for systematic review of studies on multiple pregnancy and the relationship between the question components

Structured question:

■ **Population:** Twins with features of TTTS (monochorionicity, polyhydramnios around the recipient and severe oligohydramnios surrounding the donor, and fetal size discordance with or without central fetal haemodynamic changes).

■ **Interventions:** Laser photocoagulation or serial amnioreduction.

■ **Outcomes:** Perinatal survival, neurological morbidity and complications.

■ **Study design:** Observational and randomised designs which compare the two interventions in a primary study with follow-up of twins to assess the above outcomes. Case studies without comparative information were not considered.

Step 2: Identifying relevant literature

Figure 17.3 summarises the process of literature identification and selection. The initial searching effort, covering a range of databases without any language restrictions, targeted all interventional studies on TTTS. This resulted in 831 citations from which relevant studies were selected for the review. Their potential relevance was examined and 517 citations that were only case studies were excluded and a further 290 citations

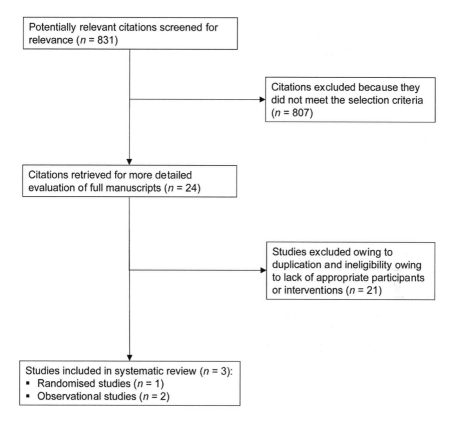

Figure 17.3.   Study selection process for systematic review of interventions for twin-to-twin transfusion syndrome

were excluded as they did not meet the selection criteria concerning population, intervention or outcome. The full papers of the remaining 24 citations were assessed, which revealed 21 that did not meet the selection criteria or were duplicates. A total of three primary studies (all in English) were selected for review, comprising one RCT (142 twins) and two observational controlled studies (272 twins).

Step 3: Assessing study quality

From the outset there was a worry that only a few studies with sound designs would be available and thus the threshold for study selection was lowered to allow observational studies to be included along with RCTs. There are many sources of bias that can invalidate observational studies. Selection bias may arise if the study groups are not similar at baseline, a problem that is less likely to occur when randomisation is used. Measurement bias may arise if observers assessing outcome measures are not kept blind to the interventions. Blinding avoids bias, as recordings made by an observer are not influenced by the knowledge of the type of intervention. Bias may also arise if data are collected retrospectively and patients are not adequately followed up. Therefore, an interventional study can be considered to be of good quality if it meets the criteria shown in Figure 17.4.

Quality assessment criteria:
- Control for confounding: Randomisation with concealment of allocation is considered ideal. In observational studies use of adjustment for confounding in analysis is considered second best.
- Data collection: Prospective collection of data is considered ideal, retrospective collection is considered second best.
- Description of interventions: Complete and transparent description to allow replication by others is considered adequate.
- Outcome ascertainment: Complete (> 90%) follow-up of the original study population is considered ideal. Blinding of carers and patients is not considered essential for quality. However, blinding of outcome assessors is considered ideal.

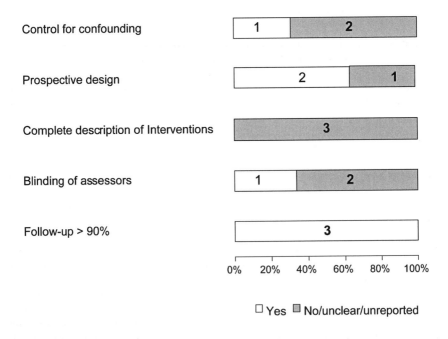

Figure 17.4.   Quality assessment of interventional studies on twin-to-twin transfusion syndrome

Step 4: Summarising the evidence

The key to summarising of evidence is adequate tabulation of the studies' character-istics and results. There are usually some differences between studies in important characteristics of their *population, intervention* and *outcome* (clinical heterogeneity) and their *study design* and quality (methodological heterogeneity). In this review the outcome measures tested were survival of both twins, survival of one twin (with differential survival for donor and recipient twin), neurological abnormalities of the surviving twin, interventional failures and complications.

The effect of an intervention may be measured in a number of ways. With regard to the pros and cons of various measures to summarise results, there is no consensus among experts and this debate is outside the remit of this chapter. Some prefer the odds ratio (OR) as it is more suitable for statistical manipulation and modelling. When there is a relative paucity of events, as is expected in studies of twins, effect estimates from individual studies computed by Peto's method for OR are considered preferable. A measure of uncertainty of effect measure may be provided with 95% confidence intervals (CI). In this review, OR values >1 indicated improvement for survival outcomes while OR values <1 indicated improvement for morbidity outcomes. Confidence intervals including 1 indicated a lack of statistical significance at $P<0.05$. Heterogeneity of effect estimates can be explored graphically using Forrest plots, as shown in Figure 17.5. Grouping studies according to study design allows qualitative inspection for methodological heterogeneity. The consistency of results from study to study may also be examined statistically using the χ^2 test for heterogeneity. As studies were clinically and methodologically heterogeneous, data from individual studies were not pooled to compute the comparative effect of interventions.

Once plots of ORs have been generated (Figure 17.5), the comparative effect of intervention on the various outcome measures can be examined. It is clear that improvement in survival of at least one twin and reduction in neurological morbidity due to laser photocoagulation (compared with serial amnioreduction) is supported by all three studies. In the RCT, overall survival and recipient survival was better with laser photocoagulation (compared with serial amnioreduction). Although not statistically significant, this trend is supported by the observational studies as well. Laser photocoagulation had slightly more spontaneous miscarriages before 24 weeks of gestation than serial amnioreduction (32/239 versus 24/218; 13.4% versus 11.0%).

Step 5: Interpreting the findings

We have the results, but first we must ascertain that the review itself has validity. The search was extensive, including contact with experts for unpublished data, giving assurance against the risk of publication bias, i.e. a tendency for studies to be selectively published if their results are significant. Exploration of study quality as a source of heterogeneity did not reveal statistically significant differences in effect estimates across studies (Figure 17.4). When considering the effect of the interventions on the outcomes in this review, laser photocoagulation conferred better overall improvements in survival and neurological outcome than amnioreduction. However, laser photo-coagulation was associated with a slightly greater number of spontaneous miscarriages than amnioreduction. Approximately 50% of affected pregnancies experience overall survival with amnioreduction. Taking the average figures and using the results from the RCT, numbers of patients needed to be treated can now be computed. If patients were treated by laser photocoagulation, for every six affected pregnancies there would be

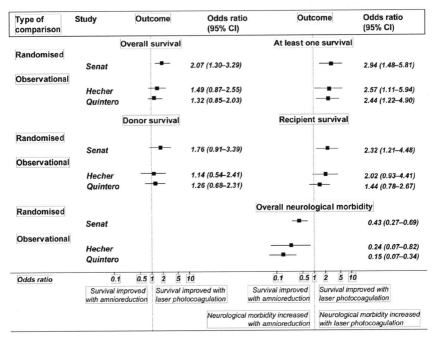

Figure 17.5. Effects of laser photocoagulation versus serial amnioreduction for twin-to-twin transfusion syndrome[7]

one additional pregnancy with overall survival. Similarly, among survivors, for every five affected pregnancies treated with laser photocoagulation there would be one additional neurologically intact outcome compared with amnioreduction.

Resolution of the scenario

After having spent some time reading and understanding the review, you know the survival and complication rates of both procedures. This systematic review revealed that for the treatment of early-onset TTTS there is a relative paucity of evidence but it seems reliable enough to inform clinical practice. The data reviewed indicate that use of laser photocoagulation in TTTS increases survival and reduces neuro-developmental morbidity but the risk of miscarriage is slightly increased. This inform-ation will help in counselling your patient appropriately. If the patient decides to pursue laser photocoagulation, you can refer her to the nearest expert centre that offers this treatment.

Methodological quality of existing systematic reviews of research on multiple pregnancies

With our understanding of the methods of a systematic review and the experience of going through an example of a systematic review on TTTS, let us examine how good existing systematic reviews on the topic of multiple pregnancy are. We found, after an extensive search, 14 systematic reviews (including the one illustrated above), comprising nine therapeutic, three prognostic and two diagnostic reviews on multiple pregnancy scattered in the medical literature.[7,10–22] Publicly available databases were searched and reviews were selected for evaluation of their methodological quality. Most of the reviews were based on observational studies. Quality assessment, based on existing checklists,[3,5,6,9,23] involved extracting information from each selected review article on framing of question, literature search and review methods, methods of literature search and data synthesis. The overall quality of the existing systematic reviews was poor, as shown in the bar chart in Figure 17.6. Only eight (60%) of the reviews had a specific question and a testable hypothesis. In seven (50%) the focus of the question was narrow. Eleven (80%) reviews described the literature search methods adequately and in 12 (90%) multiple databases were searched. However, most of them used only two databases. Two (15%) reviews searched only Medline. Seven (50%) reviews restricted their search to English language articles. A reference list to identify studies missed in electronic searches was used in 11 (80%) reviews. Assessment for risk of missing literature was adequate in only one (7%) review.[7] Quality assessment of studies included in the systematic reviews was inadequate in seven (50%) reviews. Findings were adequately tabulated in only eight (57%) reviews. Assessment for heterogeneity was not clear or inadequate in 10 (72%) reviews. Meta-analysis of data was done only in three (20%) reviews.[12,17,24]

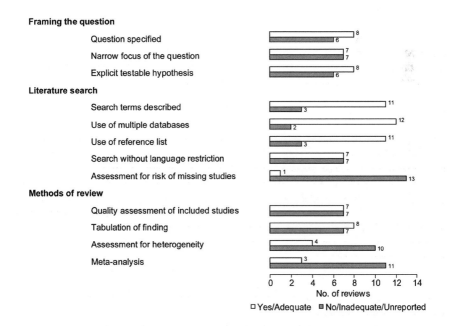

Figure 17.6.   Methodological quality of existing systematic reviews on multiple pregnancy

Reviewers and guideline makers who use research on multiple pregnancy can learn a number of lessons from this evaluation. When interrogating databases, systematic reviews are likely to be flawed if clear evidence of publication bias can be demonstrated.[25] However, lack of assessments for the risk of missing studies was an obvious deficiency in the reviews we assessed. Special efforts such as contact with experts and avoidance of language restriction are required to retrieve as many studies as possible for review. The quality of a study is defined as the degree to which it employs measures to minimise bias and error in its design, conduct and analysis and assessment for quality of the studies included in a review remains an important issue in avoiding bias. This is more challenging for reviewers of multiple pregnancy studies as the standard tools for evaluation of trials cannot be readily applied in observational research. It is important to assess the studies for their quality and heterogeneity, otherwise inferences may become weak owing to underlying weaknesses in the evidence. Despite this, quality assessment of included studies was found in only 50% of reviews. There were three reviews that included meta-analysis for summarising the evidence. However the actual need for using this statistical technique is unknown. Worryingly, data synthesis among the reviews usually ignored methods to assess heterogeneity. In this situation, the suitability of combining results in meta-analysis cannot be evaluated. This evaluation reflects the poor state of reviews of multiple pregnancy research.

Summary

This chapter has described the basic steps for conducting a systematic review to evaluate studies on multiple pregnancy. Threats to the validity of a review inherent in each step and measures to overcome them have also been described. Systematic reviews and meta-analyses are an integral part of evidence-based practice, hence the importance of collation of research evidence for scientific and clinical practice. There is a need for greater awareness about comprehensive and systematic assembly and appraisal of the relevant literature in reviews of studies of multiple pregnancy. This need is magnified in research into multiple pregnancy, since the results are based on studies of small numbers with imprecise findings, and are scattered widely across the literature. We suggest that systematic reviews of studies on multiple pregnancy should be a prerequisite for further research and clinical guidelines in this field.

References

1. Crowther CA. Multiple pregnancy. In: James DK, Steer PJ, Weiner CP, Gonic B, editors. *High Risk Pregnancy: Management Options*. North Yorkshire: WB Saunders; 1999. p. 129–52.
2. Gall SA. Ambulatory management of multiple gestation. *Clin Obstet Gynecol* 1998;41:564–83.
3. Khan KS, Kunz R, Kleijnen J, Antes G. *Systematic Reviews to Support Evidence-Based Medicine: How to Review and Apply Findings of Systematic Reviews*. London: Royal Society of Medicine; 2003.
4. Khan KS, Kunz R, Kleijnen J, Antes G. Five steps to conducting a systematic review. *J R Soc Med* 2003;96:118–21.
5. Stroup DF, Berlin JA, Morton SC, Olkin I, Williamson GD, Rennie D, et al. Meta-analysis of observational studies in epidemiology: a proposal for reporting. Meta-analysis of Observational Studies in Epidemiology (MOOSE) group. *JAMA* 2000;283:2008–12.
6. Moher D, Cook DJ, Eastwood S, Olkin I, Rennie D, Stroup DF. Improving the quality of reports of meta-analyses of randomised controlled trials: the QUOROM statement. Quality of Reporting of Meta-analyses. *Lancet* 1999;354:1896–900.
7. Fox C, Kilby MD, Khan KS. Contemporary treatments for twin–twin transfusion syndrome. *Obstet Gynecol* 2005;105:1469–77.
8. NHS Centre for Reviews and Dissemination. *Undertaking Systematic Reviews of Research on*

Effectiveness. CRD's Guidance for Carrying Out or Commissioning Reviews. CRD Report Number 4, 2nd edn. York: University of York; 2001.

9. Khan K, ter Riet G, Popay J, Nixon J, Kleijnen J, editors. *Undertaking Systematic Reviews of Research on Effectiveness*. CRD Report No. 4. York: University of York; 2001.

10. Allen VM, Windrim R, Barrett J, Ohlsson A. Management of monoamniotic twin pregnancies: A case series and systematic review of the literature. *BJOG* 2001;108:931–6.

11. Crowther CA. Caesarean delivery for the second twin. Cochrane Database Syst Rev 2000;(2):CD000047.

12. Crowther CA. Hospitalisation and bed rest for multiple pregnancy. *Cochrane Database Syst Rev* 2001;(1):CD000110.

13. Dodd JM, Crowther CA. Reduction of the number of fetuses for women with triplet and higher order multiple pregnancies. *Cochrane Database Syst Rev* 2003;(2):CD003932.

14. Dodd JM, Crowther CA. Elective delivery of women with a twin pregnancy from 37 weeks' gestation. *Cochrane Database Syst Rev* 2003;(1):CD003582.

15. Giles WB. Doppler ultrasound in multiple pregnancies. *Bailliere's Clin Obstet Gynaecol* 1998;12:77–89.

16. Helmerhorst FM, Perquin DAM, Donker D, Keirse MJN. Perinatal outcome of singletons and twins after assisted conception: A systematic review of controlled studies. *BMJ* 2004;328:261–4.

17. Hogle KL, Hutton EK, McBrien KA, Barrett JFR, Hannah ME. Cesarean delivery for twins: A systematic review and meta-analysis. *Am J Obstet Gynecol* 2003;188:220–7.

18. Roberts D, Neilson JP, Weindling AM. Interventions for the treatment of twin–twin transfusion syndrome. *Cochrane Database Syst Rev* 2001;(1):CD002073.

19. Sherer DM. First trimester ultrasonography of multiple gestations: A review. *Obstet Gynecol Surv* 1998;53:715–26.

20. Su LL. Monoamniotic twins: diagnosis and management. *Acta Obstet Gynecol Scand* 2002;81:995–1000.

21. Tan TYT, Sepulveda W. Acardiac twin: A systematic review of minimally invasive treatment modalities. *Ultrasound Obstet Gynecol* 2003;22:409–19.

22. Woo HH, Sin SY, Tang LC. Single foetal death in twin pregnancies: review of the maternal and neonatal outcomes and management. *Hong Kong Med J* 2000;6:293–300.

23. Khan KS, Bachmann LM, ter Riet G. Systematic reviews with individual patient data meta-analysis to evaluate diagnostic tests. *Eur J Obstet Gynecol Reprod Biol* 2003;108:121–5.

24. Dodd J, Crowther C. Multifetal pregnancy reduction of triplet and higher-order multiple pregnancies to twins. *Fertil Steril* 2004;81:1420–2.

25. Song F, Khan KS, Dinnes J, Sutton AJ. Asymmetric funnel plots and publication bias in meta-analyses of diagnostic accuracy. *Int J Epidemiol* 2002;31:88–95.

Chapter 18

Effects of the birth of multiples on parents' psychological wellbeing

Debbie Sen and Stephen Robson

Introduction

Parenting multiples is more complex and more difficult than parenting singleton infants and yet often more rewarding. For all first-time parents the transition to parenting has been referred to as a shift to 'living in a new and overwhelming world'.[1,2] The impact of this transition on parents of multiples is even greater. Parents of multiples report feeling unprepared for the unique experience and that information provision relating to the multiple pregnancy, birth and parenting experience is inadequate.[3,4]

The physical component (frequently termed 'care burden') of parenting multiple newborn infants results in extreme parental fatigue and consequential exhaustion.[5,6] Good organisation skills and a regulated infant care routine appear to lessen the impact of extreme carer exhaustion.[3] Anecdotal evidence suggests that this is because the carer has definite timeline boundaries to work within, ensuring that at a predetermined point 'time out' will occur.[7]

However, getting out and about with infants of multiples remains problematic. Use of public transport and negotiating a double buggy create the most difficulty, although transportation in a car is not much easier with one parent or carer alone. Difficulty with mobility and transportation increases the risk of carer isolation, usually for the mother. Physical difficulties and maternal isolation while caring for infants of multiples compounds the associated increased risk of maternal depression.[8–10] However, it is recognised that people with depression also isolate themselves as a self-protective mechanism, hence the cause and effect of isolation and depression remain unclear.[11]

Mental health states

The health states of main interest within the perinatal mental health arena are depression, anxiety and stress. However, it is important to consider positive health states and concepts, i.e. happiness, confidence, competence and self-efficacy, and to resist solely focusing on the negative. Soft markers of perinatal mental health include assessment of malaise, emotional distress and adaptation to parenthood. However, the soft marker concepts are frequently based on depression, anxiety and stress symptomatology. Perinatal mental health continues to focus predominantly on the mother during pregnancy and the first year after birth.[12] Evidence relating to impact of parenting on the father and occurrence of paternal mental ill health remains important but scarce.[13] There is evidence of a co-morbidity between maternal and paternal depression in the perinatal period[14–17] and that for fathers, pregnancy (particularly early pregnancy), rather than the postnatal period, would appear to be the most stressful period.[18] Men (as well as women) appear to be ill-prepared for the impact of parenthood on their lives, especially in terms of the sexual relationship.[19]

Negative health states

Depression

Depression is of global concern. It results in impaired personal functioning and has major psychosocial and economic resource implications. Depression has a range of meanings: from a description of normal unhappiness, through persistent and pervasive ways of feeling and thinking, to psychosis.[20] More than 20% of adults in the UK at any one time suffer mental health problems and 40% of general practice consultations involve mental health.[21] Interestingly, 10% of adults are depressed in any one week and 55% are depressed at some time in their life.[21] It has been suggested that 2% of the population suffer from pure depression (evenly distributed between mild, moderate and severe), but a further 8% suffer from mixed anxiety and depression disorder. Depression occurs in 10–14% of women during the perinatal period.[20,22] One in 20 visits to the family doctor is due to depression.[21] Worryingly, up to 50% of the population have unrecognised or undisclosed depression and 20% will develop chronic depression.[21,23,24] Most depressions have triggering life events, and this is particularly the case for the first episode.

Core features of depression include pervasive low mood, loss of interest and enjoyment (anhedonia), reduced energy and diminished activity. Other features can include poor concentration and attention, poor self-esteem and self-confidence, ideas of guilt and unworthiness, bleak or pessimistic views of the future, ideas or acts of self-harm or suicide, disturbed sleep and diminished appetite. Men are less likely than women to self-report symptoms of depression, particularly the occurrence or feelings of tearfulness.[25] Consequences of perinatal depression include cognitive impairment in infants and insecure parent–infant attachment.[26] Screening for and diagnosis of depression often relies on self-reporting of symptoms to healthcare professionals who may conduct or refer the person for a formal clinical assessment. More recently, self-completion of a depression screening tool has been used in pregnancy.[27] Treatment is based on the prescription of antidepressants or talking therapy, although a combination of the two is ideal.

Anxiety

Generalised anxiety disorder affects 2–5% of the general population,[28] with a slight female preponderance, but accounts for almost 30% of 'psychiatric' consultations in general practice.[21] Onset is usually in early adulthood and the course is often chronic, with a worse prognosis in females.[29] There appears to be a genetic predisposition and childhood traumas such as separation from parents may result in vulnerability and then be triggered and maintained by stressful life events. It is characterised by irrational worries, motor tension, hypervigilance and somatic symptoms. Anxiety is an unpleasant emotional state characterised by fearfulness and unwanted distressing symptoms. It is a normal and appropriate response to stress but becomes pathological when it is disproportionate to the severity of the stress, continues after the stressor has gone or occurs in the absence of any external stressors. Treatment includes benzo-diazepine, antidepressants and psychological treatments, including cognitive behaviour therapy.[21,29]

Stress

Stress is an important but complex concept and a number of explanatory theoretical models exist. It is important to recognise that stress is not a symptom. However, feelings of stress can be a precursor to mental ill health and excess stressors often manifest in depression, suicide and anxiety.[21] The relationship between stressor and factors affecting vulnerability, such as personality, remains unclear.[21] However, it is suspected that people low in extraversion and high in neuroticism are at increased risk for depression.[30–32] A large nationwide UK survey recently added the personality dimensions self-criticism and interpersonal dependency as additional risk factors for depression.[33]

The concept of stress is strongly correlated to the concept of control. Control is generally taken to imply power or mastery over the environment.[34] A lack of control relates to the concept of 'learnt hopelessness', which predisposes a person to depression.[35] In high-risk pregnancy and birth, such as multiple pregnancy, parents report feeling a lack of control in decision making and events. The concept of coping has been investigated but the focus has been on the strategic ways one copes (i.e. ways of coping) rather than on whether coping is successful or not. Reports have indicated that mothers use different coping strategies[36] than fathers.[37] Awareness of stressors is crucial, and relief is obtained by terminating or reducing the stressors or by the use of relaxation techniques and occasionally prescription medication. Parental stress is the prevalence and intensity of stressors relating to parenting. The most frequent reported tool to measure parental stress is the Parenting Stress Index (PSI), which also serves as a measure of family functioning. High levels of parental stress are experienced by most parents, particularly between four and 12 months following the birth of the first child, during teenage years and during periods of infant ill health or disability. Extreme and prolonged parental stress has been reported frequently by parents of multiples.[38–40]

Positive mental health states

References to positive psychological health states remain infrequent and these are in need of further study. A recent review[41] suggests that negative concept studies outweigh positive concept studies by 17 : 1. The main positive psychological health states of interest are emotional wellbeing, happiness and self-efficacy. These global concepts are used interchangeably and inconsistently. Emotional wellbeing can be described as healthy thoughts and feelings,[42] although validated tools which measure this concept are frequently based on depression and anxiety symptoms. An attempt has been made to measure global happiness, defined as a subjective transitory mood of 'gaiety and elation' that reflects how one feels at a predetermined time point.[41] Self-efficacy refers to people's assessment of their ability to cope well with a given situation − it concerns judgement of what one can do with the skills one possesses rather than the skills themselves. Self-efficacy judgements are a major determinant of how much effort people expend or sustain when dealing with stressful situations.[43]

Parenting multiples results in extreme stress for parents, but assessing and noting positive concepts and experience is equally important. One unique positive aspect reported by parents of multiples is 'specialness'. Parents report that they are made to feel special during pregnancy and after the birth as the infants, especially if identical, invite frequent attention from other people.

Prevalence of adverse perinatal mental health states

General population

Existing antenatal studies have purported that maternal depression occurs more frequently during pregnancy than after the birth.[44] This is a reflection of the psychological adjustment required in pregnancy, preoccupation with pending birth and parenting as well as maternal emotion being heightened and more labile. It has been suggested that a higher screening score threshold be used for depression during pregnancy. The prevalence of maternal depression in pregnancy is approximately 10%,[45] similar to that reported during the early postnatal period.[46] Maternal anxiety occurs frequently in pregnancy, there is comorbidity between depression and anxiety,[22,47–49] and it is associated with somatic symptoms.[50,51] Up to 30% of women have an anxiety disorder during early pregnancy.[52] Interestingly only 30% had discussed how they felt with their obstetrician, despite 82% stating they would see a mental health professional if referred. However, within a low-risk pregnancy, the intensity of maternal anxiety gradually reduces as pregnancy progresses, rising again slightly in late pregnancy, with increasing thoughts of the impending birth. Maternal anxiety during pregnancy is predictive of a 'difficult' baby temperament after birth,[53] maternal postnatal depression[54] and child behavioural problems.[55]

Approximately 20% of German mothers have depressive symptoms in the first week after birth[56] and 10–14% continue to have depression at six weeks postnatal.[57] Increased intensity of maternal depression, tearfulness and emotional lability at day five postnatal was found to be predictive of sustained maternal depression.[58] The birth of a very preterm infant predisposes mothers to depression and high stress reaction.[59] Increased maternal confidence was noted in Australian mothers receiving an intervention of counselling following a traumatic birth.[60]

Multiples population

Depression, anxiety, stress and fatigue occur more frequently and with higher intensity in parents of multiples than in parents of singletons.[39,61,62] Furthermore, for each additional child, the ability to meet care demands and the quality of life decrease while maternal depression increases.[63] All studies exploring parenting of multiples report excess parental stress and, interestingly, this excess continues to be present even when the children are three years old. However, until recently, most studies used a cross-sectional design, making it difficult to accurately assess parental stress progression. Few studies have explored prevalence and intensity of emotional wellbeing in parents of multiples during pregnancy or the first year after birth.

The authors recently conducted a randomised controlled trial (RCT), the Newcastle Twin Study, involving 182 parents expecting uncomplicated twin infants and 82 parents expecting singleton infants.[64] Parents expecting twins were randomised either to an intervention group (TI), who received a midwife-led antenatal package of care, or to the control group (TC), who received standard care and advice. Parents in the singleton control group (SC) received standard care and advice. Parents filled in a self-completion questionnaire at five time points and were interviewed at one year after birth. The hypothesis included the suggestion that mothers expecting twin infants and in receipt of the intervention would report less depression at six months after birth than mothers expecting twin infants who received standard care and advice. Secondary outcome measures included prevalence of anxiety, parental stress, parent–infant attachment, maternal confidence, happiness and satisfaction with motherhood. The prevalence of antenatal maternal probable depression and mean score (based on the Edinburgh Postnatal Depression Scale[65] was similar in all three groups (10%). The findings confirmed that mothers in the TI group were 50% less likely to have probable depression compared with mothers in the TC group at six, 12 and 26 weeks after birth (Table 18.1). However, by 52 weeks after birth prevalence of maternal probable depression was similar and in fact increased in the SC group. When comparing the mean score there was evidence of a moderate effect between mothers in the TI group and in the TC group at 26 weeks postnatal and between those in the TC group and in the SC group at 12 weeks postnatal. There was no evidence of any difference between mothers or fathers at any of the other time points.[64]

Table 18.1. Mean score and standard deviation (SD), between-group analysis and prevalence of probable[a] depression of maternal depression using the Edinburgh Postnatal Depression Scale at antenatal and 6, 12, 26 and 52 weeks postnatal (PN) time points and paternal depression at 26 weeks postnatally

Time point	Group	n	Mean score and SD	Between-group analysis			Probable depression	
				Difference between means	95% CI	P	n	%
Maternal								
Antenatal	TI	76	8.1 (5.1)	0.29	−1.3, 1.9	0.72	8	11
	TC	75	7.8 (5.0)	0.13	−1.7, 1.4	0.87	7	9
	SC	81	7.9 (4.7)				7	9
6 weeks PN	TI	69	7.0 (4.3)	0.54	−2.2, 1.1	0.52	6	8
	TC	64	7.5 (5.4)	0.32	−1.4, 2.0	0.71	13	20
	SC	72	7.2 (4.6)				9	13
12 weeks PN	TI	65	6.1 (4.4)	1.18	−3.0, 0.6	0.20	7	11
	TC	63	7.2 (5.8)	1.63	0.2, 3.4	0.08	14	22
	SC	71	5.6 (4.7)				8	12
26 weeks PN	TI	68	5.4 (4.5)	1.53	−3.3, 0.2	0.08	6	9
	TC	65	6.9 (5.5)	0.35	−0.6, 3.1	0.18	12	19
	SC	64	7.9 (5.7)				8	12
52 weeks PN	TI	63	7.2 (5.0)	0.35	−2.0, 1.3	0.68	11	18
	TC	60	7.6 (4.4)	0.35	−2.2, 1.5	0.71	12	20
	SC	64	7.9 (5.7)				12	19
Paternal								
26 Weeks	TI	54	3.8 (3.8)	0.41	−1.9, 1.1	0.60	11	20
	TC	58	4.2 (4.3)	0.61	−2.2, 0.95	0.44	14	24
	SC	69	4.8 (4.5)				20	29

TI = twin intervention group; TC = twin control group; SC = singleton control group
[a] Using the recommended cut-offs

Similar findings for maternal depression were confirmed by Thorpe *et al.* in 1995.[39] The psychological impact on fathers of multiples is broadly unknown.[66] However, the recent RCT by Sen *et al.*[67] suggests that approximately 22% of fathers of twin infants have probable depression at six months after birth compared with 29% of fathers of singleton infants, indicating a possible protective factor of twin infants for fathers.

Comorbidity between depression and anxiety is common. Maternal depression or anxiety disorder occurs in up to 25% of mothers of multiples during the perinatal period.[68,69] Anxiety occurs more frequently in mothers of multiples during pregnancy but this may be related to anticipated or actual higher maternal and fetal risk of complications.[62,70] Table 18.2 presents the mean score and prevalence of probable maternal anxiety using the Hospital Anxiety and Depression Scale (HADS)[71] in mothers of twin infants who received the antenatal intervention package compared with mothers of twins who received standard care and advice and relative to mothers of singleton infants receiving standard care and advice. No difference was found between mean score within groups at any time point. Using categorical cut-off for probable anxiety, there was evidence of a difference between mothers in the TI group and those in the TC group at 12 weeks postnatal only.

In the RCT conducted by the authors[67] there was moderate evidence of a difference in the total parenting stress and in the parental distress as measured by the PSI[72] between mothers in the TI group and those in the TC group (Table 18.3). When comparing mothers in the TC group with mothers in the SC group, there was strong evidence of a difference in difficult child subscale, indicating that mothers of twin infants perceived the infants to be more difficult than mothers of singleton infants. No differences were observed in the parent–child dysfunction subscale between any of the groups.

Table 18.2. Mean score and standard deviation (SD), between-group analysis and prevalence of probable[a] anxiety of maternal anxiety using the Hospital Anxiety and Depression Scale at antenatal and 6, 12 and 26 weeks postnatal (PN) time points

Time point	Group	*n*	Mean score and SD	Between-group analysis			Probable anxiety		
				Difference between means	95% CI	*P*	*n*	%	*P*[b]
Antenatal	TI	76	6.1 (3.6)	0.25	−0.8, 1.3	0.65	10	13	0.30
	TC	75	5.8 (3.2)	0.26	−0.8, 1.3	0.63	6	8	0.68
	SC	81	5.6 (3.5)				8	10	
6 weeks PN	TI	68	5.1 (3.3)	0.20	−1.4, 1.0	0.74	6	9	0.89
	TC	63	5.3 (3.7)	0.44	−0.7, 1.6	0.46	6	10	0.10
	SC	72	4.9 (3.2)				2	3	
12 weeks PN §	TI	65	3.5 (2.5)	0.60	−1.7, 0.5	0.26	0	0	0.04
	TC	63	4.1 (3.5)	0.20	−0.9, 1.3	0.72	4	6	0.13
	SC	71	4.1 (3.5)				1	1	
26 weeks PN	TI	67	4.5 (3.0)	0.83	−2.0, 0.39	0.18	4	6	0.93
	TC	63	5.4 (3.9)	0.26	−1.1, 1.6	0.70	4	6	0.27
	SC	67	5.1 (3.8)				8	12	

TI = twin intervention group; TC = twin control group; SC = singleton control group
[a] Using the recommended cut-offs
[b] Between-group χ^2 analysis

Impact of parenting on the marital relationship

It is widely acknowledged that the birth of a child has a large impact on the marital relationship,[73] with a decline in marital satisfaction and an increase in marital conflict. The change is particularly notable between four and 12 months after birth.[74] Relationship cohesion is important, and vulnerabilities in a relationship prior to pregnancy are likely to result in further marital conflict or distress during pregnancy, with the relationship being at significant risk after the birth. Families of multiples are at increased risk for marital separation and divorce.[75] The study recently conducted by the authors[67] reported that up to 10% of parents of twin infants consider or actually separate during the first year after the birth, compared with 6% of parents of singleton infants.

Impact of adverse mental health states

Mental ill health results in psychosocial and cognitive dysfunction, impacting on the relationship between mother and father and the parenting experience. Successful role adaptation and adjustment from partner to parent is crucial. In particular, an expectation of traditional female roles involving household tasks and childcare often results in increased dissatisfaction for the woman within the relationship.[76] It is widely recognised that parental mental ill health results in less favourable parent–infant attachment[77] and cognitive impairment in infants,[78] with this being particularly notable in triplet infants.[79] Interestingly, despite increased levels of anxiety, similar levels of parent–infant attachment occur between high-risk and low-risk pregnancies.[80] The prevalence of post-traumatic stress disorder in multiple-birth parents is not known. However, symptoms associated with post-traumatic stress disorder occur during the first year after birth in mothers of preterm infants and in mothers who perceived low control during delivery.[81,82]

Table 18.3. Mean score and standard deviation (SD) and between-group analysis of parenting stress, parental distress subscale, difficult child subscale and parent–child dysfunction subscale using the Parenting Stress Index (PSI) at 26 weeks post birth

Time point	Group	n	Mean score and SD	Between-group analysis		
				Difference between means	95% CI	P
Parenting stress	TI	64	64.2 (11.9)			0.07
	TC	58	68.4 (13.2)	4.2	–8.7, 0.3	0.33
	SC	66	67.0 (14.8)	2.6	–2.6, 7.8	
Parental distress subscale	TI	64	26.1 (5.9)			0.06
	TC	58	28.1 (5.7)	2.0	–4.1, 0.1	0.75
	SC	66	27.8 (6.6)	0.4	–1.9, 2.6	
Difficult child subscale	TI	63	23.6 (7.3)			0.66
	TC	55	24.2 (7.6)	0.6	–3.3, 2.1	0.03
	SC	65	21.7 (4.9)	2.5	0.2, 4.8	
Parent–child dysfunction subscale	TI	63	16.1 (4.5)			0.17
	TC	57	17.3 (5.2)	1.2	–2.9, 5.4	0.56
	SC	62	17.9 (5.2)	0.6	–2.4, 1.3	

TI = twin intervention group; TC = twin control group; SC = singleton control group

Parent–infant attachment

Parent–infant attachment in multiples is interesting. It is recognised that it is difficult for parents to attach equally to newborn multiple birth infants at the same time and the theory of monotropy is widely acknowledged and recognised.[83] Monotropy is the attachment of only one infant to a parent at any one time. Alternative theories about parent–infant attachment in multiples are complex. There is debate about the theory that attachment between a parent and one particular infant continues at the expense of the other infant, with preference for an infant being based on physical or temperament characteristics.[84] However, parental attachment frequently alternates between infants.[84] Depressed mothers (of singleton and of multiple infants) tend to be less sensitively attuned to their baby's needs, which impacts on the security of the attachment relationship.[85] There is concern about the substantial increased risk of physical and mental child abuse in families with multiples.[66,86–88] This increased risk usually applies to siblings of multiples but in some cases to the twin or triplet infants themselves. Interestingly, the abuser is usually the mother.

Because of the impact of mental ill health in parents of multiples, it is important to note the factors that are different between the parenting of multiples and the parenting of singleton infants. Fortunately, it is not all bad news. One benefit is the development of a secure attachment between the infants themselves.[83,89] In a recent study conducted by the author,[90] compared with parents of singleton infants, parents of multiples reported feeling more assured about leaving twin infants in a room by themselves while a parent completed a task, as they felt the infants had each other for company. This particular benefit appears to be unique to families with multiples. Within the Newcastle Twin Study[90] there was some anecdotal suggestion that 'turn taking' was optimised from an early age in children from multiples compared with singleton children. Infant temperament and infant health are important factors to consider and can influence the risk of perinatal mental ill health. Parental perception of infant temperament is important and may reflect some aspect of parent–infant attachment.[91]

Negative impact of multiples

However, reports of the negative impact of multiples are frequent. During pregnancy, mothers expecting multiples experience emotional trauma and high anxiety.[40] There are tremendous physical childcare needs in families of multiples over and above that of families with singleton infants.[66] Meeting these physical care needs of infants of multiples has been termed 'care burden.' There is no doubt that caring for multiples results in extreme fatigue for both parents. Organisation of tasks and a strict routine appear to limit the impact of extreme fatigue in parents of singletons. In the recent Newcastle Twin Study conducted by the authors,[90] parents who self-reported good or excellent organisation skills and a regimented routine pattern felt they coped better because they could anticipate their next rest period. Similar considerations were not reported by parents of singleton infants. However, parents of twin infants frequently reported restriction due to mobility issues, often leading to parental isolation. Parents of singleton infants did not self-report restriction due to mobility issues.

Influencing and protective factors

Parental personality

There are a number of influences and protective factors that may increase or decrease the risk of perinatal mental ill health. These include personality (sometimes referred to as temperament) of the mother or the father, in particular the degree of extraversion, neuroticism and self-criticism traits.[33] Positive self-concept is important in the prevention of perinatal mental ill health.[92] Self-concept consists of our thoughts and feelings about ourselves, both as individuals and in relation to others. The presence of resilience, optimism and hope as personality characteristics is important.[93] Bandura's explanatory model[43] regarding self-efficacy is important as it relates to the way one copes in the presence of extreme stresses. It is widely acknowledged that the birth of a child impacts on the relationship between the mother and father. However, for fathers the impact of pregnancy is perceived as more stressful than the impact after birth.[19]

Support

The concept of support is important and widely acknowledged within the perinatal arena. There are three main types of support: physical, emotional and social. The Newcastle Twin Study[90] found that it was the provision of support rather than the type of provider that was important. A lack of support has consistently been shown to be one of the most important factors that contribute to a negative parenting experience.[94] Provision of social support from family and/or friends allows time out to focus on the partner relationship. However, accessing and asking for help can be problematic for some families of multiples. In the Newcastle Twin Study parents reported that accessing and asking for help was vital. Parents of multiples often cared for the infants as a unit rather than as individuals.[95] The Newcastle Twin Study reported that grandparents and friends were often reluctant to take on the responsibility of more than one infant at one time. Parents should be informed that assistance with one of the infants, at one time, fosters individuality and may be more acceptable to family and friends. The study found that care crises occurred more frequently in families of multiples than in families of singleton infants. Care crises were associated with maternal or infant ill health rather than with an inability to cope with infant care in general.

Finance

In multiple birth families financial constraints are more of an issue than in families with singleton infants.[96,97] Not only is the purchasing of two sets of equipment such as cots and car seats and a double buggy essential, the mother is more likely to leave paid work earlier in pregnancy and less likely to return to paid work after the birth.[38] Financial responsibility for the family usually, but not always, falls to the father. Fathers of multiples have additional stressors compared with fathers of singleton infants. Not only is he the financial provider, but he is often acutely aware of the difficulties the mother is experiencing. The father may thus experience internal conflict from the need to provide support to the mother and from having responsibility as the financial provider.

Life events

The impact of life events before, during and after the birth of infants should never be underestimated. The experience of life events is interrelated with psychological vulnerability and strength.[98,99] The impact of life events may be positive or negative. Negative life events increase vulnerability for mental ill health, but the experience may also have positive effects such as increased resilience, self-efficacy and/or improved self-concept. The birth experience itself is indeed a life event. Multiple pregnancy and birth is identified appropriately as high risk.[100] Loss of control during the birthing process is associated with maternal psychological distress after birth.[91] Unexpected childbirth events such as emergency caesarean section are more likely to result in the mother's feeling a loss of control during the birthing process.

The birthing experience itself may be more traumatic for the father, as he observes the process directly and witnesses any untoward events that occur. In the Newcastle Twin study fathers and mothers of twin infants reported feelings of fear that the mother and/or infants would die.[67] These feelings were associated with emergency caesarean section, postpartum haemorrhage and prematurity.

Planned pregnancy

Planning or intention of pregnancy is an important consideration.[101] It is widely accepted that the planning of pregnancy influences the risk of perinatal mental ill health. Ease of conception is also an important factor to consider. Women undergoing fertility treatment are reported to perceive 'compound losses' and social stigma:[102] these feelings are long-lasting and continue even following a successful pregnancy and the birth of a healthy infant.[103] Mothers who required assisted conception are at an increased risk of perinatal mental ill health after the birth when compared with mothers who conceived twin infants spontaneously.[38,104] Although there remains uncertainty regarding causation, the best predictor of mental ill health during and/or after fertility treatment is pretreatment mental health state.[105] Couples undergoing assisted conception frequently 'desire' twin infants and sometimes consider the resultant multiple pregnancy as a 'benefit' or 'double bonus'.[61,106] The assisted conception process itself is often referred to as a 'roller coaster ride'.[107,108] The desire in these families to have and hold a baby is immense. Potential parents invest financially, physically and emotionally and will often go to any lengths to achieve and take home a baby. During the process of fertility treatment, women idealise motherhood, contemplating an emotional vision of a happy, smiling mother with an equally happy, smiling infant. This leads to high and unrealistic expectations of what 'being a parent' is like and this discrepancy between expectation and reality contributes to maternal depression after birth.[109] Interestingly, the expectation of being a parent is interlinked with preconceived ideas and ideology of self as mother and self as father.[110] Some parents manage a seamless transition to parenthood with ease and confidence regardless of adverse previous and concurrent life events, increased risk and a complex birthing experience. It would appear that, despite adversity, they would always have been 'natural' and 'good' parents.[111,112]

The greatest risk of perinatal mental ill health is following a multiple pregnancy where one or more infant dies during pregnancy or after the birth. The second highest risk for parental perinatal mental ill health occurs in families with multiple pregnancies following an assisted conception, and this is followed by families with multiple pregnancies conceived naturally. The risk factors continue to increase in families with siblings or children with a close gap (within two years).[113] It would appear that there is some correlation between maternal emotional distress during the transition to parenting and quantity and/or complexity of infant care burden.

Fetal and infant death

There are substantial differences in the mortality and morbidity outcomes of triplet or higher order pregnancies compared with twin pregnancies,[78,114,115] and also in twin pregnancies compared with singleton pregnancies.[116,117] The issue of fetal or infant death in one of a multiple birth results in a complex grief reaction, particularly in the event of one survival and one death.[86,118,119] The birth date often serves as a reminder to parents of the birth of one infant and the death of another.[120] These issues are further compounded as the infant grows and their presence results in reminders of the dead sibling. These feelings are particularly complex and difficult for parents of identical infants.[120] To grieve for one child, at the same time as celebrate the birth of another is difficult and increases the risk of maternal and paternal anxiety and depression. In the UK, the Multiple Birth Foundation (MBF) and the Twins and Multiple Births Association (TAMBA) provide essential educational material, both for health professionals and for parents when dealing with this emotional and distressing circumstance. The intensities of mothers' and fathers' grief reaction to infant loss are reported to be similar, although gender differences in the way parents cope have been noted.[118]

Implications for practice

It is important that parents expecting multiples have realistic expectations of both the birthing process and the parenting experience. Mothers and fathers of multiples remain ill-prepared for their unique and special role. The provision of educational sessions during multiple pregnancy informs parents, assists in the generation of realistic expectations and provides a valuable opportunity to share experience. Fathers should be involved in these sessions as well as in the care and decision-making process. It is important that during pregnancy parents have access to a midwife and health visitor, as well as to the obstetrician. Provision of care within an antenatal twin clinic provides continuity of care and carer.

There is some evidence from the recent Newcastle Twin Study[64] that attending sessions on preparation for parenting of multiples improves the psychological outcome of the parents after the birth, particularly in respect to father support and relationship cohesion. The levels of parental distress were also reduced in mothers at six months post birth.

Parenting multiples remains more difficult and complex than parenting singleton infants. However, it is important to recognise that, despite frequent reports of negative impact, parenting multiples is often positive, special and unique.

Another implication for practice is the assessment of risk for perinatal mental ill health. It is important that potential parents be screened for psychological vulnerability as unidentified parental anxiety, depression and/or stress result in relationship conflict, child abuse, poor parent–infant attachment and negative parenting experience. Such assessments should consider the level of availability support, relationship vulnerability, the presence of a pre-existing anxiety trait disorder, concurrent and previous life events, type and ease of conception as well as expectations of being a parent. In the current climate of limited health service provision, assessment and identification of at-risk status for perinatal mental ill health would enable the appropriate resources to be directed at those most at need.

Information is available online from the Multiple Births Foundation and the Twins and Multiple Births Association.

References

1. Nystrom K, Ohrling K. Parenthood experiences during the child's first year: literature review. *J Adv Nurs* 2004;46:319–30.
2. Robin M, Josse D, Tourrette C. Mother–twin interaction during early childhood. *Acta Genet Med Gemellol* 1988;37:151–9.
3. Nys K, Colpin H, De Munter A, Vandemeulebroecke L. Feelings and the need for information and counselling of expectant parents of twins. *Twin Res* 1998;1:142–9.
4. Bryan E. Educating families, before, during and after a multiple birth. *Semin Neonatol* 2002;7:241–6.
5. Robin M, Kheroua H, Casati I. Effects of early mother–twin relationships from birth to age 3, on twin bonding. *Acta Genet Med Gemellol* 1992;41:143–8.
6. Yokoyama Y, Shimizu T, Hayakawa K. [Childcare problems and maternal fatigue symptoms in families with twins and triplets]. *Nippon Koshu Eisei Zasshi* 1995;42:187–93.
7. Ford G. *The New Contented Baby Book.* London: Vermilion Publishing; 2002.
8. Nielsen Forman D, Videbech P, Hedegaard M, Dalby Salvig J, Secher NJ. Postpartum depression: identification of women at risk. *BJOG* 2000;107:1210–17.
9. Sakado K, Sato T, Uehara T, Sakado M, Someya T. Perceived parenting pattern and response to antidepressants in patients with major depression. *J Affect Disord* 1999;52:59–66.
10. Sharp LK, Lipsky MS. Screening for depression across the lifespan: a review of measures for use in primary care settings. *Am Fam Physician* 2002;66:1001–8.
11. Whiffen VE, Kerr MA, Kallos-Lilly V. Maternal depression, adult attachment, and children's emotional distress. *Fam Process* 2005;44:93–103.
12. Austin MP. Antenatal screening and early intervention for 'perinatal' distress, depression and anxiety: where to from here? *Arch Women Ment Health* 2004;7:1–6.
13. Currid TJ. Psychological issues surrounding paternal perinatal mental health. *Nurs Times* 2005;101:40–2.
14. Goodman JH. Paternal postpartum depression, its relationship to maternal postpartum depression, and implications for family health. *J Adv Nurs* 2004;45:26–35.
15. Morse CA, Buist A, Durkin S. First-time parenthood: influences on pre- and postnatal adjustment in fathers and mothers. *J Psychosom Obstet Gynaecol* 2000;21:109–20.
16. Matthey S, Barnett B, Ungerer J, Waters B. Paternal and maternal depressed mood during the transition to parenthood. *J Affect Disord* 2000;60:75–85.
17. Areias ME, Kumar R, Barros H, Figueiredo E. Correlates of postnatal depression in mothers and fathers. *Br J Psychiatry* 1996;169:36–41.
18. Buist A, Morse CA, Durkin S. Men's adjustment to fatherhood: implications for obstetric health care. *J Obstet Gynecol Neonatal Nurs* 2003;32:172–80.
19. Condon JT, Boyce P, Corkindale CJ. The First-Time Fathers Study: a prospective study of the mental health and wellbeing of men during the transition to parenthood. *Aust N Z J Psychiatry* 2004;38:56–64.
20. Williamson V, McCutcheon H. Postnatal depression: a review of current literature. *Aust J Midwifery* 2004;17:11–16.
21. Davies T, Craig T. *ABC of Mental Health (ABC's).* London: BMJ Publishing; 1998. p. 120.
22. Perfetti J, Clark R, Fillmore CM. Postpartum depression: identification, screening, and treatment. *WMJ* 2004;103:56–63.
23. Sheehan DV. Depression: underdiagnosed, undertreated, underappreciated. *Manag Care* 2004;13(6 Suppl Depression):6–8.
24. Coates AO, Schaefer CA, Alexander JL. Detection of postpartum depression and anxiety in a large health plan. *J Behav Health Serv Res* 2004;31:117–33.
25. Matthey S, Barnett B, Kavanagh DJ, Howie P. Validation of the Edinburgh Postnatal Depression Scale for men, and comparison of item endorsement with their partners. *J Affect Disord* 2001;64:175–84.
26. Ryan D, Milis L, Misri N. Depression during pregnancy. *Can Fam Physician* 2005;51:1087–93.
27. Clark G. Discussing emotional health in pregnancy: the Edinburgh Postnatal Depression Scale. *Br J Community Nurs* 2000;5:91–8.

28. Stein MB. Public health perspectives on generalized anxiety disorder. *J Clin Psychiatry* 2004;65 Suppl 13:3–7.

29. Wittchen HU. Generalized anxiety disorder: prevalence, burden, and cost to society. *Depress Anxiety* 2002;16:162–71.

30. Ranjith G, Farmer A, McGuffin P, Cleare AJ. Personality as a determinant of social functioning in depression. *J Affect Disord* 2005;84:73–6.

31. Eysenck HJ. Comments on "The orthogonality of extraversion and neuroticism scales". *Psychol Rep* 1987;61:50.

32. Roberts SB, Kendler KS. Neuroticism and self-esteem as indices of the vulnerability to major depression in women. *Psychol Med* 1999;29:1101–9.

33. Cox BJ, McWilliams LA, Enns MW, Clara IP. Broad and specific personality dimensions associated with major depression in a nationally representative sample. *Compr Psychiatry* 2004;45:246–53.

34. Fisher S. *Stress and Strategy*. London: Lawrence Erlbaum Associates; 1986.

35. Thackston-Hawkins L, Compton WC, Kelly DB. Correlates of hopelessness on the MMPI-2. *Psychol Rep* 1994;75(3 Pt 1):1071–4.

36. Huizink AC, de Medina PG, Mulder EJ, Visser GH, Buitelaar JK. Coping in normal pregnancy. *Ann Behav Med* 2002;24:132–40.

37. Johnson MP, Baker SR. Implications of coping repertoire as predictors of men's stress, anxiety and depression following pregnancy, childbirth and miscarriage: a longitudinal study. *J Psychosom Obstet Gynaecol* 2004;25:87–98.

38. Glazebrook C, Sheard C, Cox S, Oates M, Ndukwe G. Parenting stress in first-time mothers of twins and triplets conceived after *in vitro* fertilization. *Fertil Steril* 2004;81:505–11.

39. Thorpe K, Greenwood R, Goodenough T. Does a twin pregnancy have a greater impact on physical and emotional well-being than a singleton pregnancy? *Birth* 1995;22:148–52.

40. Robin M, Cahen F, Pons J. Maternal adjustment to a multiple birth. *Early Child Dev Care* 1992;79:1–11.

41. Myers DG, Diener E. Who is happy? *Psychol Sci* 1995;6:10–19.

42. Colman AM. *Oxford Dictionary of Psychology*. Oxford: Oxford University Press; 2003.

43. Bandura A. Self-Efficacy: Towards a unifying theory of behavioural change. *Psychol Rev* 1977;84:191–215.

44. Hayes BA, Muller R. Prenatal depression: a randomized controlled trial in the emotional health of primiparous women. *Res Theory Nurs Pract* 2004;18:165–83.

45. Thoppil J, Riutcel TL, Nalesnik SW. Early intervention for perinatal depression. *Am J Obstet Gynecol* 2005;192:1446–8.

46. Austin MP. Psychosocial assessment and management of depression and anxiety in pregnancy. Key aspects of antenatal care for general practice. *Aust Fam Physician* 2003;32:119–26.

47. Da Costa D, Larouche J, Dritsa M, Brender W. Psychosocial correlates of prepartum and postpartum depressed mood. *J Affect Disord* 2000;59:31–40.

48. Ross LE, Gilbert Evans SE, Sellers EM, Romach MK. Measurement issues in postpartum depression Part 1. anxiety as a feature of postpartum depression. *Arch Women Ment Health* 2003;6:51–7.

49. Noyes R, Jr. Comorbidity in generalized anxiety disorder. *Psychiatr Clin N Am* 2001;24:41–55.

50. Kelly RH, Russo J, Katon W. Somatic complaints among pregnant women cared for in obstetrics: normal pregnancy or depressive and anxiety symptom amplification revisited? *Gen Hosp Psychiatry* 2001;23:107–13.

51. Maldonado-Duran JM, Lartigue T, Feintuch M. Perinatal psychiatry: infant mental health interventions during pregnancy. *Bull Menninger Clin* 2000;64:317–43.

52. Birndorf CA, Madden A, Portera L, Leon AC. Psychiatric symptoms, functional impairment, and receptivity toward mental health treatment among obstetrical patients. *Int J Psychiatry Med* 2001;31:355–65.

53. Austin MP, Hadzi-Pavlovic D, Leader L, Saint K, Parker G. Maternal trait anxiety, depression and life event stress in pregnancy: relationships with infant temperament. *Early Hum Dev* 2005;81:183–90.

54. Heron J, O'Connor TG, Evans J, Golding J, Glover V. The course of anxiety and depression through pregnancy and the postpartum in a community sample. *J Affect Disord* 2004;80:65–73.

55. O'Connor TG, Heron J, Golding J, Beveridge M, Glover V. Maternal antenatal anxiety and children's behavioural/emotional problems at 4 years. Report from the Avon Longitudinal Study of Parents and Children. *Br J Psychiatry* 2002;180:502–8.

56. Bergant A, Nguyen T, Moser R, Ulmer H. [Prevalence of depressive disorders in early puerperium]. *Gynakol Geburtshilfliche Rundsch* 1998;38:232–7.

57. Buist A. Promoting positive parenthood: emotional health in pregnancy. *Aust J Midwifery* 2003;16:10–14.

58. Kendell RE, McGuire RJ, Connor Y, Cox JL. Mood changes in the first three weeks after childbirth. *J Affect Disord* 1981;3:317–26.

59. Hagan R, Evans SF, Pope S. Preventing postnatal depression in mothers of very preterm infants: a randomised controlled trial. *BJOG* 2004;111:641–7.

60. Gamble JA, Creedy DK, Webster J, Moyle W. A review of the literature on debriefing or non-directive counselling to prevent postpartum emotional distress. *Midwifery* 2002;18:72–9.

61. Klock SC. Psychological adjustment to twins after infertility. *Best Pract Res Clin Obstet Gynaecol* 2004;18:645–56.

62. Yokoyama Y. [Childcare problems in mothers with twins as compared with children born singly]. *Nippon Koshu Eisei Zasshi* 2002;49:229–35.

63. Ellison MA, Hotamisligil S, Lee H, Rich-Edwards JW, Pang SC, Hall JE. Psychosocial risks associated with multiple births resulting from assisted reproduction. *Fertil Steril* 2005;83:1422–8.

64. Sen D, Robson S, Bond S. Peripartum depression. and anxiety in mothers expecting uncomplicated twin infants – an antenatal model of care in the north east of England. *J Reprod Infant Psychol* 2004;22:138.

65. Cox JL, Holden JM, Sagovsky R. Detection of postnatal depression. Development of the 10-item Edinburgh Postnatal Depression Scale. *Br J Psychiatry* 1987;150:782–6.

66. Fisher J, Stocky A. Maternal perinatal mental health and multiple births: implications for practice. *Twin Res* 2003;6:506–13.

67. Sen DM, Robson SC, Bond S. Newcastle Twin Study. – A midwife-led RCT to reduce maternal emotional distress when parenting twin infants. *J Obstet Gynaecol* 2005;25 Suppl 1:S21

68. Leonard LG. Depression and anxiety disorders during multiple pregnancy and parenthood. *J Obstet Gynecol Neonatal Nurs* 1998;27:329–37.

69. Thorpe K, Golding J, MacGillivray I, Greenwood R. Comparison of prevalence of depression in mothers of twins and mothers of singletons. *BMJ* 1991;302:875–8.

70. Dulude D, Gollapalli A, Mitchell A, Stanko S. High-risk pregnancies, psychological distress, and dyadic adjustment. *J Reprod Infant Psychol* 2002;20:101–23.

71. Zigmond AS, Snaith RP. The hospital anxiety and depression scale. *Acta Psychiatr Scand* 1983;67:361–70.

72. Abidin RR. *Parenting Stress Index – Professional Manual*, 3rd ed. Odessa, FL: Psychological Assessment Resources; 1995.

73. Terry DJ, McHugh TA, Noller P. Role dissatisfaction and the decline in marital quality across the transition to parenthood. *Aust J Psychol* 1991;43:129–32.

74. Elek SM, Hudson DB, Bouffard C. Marital and parenting satisfaction and infant care self-efficacy during the transition to parenthood: the effect of infant sex. *Issues Compr Pediatr Nurs* 2003;26:45–57.

75. Hay DA, Gleeson C, Davies C, Lorden B, Mitchell D, Paton L. What information should the multiple birth family receive before, during and after the birth? *Acta Genet Med Gemellol* 1990;39:259–69.

76. Belsky J, Lang M, Huston TL. Sex typing and division of labor as determinants of marital change across the transition to parenthood. *J Pers Soc Psychol* 1986;50:517–22.

77. Righetti-Veltema M, Bousquet A, Manzano J. Impact of postpartum depressive symptoms on mother and her 18-month-old infant. *Eur Child Adolesc Psychiatry* 2003;12:75–83.

78. Cogill SR, Caplan HL, Alexandra H, Robson KM, Kumar R. Impact of maternal postnatal depression on cognitive development of young children. *Br Med J (Clin Res Ed)* 1986;292:1165–7.

79. Feldman R, Eidelman AI. Does a triplet birth pose a special risk for infant development? Assessing cognitive development in relation to intrauterine growth and mother–infant interaction across the first 2 years. *Pediatrics* 2005;115:443–52.

80. Mercer RT, Ferketich SL. Stress and social support as predictors of anxiety and depression during pregnancy. *ANS Adv Nurs Sci* 1988;10:26–39.

81. Czarnocka J, Slade P. Prevalence and predictors of post-traumatic stress symptoms following childbirth. *Br J Clin Psychol* 2000;39(Pt 1):35–51.

82. Holditch-Davis D, Bartlett TR, Blickman AL, Miles MS. Posttraumatic stress symptoms in mothers of premature infants. *J Obstet Gynecol Neonatal Nurs* 2003;32:161–71.

83. Thomas JG. The early parenting of twins. *Mil Med* 1996;161:233–5.

84. Yokoyama Y, Simizu T. [Maternal partiality in attachment with multiple birth children and the related factors]. *Nippon Koshu Eisei Zasshi* 2001;48:85–94.

85. Austin J, McGuinness M, Hever T. Developing a baby bonding group to reduce parenting stress and improve mother–baby bonding. *J Reprod Infant Psychol* 2005;23:253.

86. Bryan E. The impact of multiple preterm births on the family. *BJOG* 2003;110 Suppl 20:24–8.

87. Nelson HB, Martin CA. Increased child abuse in twins. *Child Abuse Negl* 1985;9:501–5.

88. Groothuis JR, Altemeier WA, Robarge JP, O'Connor S, Sandler H, Vietze P, *et al*. Increased child abuse in families with twins. *Pediatrics* 1982;70:769–73.

89. Gottfried NW, Seay BM, Leake E. Attachment relationships in infant twins: the effect of co-twin presence during separation from mother. *J Genet Psychol* 1994;155:273–81.

90. Sen DM. *A Randomised Controlled Trial of a Twin Antenatal Programme – Newcastle Twin Study*. PhD Thesis, Newcastle University, 2006.

91. Green JM, Coupland VA, Kitzinger JV. *Great Expectations: a Prospective Study of Women's Expectations and Experiences of Childbirth*. 2nd ed. Hale: Books for Midwives Press; 1998.

92. Fowles ER. The relationship between maternal role attainment and postpartum depression. *Health Care Women Int* 1998;19:83–94.

93. Scioli A, Chamberlin CM, Samor CM, Lapointe AB, Campbell TL, MacLeod AR, *et al*. A prospective study of hope, optimism, and health. *Psychol Rep* 1997;81(3 Pt 1):723–33.

94. Heh SS. Relationship between social support and postnatal depression. *Kaohsiung J Med Sci* 2003;19:491–6.

95. Robin M, Corroyer D, Casati I. Childcare patterns of mothers of twins during the first year. *J Child Psychol Psychiatry* 1996;37:453–60.

96. Chang C. Raising twin babies and problems in the family. *Acta Genet Med Gemellol (Roma)* 1990;39:501–5.

97. Malmstrom PM, Biale R. An agenda for meeting the special needs of multiple birth families. *Acta Genet Med Gemellol (Roma)* 1990;39:507–14.

98. Dennis CL, Janssen PA, Singer J. Identifying women at-risk for postpartum depression in the immediate postpartum period. *Acta Psychiatr Scand* 2004;110:338–46.

99. Bebbington PE, Brugha T, MacCarthy B, Potter J, Sturt E, Wykes T, *et al*. The Camberwell Collaborative Depression Study. I. Depressed probands: adversity and the form of depression. *Br J Psychiatry* 1988; 152:754–65.

100. Crowther CA. Multiple pregnancy. In: James D, Weiner C, Gonik B, editors. *High Risk Pregnancy – Management Options*. 2nd ed. London: WB Saunders; 1999. p. 129–51.

101. Wikman M, Jacobsson L, Joelsson I, von Schoultz B. Ambivalence towards parenthood among pregnant women and their men. *Acta Obstet Gynecol Scand* 1993;72:619–26.

102. Ellison MA, Hall JE. Social stigma and compounded losses: quality-of-life issues for multiple-birth families. *Fertil Steril* 2003;80:405–14.

103. Sheard C, Glazebrook C, Cox S, Oates M, Ndukwe G. The impact of parenting multiples on first-time mothers conceiving following in-vitro fertilisation (IVF). *J Reprod Infant Psychol* 2005;23:251–97.

104. Yokoyama Y. Comparison of child-rearing problems between mothers with multiple children who conceived after infertility treatment and mothers with multiple children who conceived spontaneously. *Twin Res* 2003;6:89–96.

105. Khademi A, Alleyassin A, Aghahosseini M, Ramezanzadeh F, Abhari AA. Pretreatment Beck Depression Inventory score is an important predictor for post-treatment score in infertile patients: a before–after study. *BMC Psychiatry* 2005;5:25.

106. Child TJ, Henderson AM, Tan SL. The desire for multiple pregnancy in male and female infertility patients. *Hum Reprod* 2004;19:558–61.

107. Devine KS. Caring for the infertile woman. *MCN Am J Matern Child Nurs* 2003;28:100–5.

108. Mahlstedt PP, Macduff S, Bernstein J. Emotional factors and the *in vitro* fertilization and embryo transfer process. *J In Vitro Fert Embryo Transf* 1987;4:232–6.

109. Tammentie T, Paavilainen E, Astedt-Kurki P, Tarkka MT. Family dynamics of postnatally depressed mothers – discrepancy between expectations and reality. *J Clin Nurs* 2004;13:65–74.

110. Pancer SM, Pratt M, Hunsberger B, Gallant M. Thinking ahead: complexity of expectations and the transition to parenthood. *J Pers* 2000;68:253–80.

111. Willinger U, Diendorfer-Radner G, Willnauer R, Jorgl G, Hager V. Parenting stress and parental bonding. *Behav Med* 2005;31:63–9.

112. Kendler KS. Parenting: a genetic-epidemiologic perspective. *Am J Psychiatry* 1996;153:11–20.

113. Colpin H, Munter AD, Nys K, Vandemeulebroecke L. Parenting stress and psychosocial well-being among parents with twins conceived naturally or by reproductive technology. *Hum Reprod* 1999;14:3133–7.

114. Wen SW, Demissie K, Yang Q, Walker MC. Maternal morbidity and obstetric complications in triplet pregnancies and quadruplet and higher-order multiple pregnancies. *Am J Obstet Gynecol* 2004;191:254–8.

115. Dafallah SE, Yousif EM. A comparative study of twin and triplet pregnancy. *Saudi Med J* 2004;25:502–6.

116. Rao A, Sairam S, Shehata H. Obstetric complications of twin pregnancies. *Best Pract Res Clin Obstet Gynaecol* 2004;18:557–76.

117. Ochsenkuhn R, Strowitzki T, Gurtner M, Strauss A, Schulze A, Hepp H, *et al.* Pregnancy complications, obstetric risks, and neonatal outcome in singleton and twin pregnancies after GIFT and IVF. *Arch Gynecol Obstet* 2003;268:256–61.

118. Harrigan R, Naber MM, Jensen KA, Tse A, Perez D. Perinatal grief: response to the loss of an infant. *Neonatal Netw* 1993;12:25–31.

119. Pector EA, Smith-Levitin M. Mourning and psychological issues in multiple birth loss. *Semin Neonatol* 2002;7:247–56.

120. Bryan EM. The death of a twin. *Palliat Med* 1995;9:187–92.

Chapter 19

Consensus views arising from the 50th Study Group: Multiple Pregnancy

Consensus expert views relating to clinical practice

1. The risk of multiple pregnancy should be reduced by conservative use of ovarian stimulation with careful monitoring according to published guidelines (RCOG, 1999; NICE, 2004; Grade A).

2. In view of the risks associated with multiple pregnancy, consideration should be given to transferring only a single embryo in women undergoing *in vitro* fertilisation (Grade A).

3. In view of the changing effects of maternal age and fertility treatment on multiple pregnancy rates, there needs to be a mechanism for recording their impact on the rates of multiple pregnancy.

4. Prepregnancy counselling regarding the risks of multiple pregnancy should be given to a woman undergoing fertility treatment (Grade C).

5. Parents of high order multiple pregnancies (≥3) should be counselled and offered multifetal pregnancy reduction (MFPR) to twins in specialist centres (Grade B).

6. Long-term neurodevelopmental follow-up studies are needed of survivors of multiple pregnancies who have undergone MFPR (Grade C).

7. All women with a multiple pregnancy should be offered an ultrasound examination at 10–13 weeks of gestation (Grade B) to assess:
   (a) viability
   (b) chorionicity
   (c) major congenital malformation
   (d) nuchal translucency for designation of risk of aneuploidy and twin-to-twin transfusion syndrome.

8. All monochorionic twins should have a detailed ultrasound scan which includes extended views of the fetal heart (Grade B).

9. Monochorionic twins require increased ultrasound surveillance from 16 weeks of gestation onwards to detect twin-to-twin transfusion syndrome and growth discordance. This should be offered at an interval of 2 weeks (Grade C).

10. Nuchal translucency based screening should be offered as the preferred method of aneuploidy screening in women with multiple pregnancy (Grade B).

11. Monochorionic twins that are discordant for fetal anomaly must be referred at an early gestation for assessment and counselling in a regional fetal medicine centre (Grade B).

12. Twins that are discordant for fetal anomaly should be managed in fetal medicine centres with specific expertise (Grade C).

13. Hospitals should organise antenatal and postnatal care around specialist-led, multidisciplinary multiple pregnancy clinics (Grade C).

14. The organisation of antenatal twin clinics should be facilitated by care pathways and allow referral to regional fetal medicine centres when appropriate (Grade C).

15. The lead clinician for multiple pregnancy clinics should have expertise in ultrasound and in the intrapartum care of multiple pregnancies (Grade C).

16. Twin-to-twin transfusion syndrome should be managed in conjunction with regional fetal medicine centres with recourse to specialist expertise (Grade C).

17. Fetoscopic laser ablation is the treatment of choice in severe twin-to-twin transfusion syndrome presenting prior to 26 weeks of gestation (Grade A).

18. Single-twin demise in a monochorionic twin pregnancy should be referred and assessed in a regional fetal medicine centre (Grade B).

19. The survivor after single-twin demise in monochorionic twins should have follow-up ultrasound and, if normal, an MRI examination of the fetal brain 2–3 weeks after the co-twin death. Counselling should include the long-term morbidity in this condition (Grade C).

20. Vaginal delivery of twins should be performed in a setting with continuous intrapartum monitoring, immediate recourse to caesarean section, appropriate analgesia and an obstetrician experienced in twin delivery (Grade B).

21. In view of the increased risk of stillbirth in twin pregnancy, elective delivery is recommended between 37 and 38 weeks of gestation (Grade C).

22. Mothers with a multiple pregnancy have a need for specific information, including discussion of delivery and postnatal wellbeing, including breastfeeding (Grade C).

23. The role of midwives and other healthcare specialists is integral to the management of multiple pregnancies within specialist clinics (Grade C).

24. Additional support to women is available from TAMBA and the Multiple Births Foundation, and this should be encouraged (Grade C).

25. There is a need to support women emotionally with multiple pregnancies (Grade A).

26 There is a need to recognise early signs of perinatal psychological disturbance, which is increased after multiple births, and to offer treatment (Grade A).

Consensus expert views relating to future research

1. The optimum method of delivery of twins at greater than 32 weeks of gestation is unknown. Continuing research may inform this uncertainty.

2. The optimum treatment of early-stage twin-to-twin transfusion syndrome is unclear. This needs to be informed by further research, preferably in the form of a randomised trial investigating conservative management, amnioreduction or laser ablation and their effects on disease progression.

3. There is a need for further multicentre randomised controlled trials evaluating effectiveness and cost effectiveness of a single-embryo transfer policy in *in vitro* fertilisation.

4. Further research is required to assess the outcome of the single surviving fetus in a monochorionic twin set where *in utero* therapy has been instigated.

5. Because most epidemiological studies on cerebral palsy were performed before the impact of fertility treatment on multiple births, there is a need for updated surveys to establish the current prevalence of cerebral palsy following assisted conception.

7. There is a need to understand mechanisms of prematurity in multiple pregnancies.

8. There is a need to explore other interventions with the aim of reducing maternal psychological distress.

9. Given the uncertainties about many interventions during multiple pregnancy, it is important to encourage clinical research aimed at improving pregnancy outcome.

Consensus expert views relating to health education/policy

1. There is an urgent need for the establishment of a prospective registry of multiple pregnancies that relates chorionicity to outcome.

2. A prospective cohort registry should evaluate the risks mediating neurological morbidity in multiple pregnancy.

3. The UK regional congenital anomaly registers should collect information regarding plurality and chorionicity.

4. The general health problems related to twinning should be brought more widely into the public domain.

5. There is a need to enhance the provision of antenatal education for multiple pregnancies. This should facilitate realistic preparation for birth and parenting, and should aim to meet the needs of the father as well as the mother.

Key pre- and postnatal events to be offered in pregnancy

Dichorionic twins

- Multiples clinic: lead clinician with multidisciplinary team.
- Ultrasound at 10–13 weeks: (a) viability; (b) chorionicity; (c) NT: aneuploidy
- Structural anomaly scan at 20–22 weeks.
- Serial fetal growth scans e.g 24, 28, 32 and then two- to four-weekly.
- BP monitoring and urinalysis at 20, 24, 28 and then two-weekly.
- Discussion of woman's/family needs relating to twins.
- 34–36 weeks: discussion of mode of delivery and intrapartum care.
- Elective delivery at 37–38 completed weeks.
- Postnatal advice and support (hospital- and community-based) to include breastfeeding and contraceptive advice.

Monochorionic twins

- Multiples clinic: lead clinician with multidisciplinary team.
- Ultrasound at 10–13 weeks: (a) viability; (b) chorionicity; (c) NT: aneuploidy/TTTS
- Ultrasound surveillance for TTTS and discordant growth: at 16 weeks and then two-weekly.
- Structural anomaly scan at 20–22 weeks (including fetal ECHO).
- Fetal growth scans at two-weekly intervals until delivery.
- BP monitoring and urinalysis at 20, 24, 28 and then two-weekly.
- Discussion of woman's/family needs relating to twins.
- 32–34 weeks: discussion of mode of delivery and intrapartum care.
- Elective delivery at 36–37 completed weeks (if uncomplicated).
- Postnatal advice and support (hospital- and community-based) to include breastfeeding and contraceptive advice.

Index